PEDIATRIC PHYSICAL THERAPY STRENGTHENING EXERCISES OF THE HIPS

PEDIATRIC PHYSICAL THERAPY STRENGTHENING EXERCISES OF THE HIPS

Treatment Suggestions
by
Muscle Action

Amy E. Sturkey, PT

Pediatric Physical Therapy Strengthening Exercises of the Hips

For information contact:
Amy E. Sturkey, PT
amysturkey@gmail.com
www.igotchaapps.com

Book and Cover design by Guy Bryant
Edited by Amy Plyer

ISBN-13: 978-0-9981567-3-6
First Edition: May 2020

DEDICATION

This book is dedicated to all PT students who asked for treatment ideas and every mother who wanted help for her child.

CONTENTS

I. HIP FLEXION

THE HIP FLEXORS MOVE THE femur toward the pelvis and the lower back or conversely the pelvis and the lower spine toward the femur if the femur is stabilized. This movement is in the sagittal plane. The hip flexors are powerful lower body stabilizers. Weakness or tightness in the hip flexors will affect gait, sitting and standing posture. This chapter includes a wide variety of exercises to improve hip flexor strength.

* * *

1. HIP/KNEE FLEXION SUPINE ON THE BALL

I tend to use this exercise on clients who have either little idea or capability of pulling with hip and knee flexion. If you carefully balance the client, then a small pull from the client can produce a big and rewarding movement. I often end up taking this kind of client through the movement so she can get the feel of the motion or so that the client will be motivated by the motion and want to repeat it.

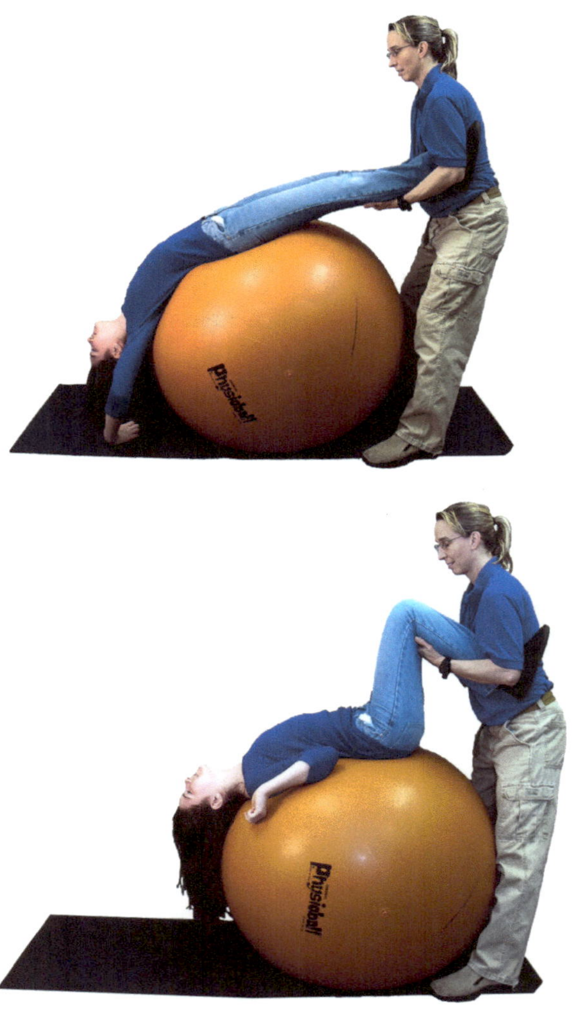

2. SUPINE BICYCLE

Want a greater step length or pelvic disassociation? In many of my clients with low tone or increased stiffness I have trouble getting one leg to move significantly differently than the other for crawling without bunny hopping, longer step length, or half kneel to stand. Here is a wonderful way to strengthen hip flexors and increase pelvic disassociation.

I use this exercise with manual assistance when my client is really clueless about how to perform the movement. I use elastic bands or manual resistance when a child has more strength and a high level of cooperation. I have found this a really good exercise particularly after the Selective Dorsal Rhizotomy. Pelvic disassociation is always tricky for my clients with quadriplegic or diplegic cerebral palsy, so this is a great activity to encourage it. This exercise technically works hip flexion on one leg with hip extension on the other leg, reciprocally and alternating.

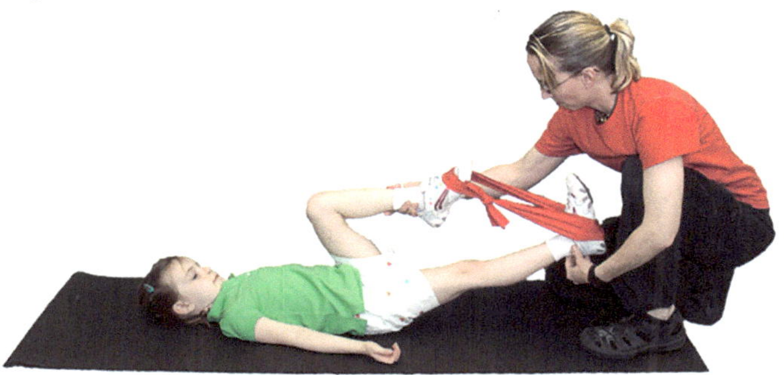

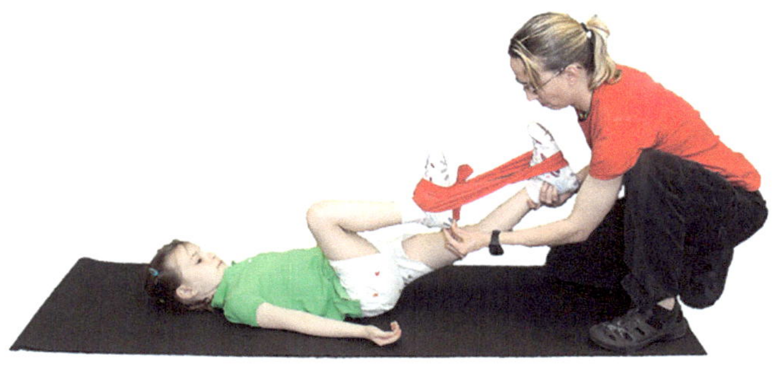

3. STAMP IN BRIDGE

This exercise works flexion of one hip and extension of the other. It is a good activity to work on strength as well as balance and weight shift for some clients. You can have your client stamp the same foot over and over or alternate legs. I always find my clients do best if I tell them up front how many stamps I am expecting before they can be done. Sometimes I put squeak toys down under the foot to stamp for auditory confirmation of the stamp-but mostly for fun. I also have a relatively flat keyboard that I put under the client's hips. I tell my client that she is to stamp the squeak toy but not play the piano with her "bohonkas!" This makes an otherwise boring activity fun. If you want hilarity, put a whoopee cushion underneath the hips and tell her to stamp the squeak toy, but don't "toot." This is perfect for a boy of any age and certain girls.

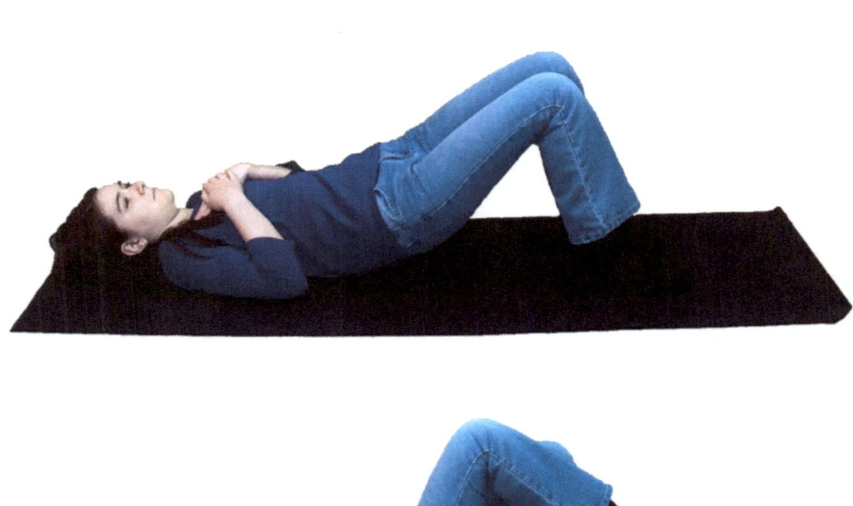

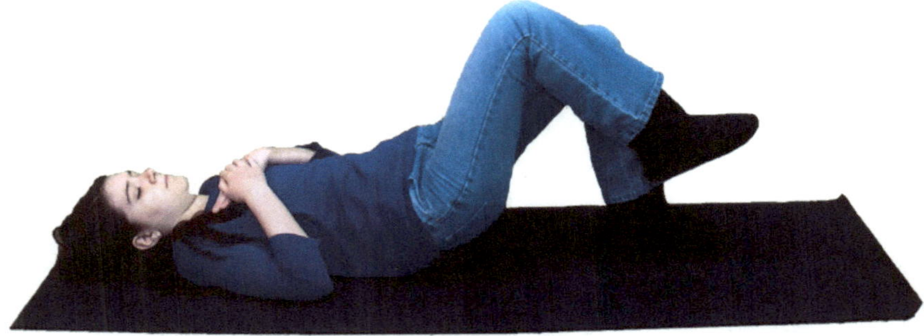

4. LATERAL FLEXION PRONE

The child lies prone and laterally flexes to one side. He flexes his hip and touches his elbow to his knee on the same side. Then he laterally flexes the other direction with unilateral hip flexion to touch the other elbow to his other knee. In order to laterally flex prone like this, I get a great deal of back extension activation, as well as lateral flexion and hip flexion. I really like this exercise! It is terrific for clients with diplegia and hemiplegia, and it is also great for the really common child with core and proximal hip weakness.

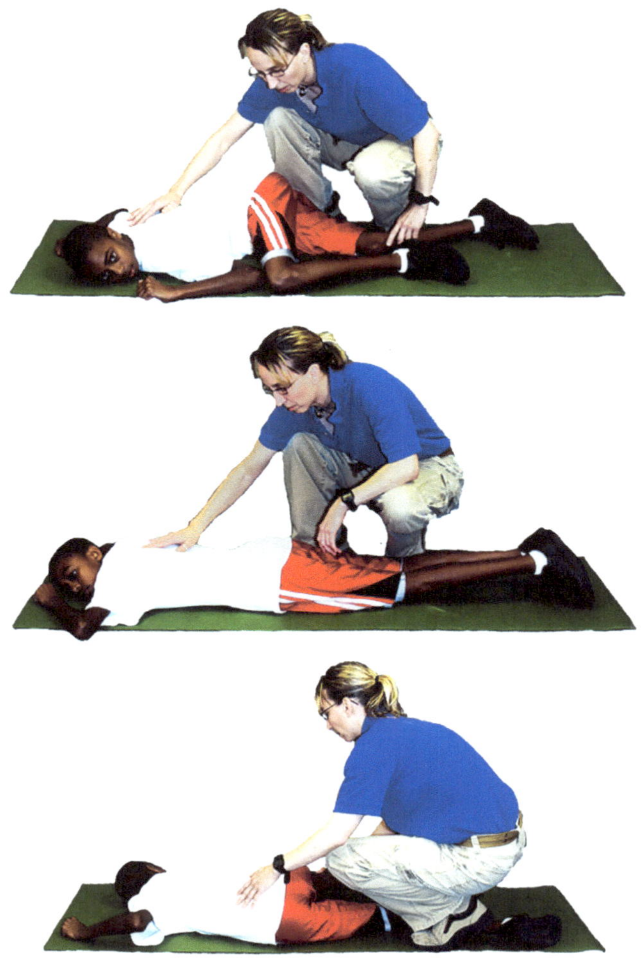

5. STANDING HIP FLEXION/MARCHING

Pelvic disassociation is almost always tricky for my clients with quadriplegic or diplegic cerebral palsy. This exercise technically works hip flexion on one leg with hip extension on the other leg, reciprocally and alternating. Here I am using my hand as a target to help the client know how high I expect her to elevate her knee. I may also use the ever-popular electric piano for a client to bring her knees up to hit. When having the client use her own hands to touch, the tendency is for the client to progressively lower her own hands to her knees, instead of raising her knees to her hands. You can add weight to the ankles to add more resistance. To challenge balance, provide less to no upper extremity support and ask the client to hold end range hip flexion for a specified amount of time. Document the weight used, the angle of hip flexion achieved, the support provided, the repetitions, and the duration of end range hip flexion performed.

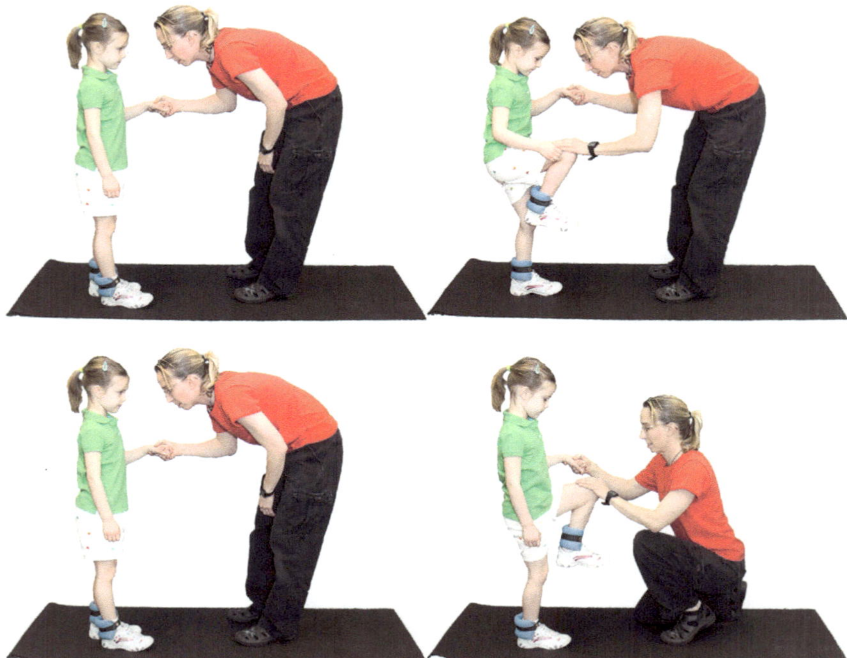

6. POSTERIOR TILT WITH PT POSTERIORLY

I actually perform this activity with me either behind or in front. From behind I am in an excellent position to catch my client if he falls. I am also in a very good position to really pull down the hips relative to the knees to encourage the forward hip flexion.

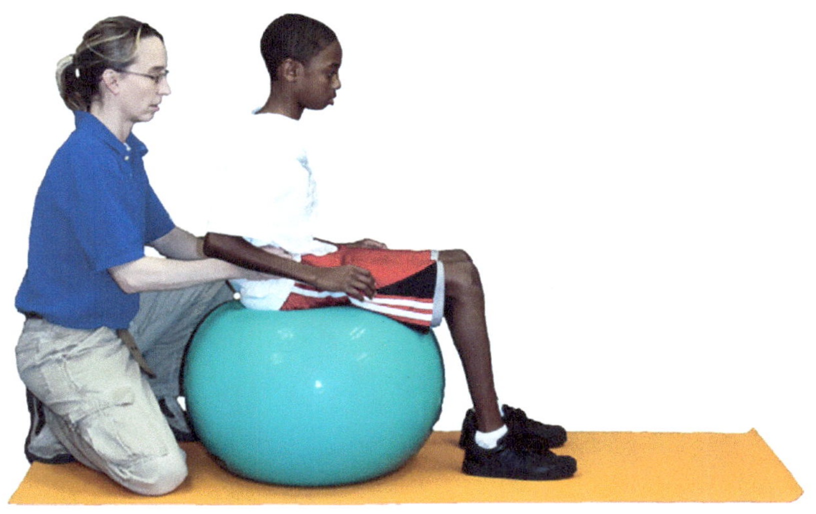

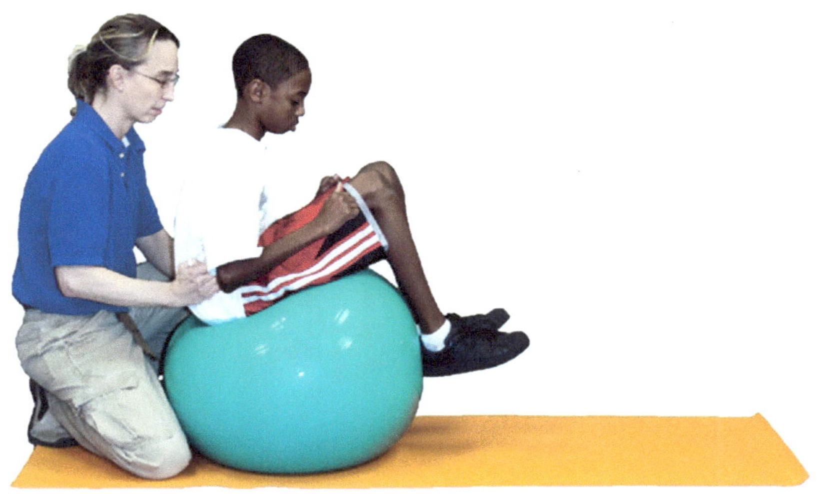

7. BALL LEG LIFTS

This is one of my clients' all time favorites. Something about getting to put their smelly feet on my head never loses its fun! There is a quick switch right at the end of this move where the therapist switches her hands from trunk support to grabbing the shins. That is critical! Otherwise you really could get whacked HARD. I have children who cannot do a sit-up flat on the floor, but can do leg lifts on the large ball. I may need the parent to help lift up the legs initially to get the feel for the activity. I use the ball to give more momentum or gravity assistance if needed to make this activity easier. If I want to make it harder, I hang the child off the far side of the ball.

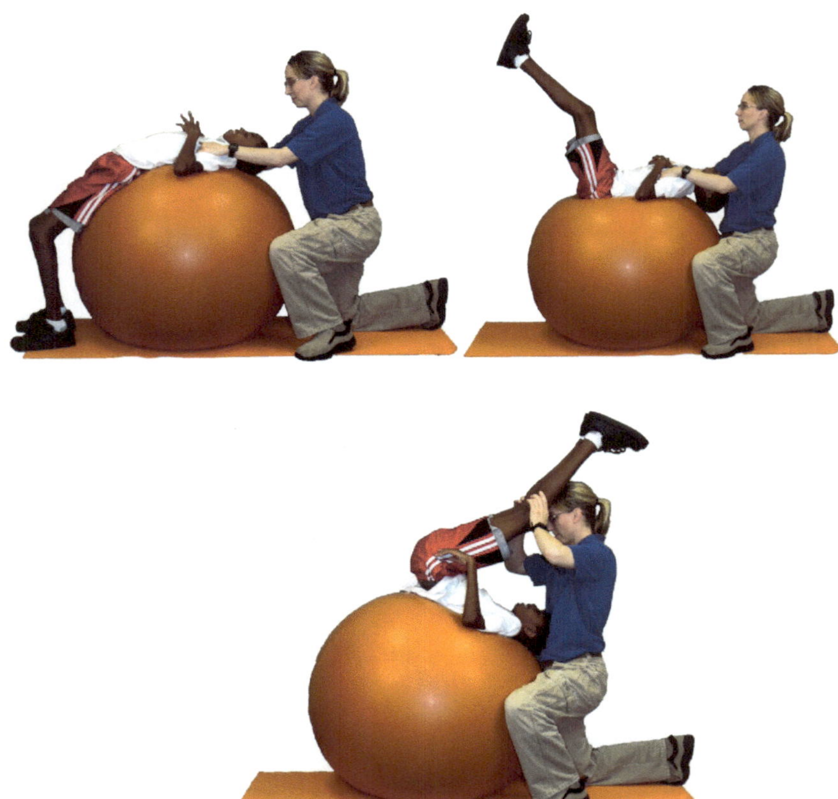

8. BALL SITTING-HIP FLEXION/MARCHING

There is nothing like a ball to add a little more fun! The smaller the ball, the closer to end range this will be for the child. I usually get a ball that is about the height of the back of the child's knees when sitting on it. If she continues to have a hard time I get a larger ball for her to sit on. If I don't have a large enough ball, then I simply put a mat of single, double thickness, whatever is needed under the ball, but not under her feet, to magically elevate the ball underneath her. I use my hand as a target for end range hip flexion.

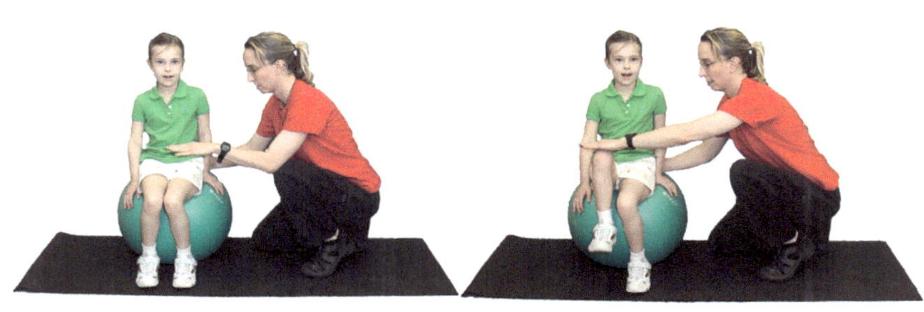

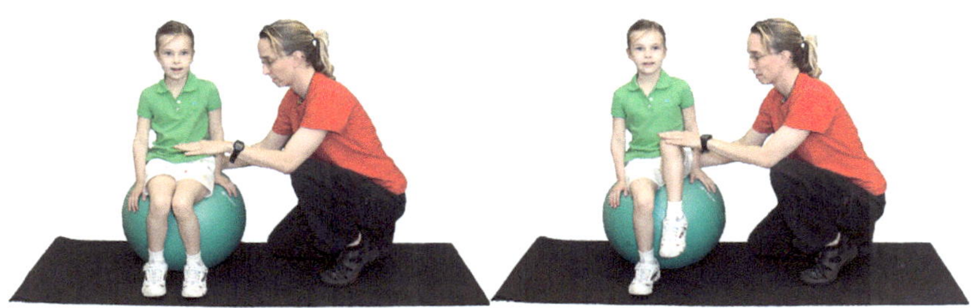

9. PLACE/REMOVE ONE FOOT ON BENCH

I don't know if my clients love this activiy, but I do! It is one of my staples. You can give a variety of support at the trunk or hips, by holding two or one hand, or having the client hold one or two Kaye Products Upright poles. Obviously the higher the bench, the harder this activity is for the client. I love the Kaye Products benches because I can easily raise and lower the height of the bench. If the bench I am using is not adjustable, I simply put a mat under the bench in single, double or triple thickness to raise or lower the bench relative to the child.

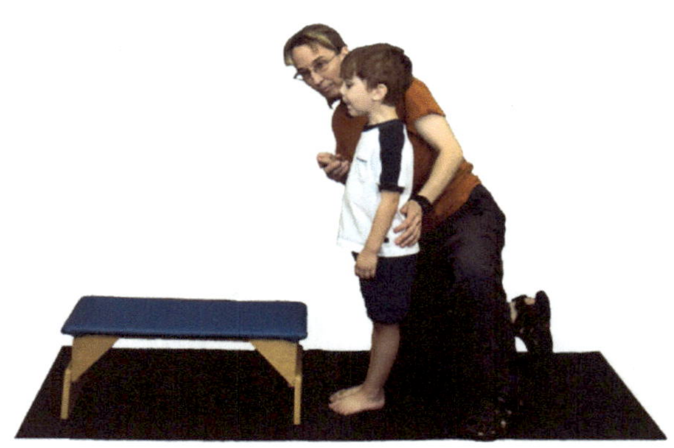

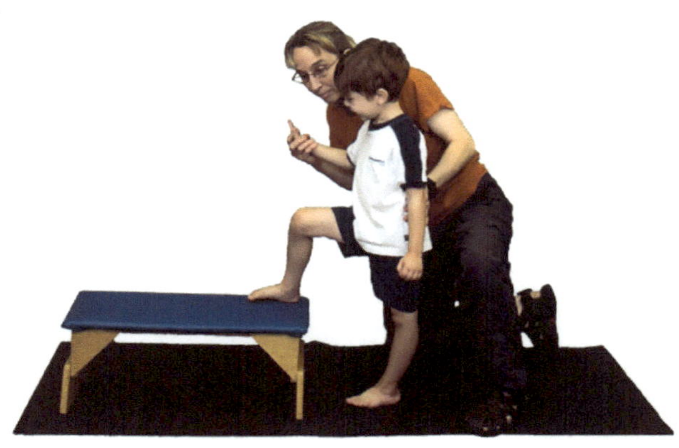

10. SIT-UPS, ARMS AND LEGS STRAIGHT

As long as the legs are straight and stabilized, this form of sit-up strongly relies on the hip flexors. Once clients are strong enough to perform a bench sit-up, I start trying sit-ups on the floor. I always stabilize the legs. Sometimes I put a 10" (25 cm) bench down over their legs so they can still interact with a toy-like a puzzle. But usually I just try to get the client to perform 10 repetitions to earn a reward afterward. I may need to coach clients on how to use their arms to help get the momentum to sit-up.

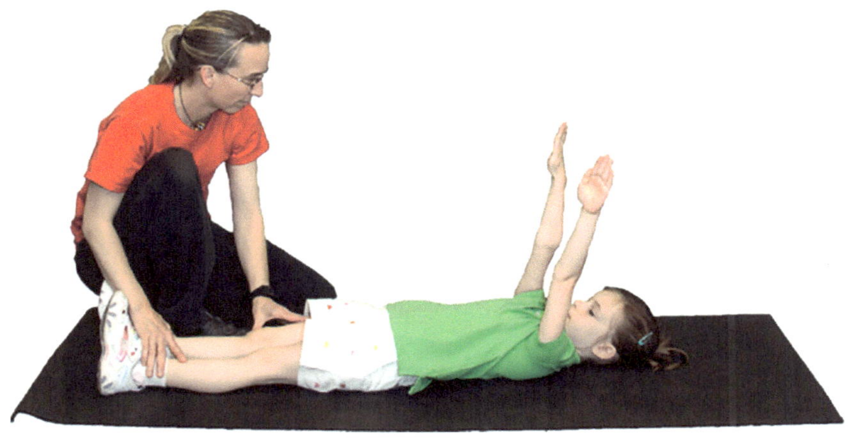

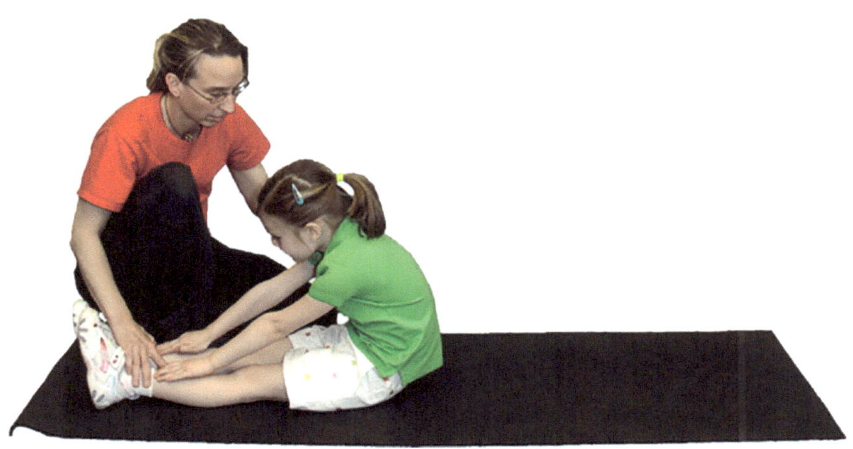

11. NET SWING SIT, KNEES TUCKED

With a rare exception, when I can use a swing, I almost always have a motivated child. The concept is easy. The child sits in a low swing. Typically I use in the clinic a net swing attached at one point, but really any swing that does not support the legs would do. Put the swing as low as you can to the floor. Tell your client to keep her legs up and not drag them. This usually takes some experimentation with height, usually accompanied by me saying something like, "Oh yeah, I bet you can't keep your feet up if I put the swing this low."

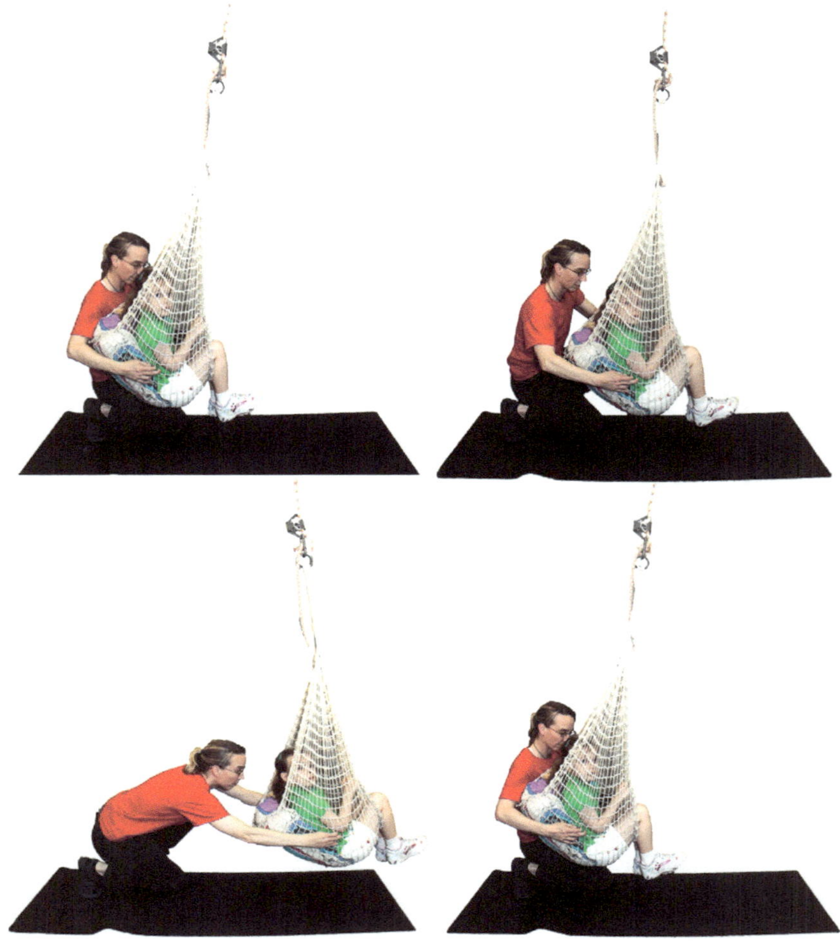

12. HIGH FRONT KNEE KICK

I usually do this game with a tether ball but any target will do. I ask my child to keep her leg cocked up, and as the tether ball comes back, she kicks it again. If a client can't keep her leg up in hip flexion, I allow the child to put her leg down on the floor between each repetition. The higher the tether ball/target, the harder this is. When using a tether ball I like to have the parent help me. In which case I have the parent stand on one end of the arc of the tether ball, and the client and I stand at the other end of the arc. I have the mother hold the tether ball with the rope pulled taut, and release it on cue. If she pulls the tether ball rope tight between repetitions, then the arch of the tether ball swing is more regular and the exercise seems to go more smoothly.

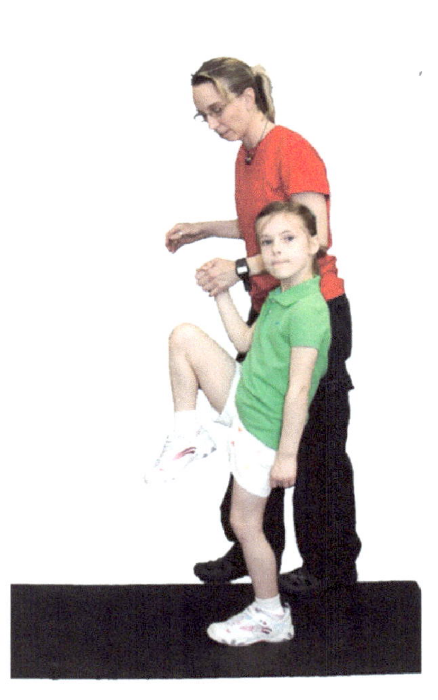

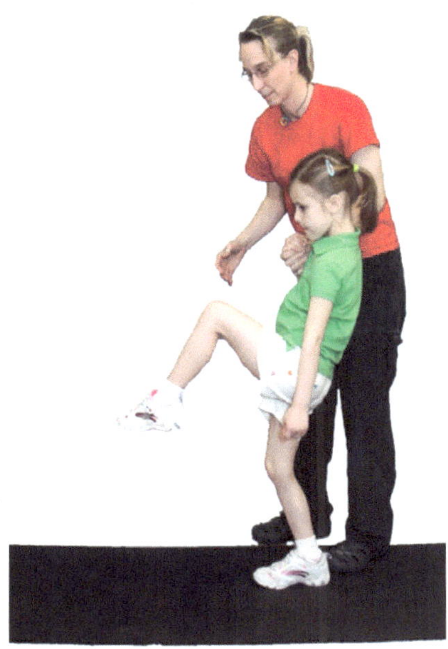

13. KICK BALL HIGH AND HARD

For clients who have a little more control-both impulse control and motor control; you can have the client kick a ball that you hold up. I like to tell them to kick it hard enough to kick it out of my hand. For your safety, you might want a slightly larger ball than I have pictured here and position yourself to the side. I make it difficult to kick the ball out of my hand, ensuring multiple powerful repetitions.

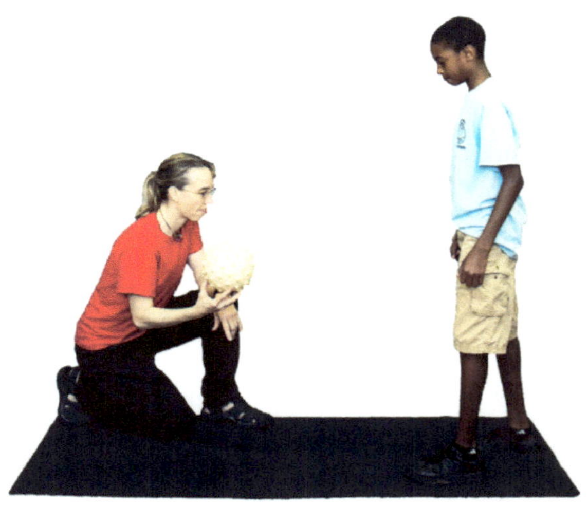

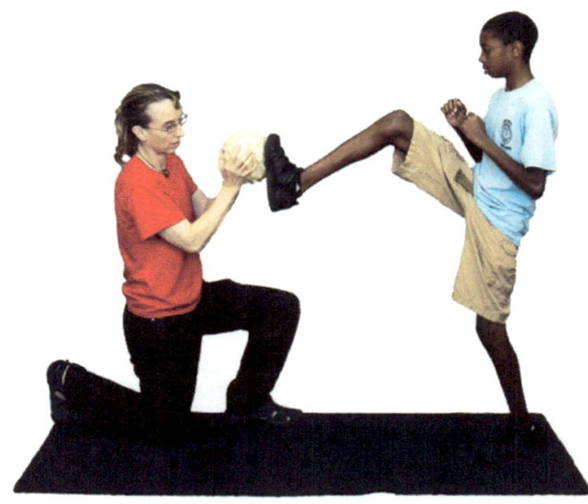

14. TUCK KNEES ON BALL, HANDS ON BENCH

This is a hard activity. The ball has a great deal of degrees of freedom of movement, so spot your client closely if you have any concerns regarding their safety. Make sure you start with the ball under the knees in the quadruped position. This will make sure the client has room to go from prone to quadruped.

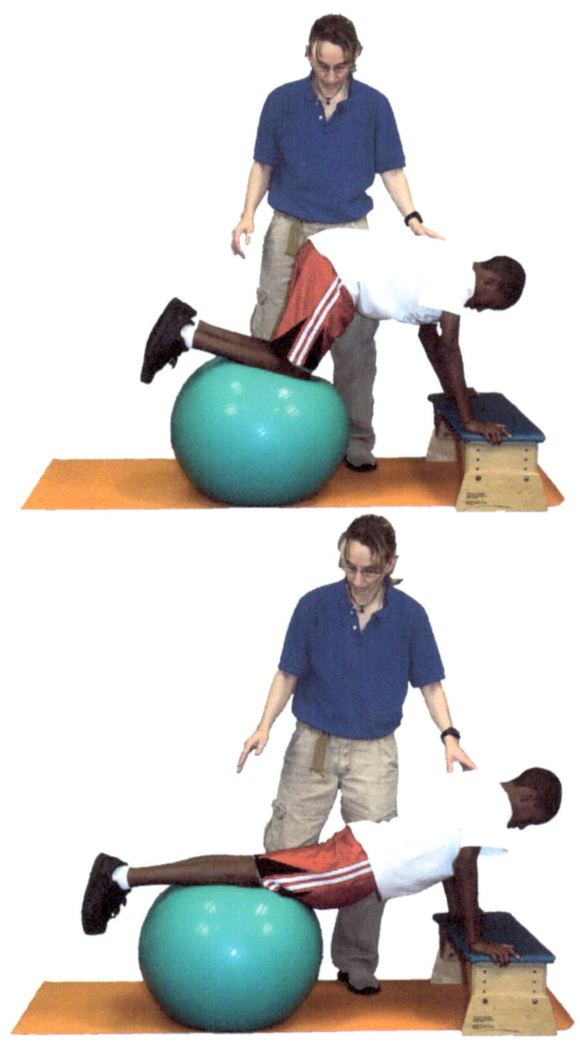

15. SUPINE LEG LIFTS HOLDING PT'S ANKLES

Great exercise-just take care not to step on the child's hair! I really have to emphasize legs straight if they are capable. Sometimes the child is unable to lift both legs at a time. If this is the case, then I will let her lift one leg and I'll hold it for the other leg to come up.

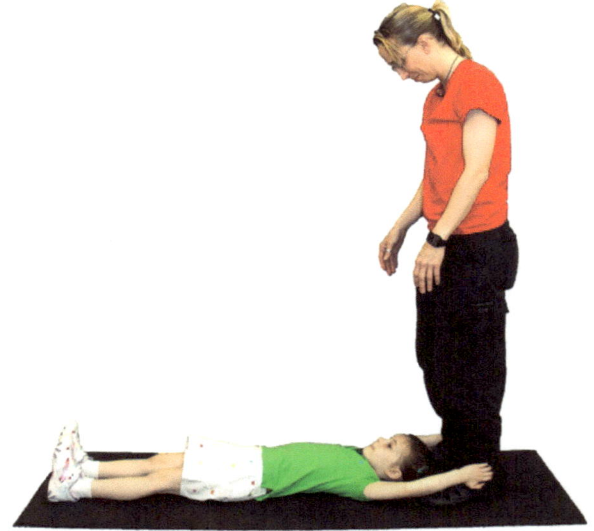

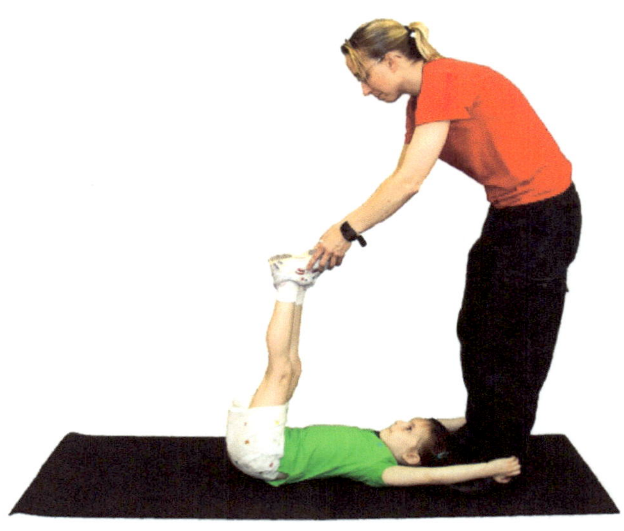

16. SUPINE BALL LIFTS, PT AT HEAD

Stand at the child's head, taking care not to step on her hair. The client lifts the ball to me and I take the ball. I hold the ball until she can take it from me again, and set it down on the floor without losing the ball. This always takes some control. Clearly a beach ball is easier than a playground ball but either way this is still a tough game.

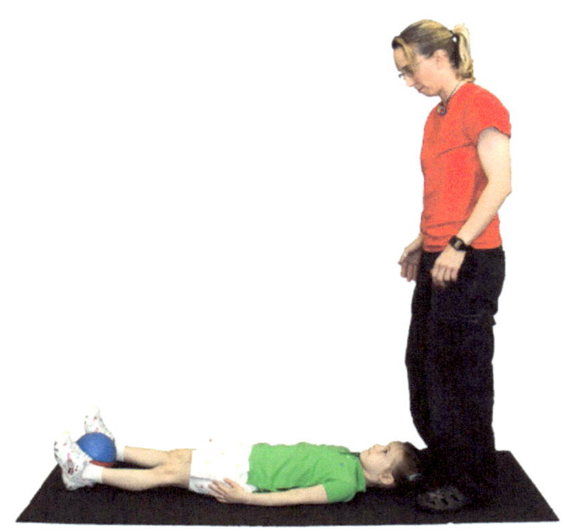

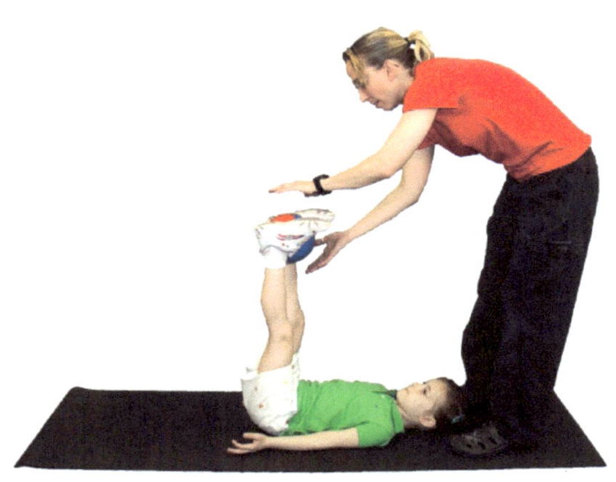

17. KNEEL TO HALF KNEEL WITH TWO POLES

Moving from kneel to half kneel requires hip extension on the stabilizing side, and it also requires hip flexion on the moving side. I love doing this exercise in the vertical poles. We have several sets of Kaye Product poles at our clinic. I love them. This is one of those exercises that my kids with diplegia need to practice and practice. I find I need to keep returning to it even after it is mastered. This pelvic disassociation is so hard for them to attain and maintain.

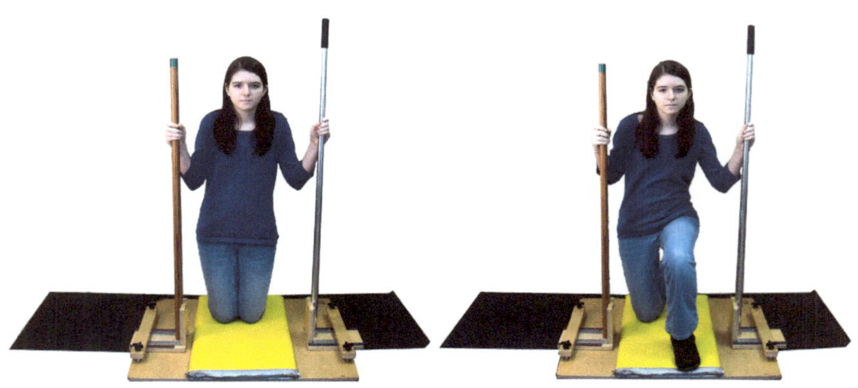

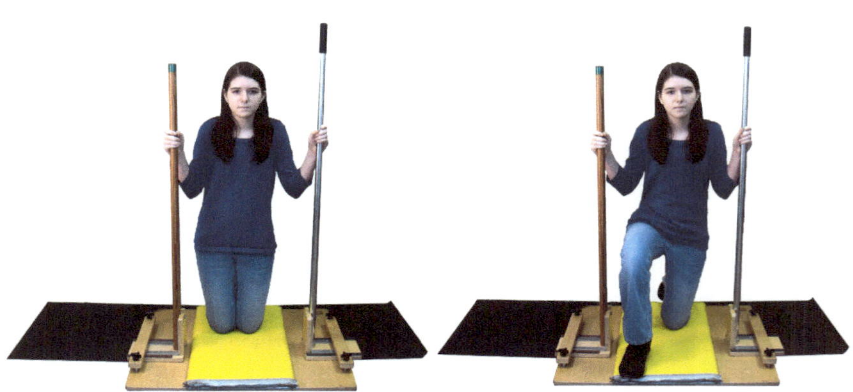

18. KNEEL TO HALF KNEEL WITH ONE HAND HELD

One hand held gives significantly less stable support than the upright poles. My diplegic kids all want to skip from tall kneel up to standing at a support. They need to practice this work until they can do it on both sides in their sleep!

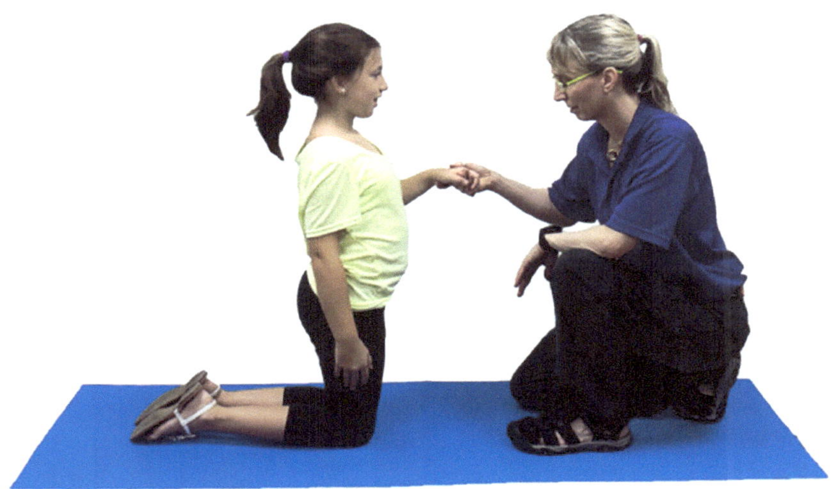

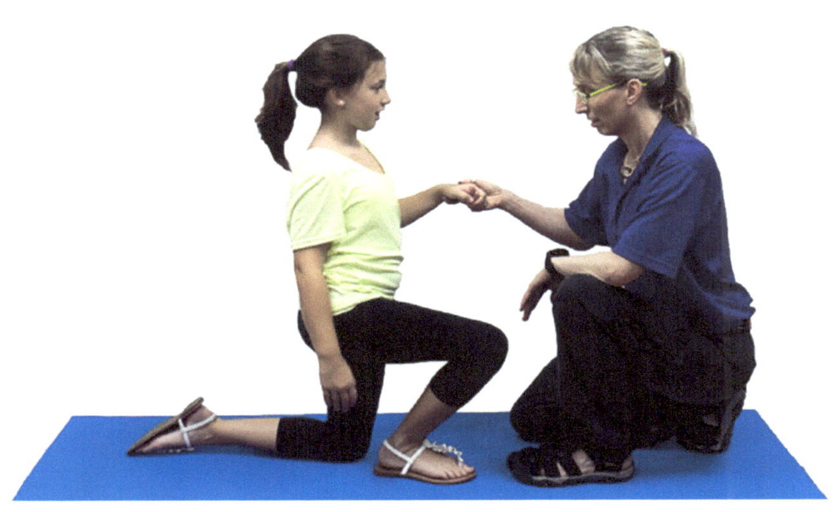

19. HALF KNEEL TOSS AND CATCH

Maintenance of this position with one leg flexed and one leg extended is certainly a hip strength issue. I particularly like this activity with my higher functioning children with diplegia and quadriplegia. In a progression, reading books and turning pages while in half kneel would be easiest, followed by placing puzzle pieces or stacking cups, then rolling a ball back and forth on a counter top, culminating in the pictured throw and catch.

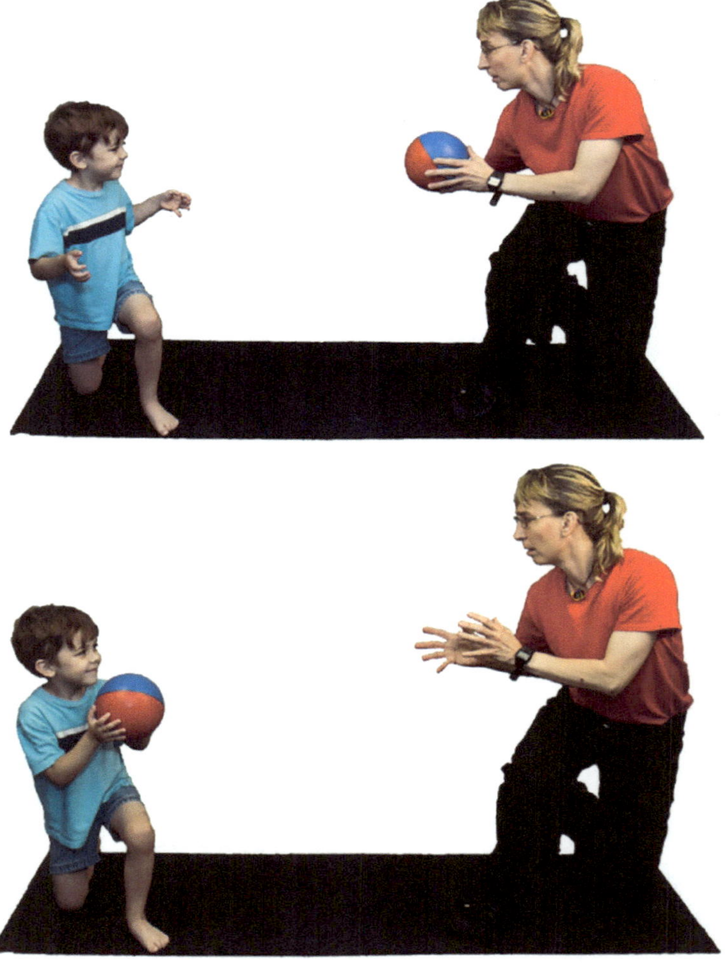

20. STAMP IN 1/2 KNEEL

This exercise is in both the hip flexion and hip extension sections. It requires both to perform this activity well. Hip stability work is often desperately needed in children with cerebral palsy.

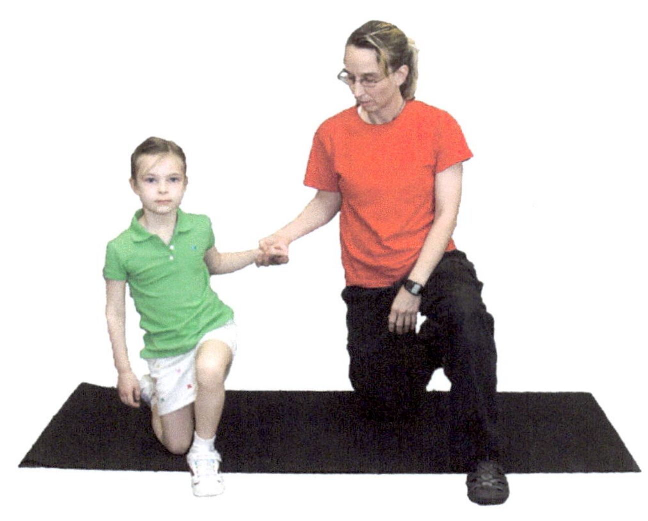

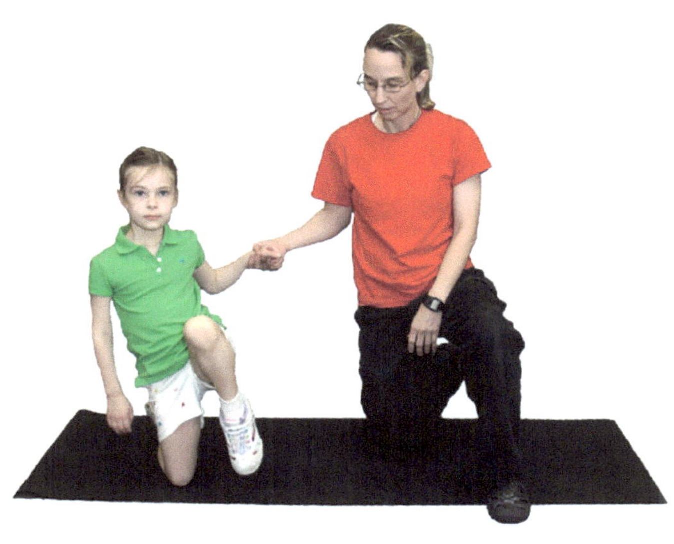

21. STAMP SQUEAK TOYS IN HALF KNEEL

I've always found that exercises with noise-making toys help the exercise work better. This can be hard to very difficult depending on the placement of the toys. You can give more support with one or two hands held or one hand on the wall. The upright poles unilaterally or bilaterally are also a great option for support here.

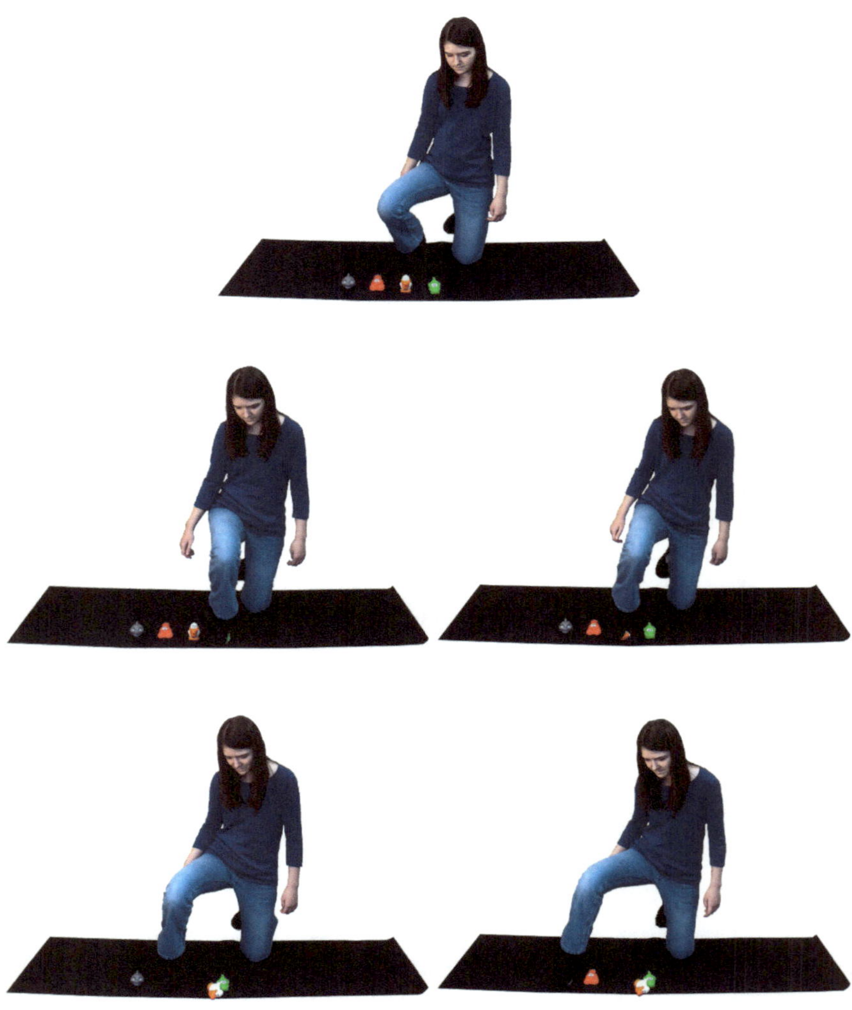

22. KICK CONES IN HALF KNEEL

This can be a very hard activity based both on the placement and the number of the cones. This can be easier if you allow your client to put her foot down between kicking each object. Or it can be very difficult if you require her to keep her foot up until she has kicked down a specified number of the cones. Obviously, kicking down more cones is harder. You can give one or two hand support or no support according to the difficulty you desire.

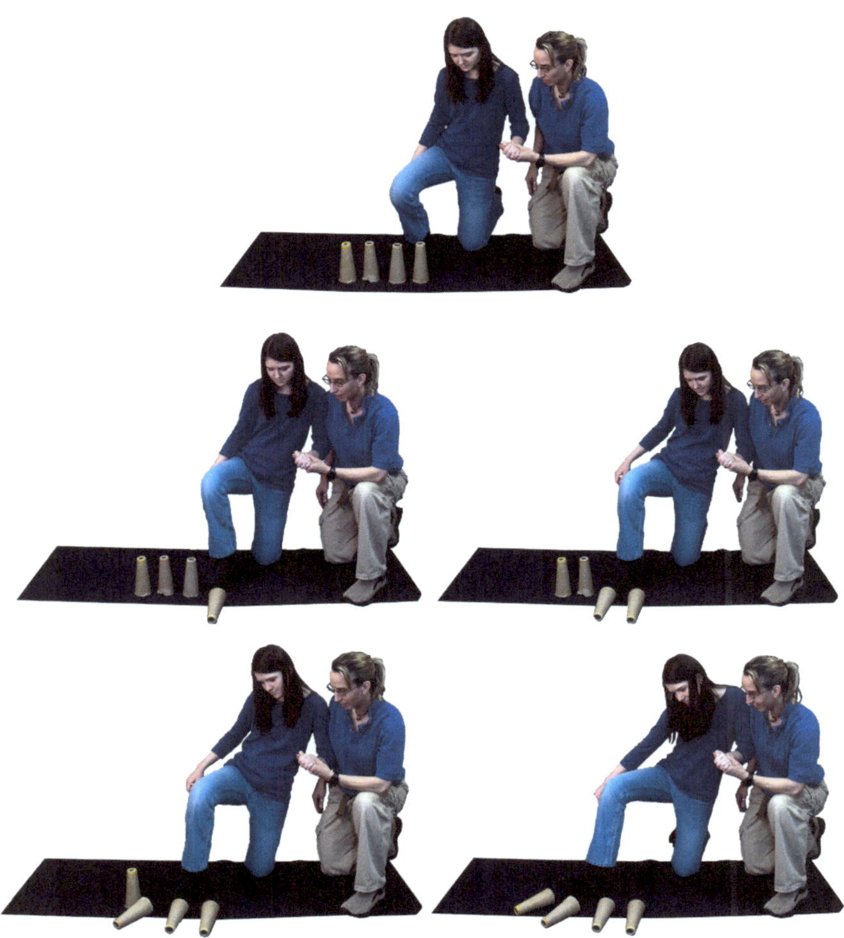

23. BENCH KNEEL STEP OVER AND BACK

This activity requires a lot of balance, pelvic disassociation and control, and hip flexion strength. I like using a padded bench that is around the height of the client's knees. You can provide one hand held, two hands held, or spot closely for safety. This activity can be challenging on the moving side leg or on the stable side leg. I try to let the client practice first on whatever side I think will be the easiest.

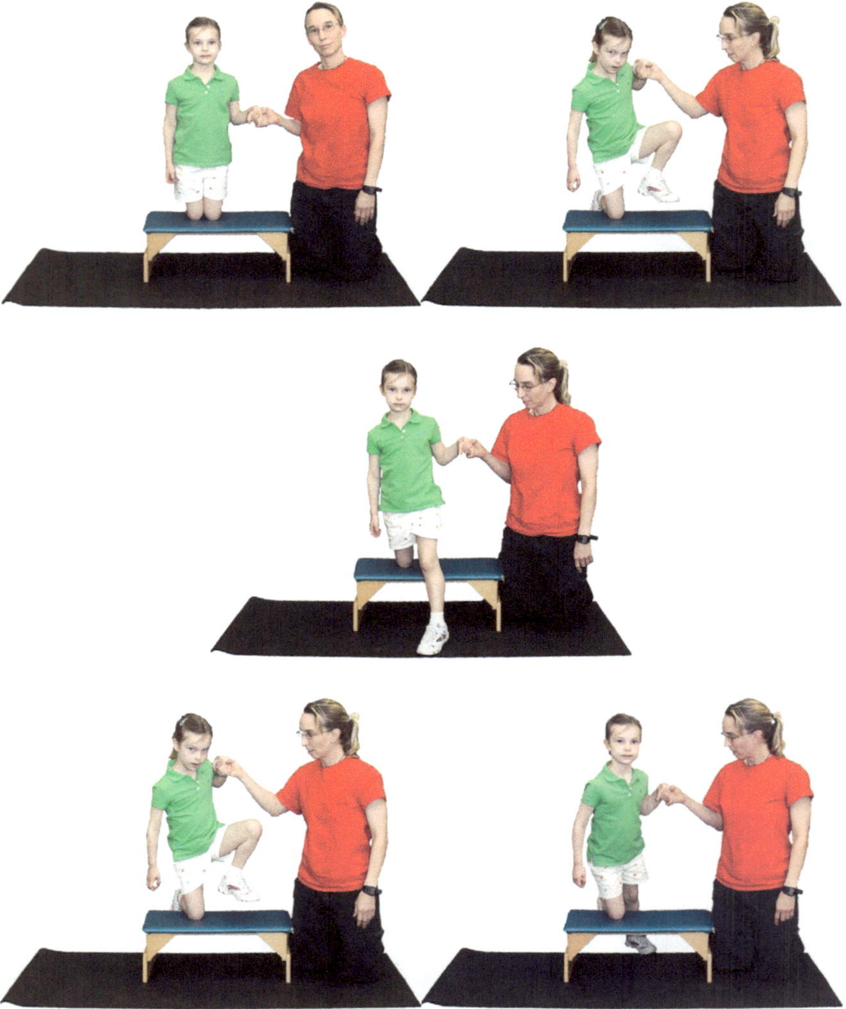

24. BENCH KNEEL TO HALF KNEEL WITH TRAY

Here I have made this exercise quite difficult. Holding the tray -especially with food on it, prevents her from using her arms significantly to counter-balance as she brings her leg from behind the bench to foot up on top of the bench, then to foot in front of the bench and back posteriorly again.

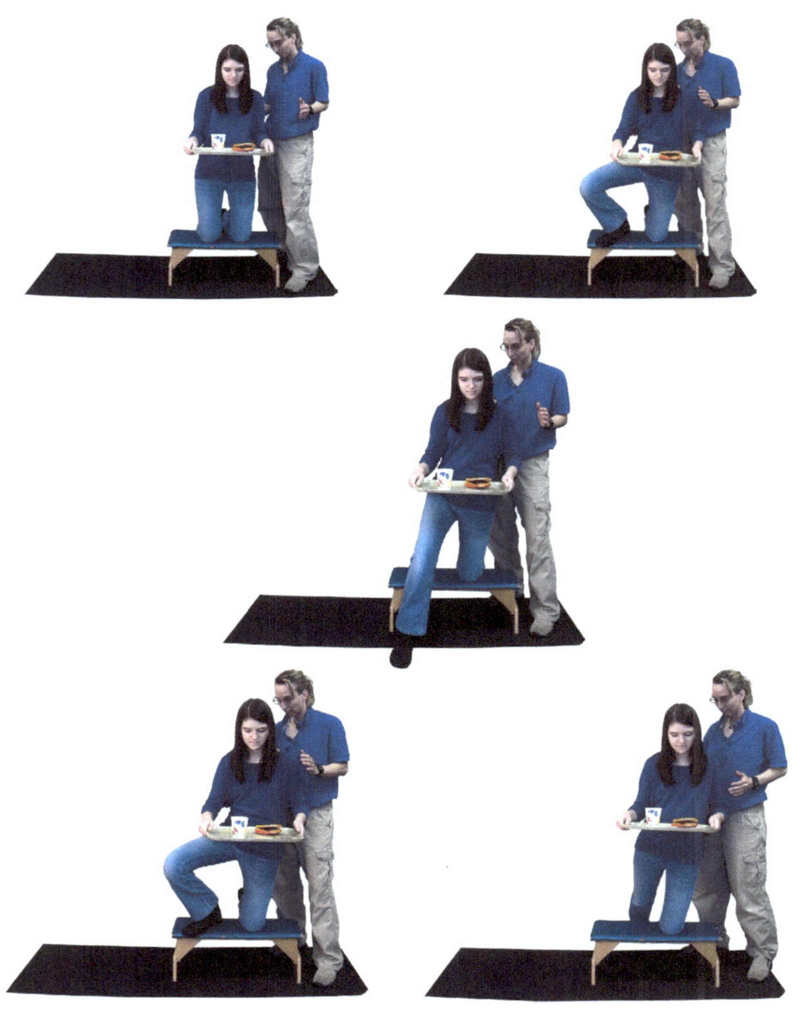

25. SQUAT WALK

This is a wonderful end range hip flexor exercise. Sometimes I have to hold one or two hands for success with this activity. As the child gets stronger, I fade out my support.

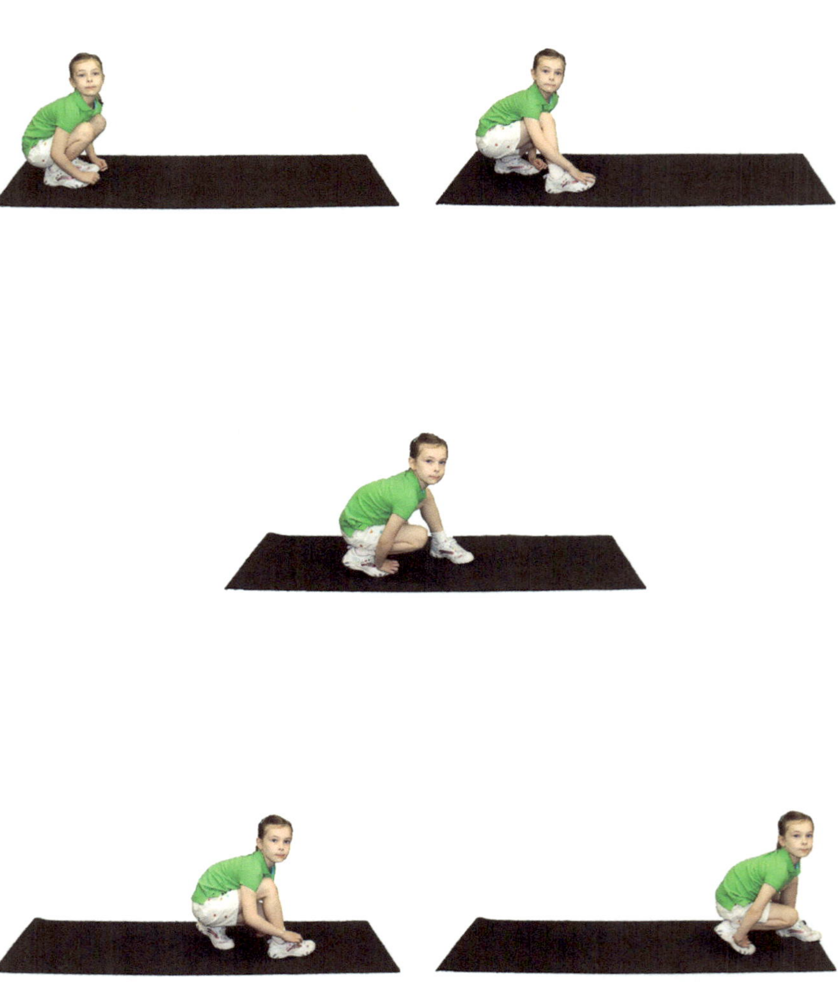

26. STAMP A FOOT IN VAULT POSITION

This works end range hip flexion. This is extremely hard for even my high-functioning clients with cerebral palsy. If this is too hard, have the child in vault position on a single, double or triple thick mat; with only the foot to be stamped off the mat on the floor.

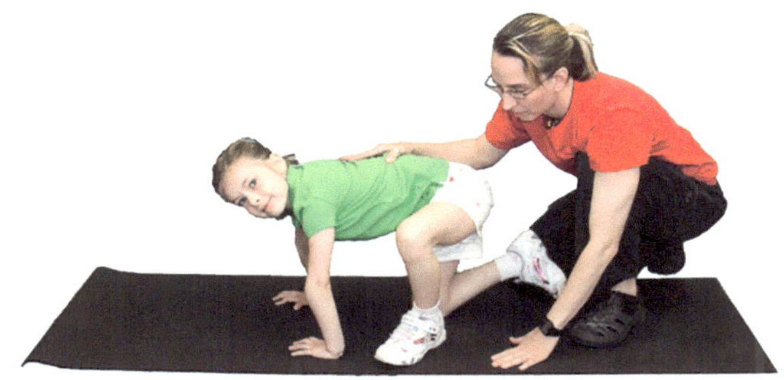

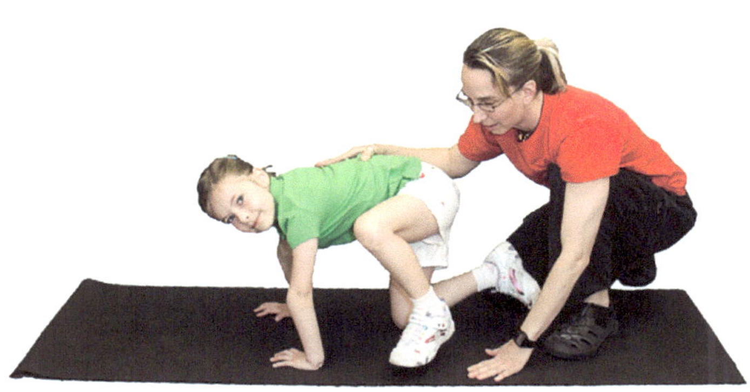

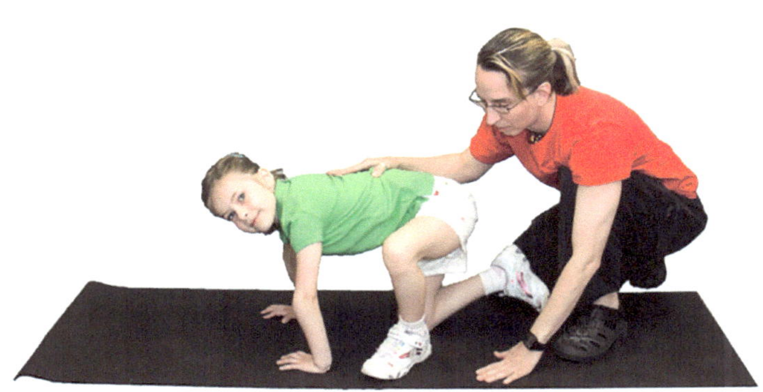

27. KICK IN VAULT A ROLLED BALL

Add in a ball and most activities become more fun. I roll the ball and the client kicks it. Again, this is extremely hard for even my high-functioning clients with cerebral palsy. To make it easier, have the child in vault on a single, double or triple thick mat; with the foot off the mat on the floor.

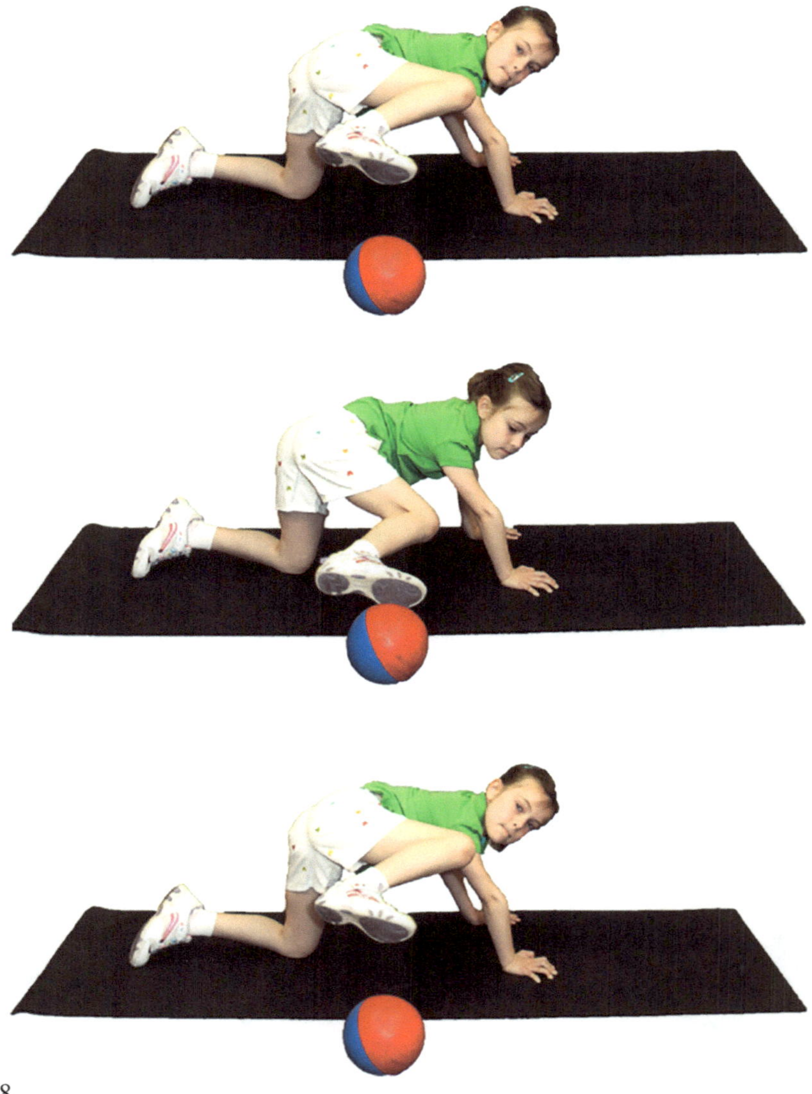

28. MOUNTAIN CLIMBERS

Combine end range hip flexion, extreme pelvic disassociation, quick timing requirements and voila! You have mountain climbers. I often have to start clients with two hands on a bench or a chair and work progressively lower until they can make it all the way down to the floor. I am not sure in this picture that it is clear but the client is jumping and clearing her legs from one position to the next. Technically you could do this activity without a jump if your client was in socks on a slippery floor or her feet were on sliding disks, but then this already hard activity would be even more difficult!

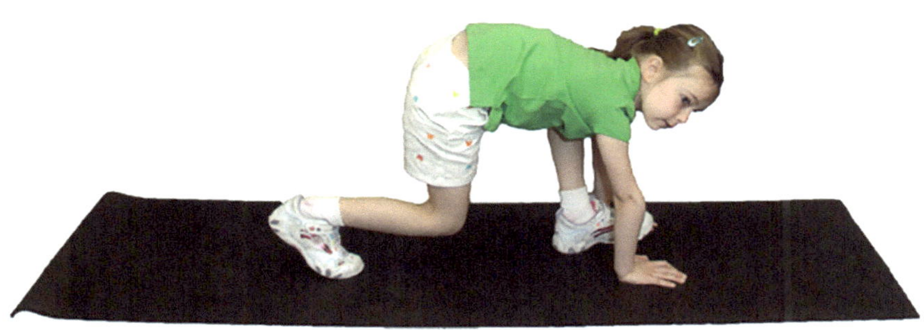

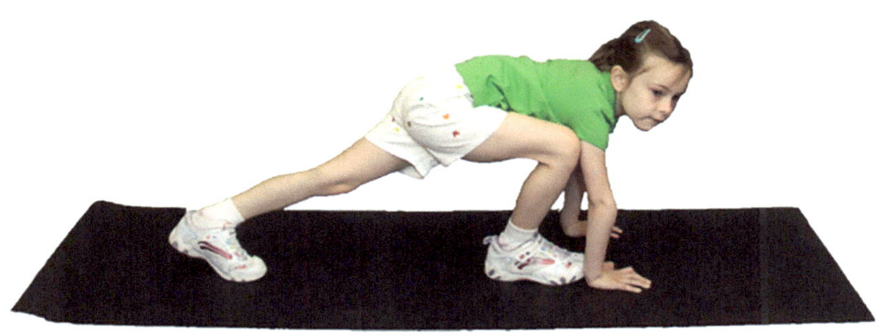

29. TUCK JUMPS, HANDS TO KNEES

It is the quick timing of this activity that makes it hard. My clients have a tendency to cheat by lowering their hands to the knees so watch out for this. I usually start this on the trampoline. If my client is successful, then I try the floor.

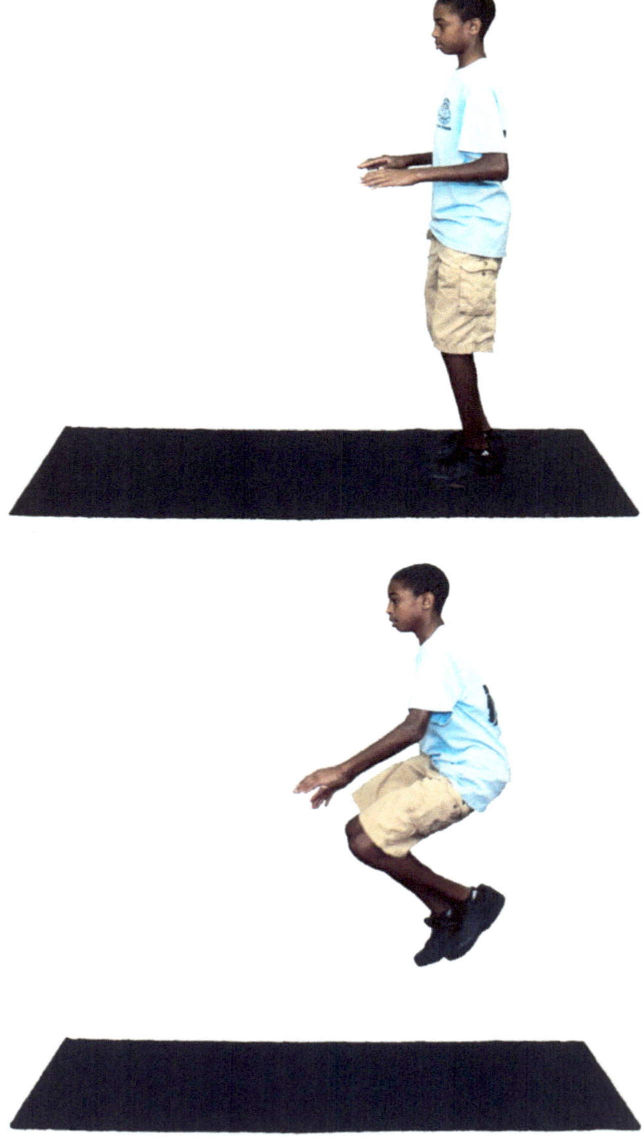

30. TUCK JUMPS, KNEES TO CHEST

I start by allowing the client to simply encircle his knees with his arms without having to bring the knees totally to his chest. Then I push for knees to chest. I usually start this activity on the trampoline to get a little more hang time to complete the move. If successful, then I go to the floor.

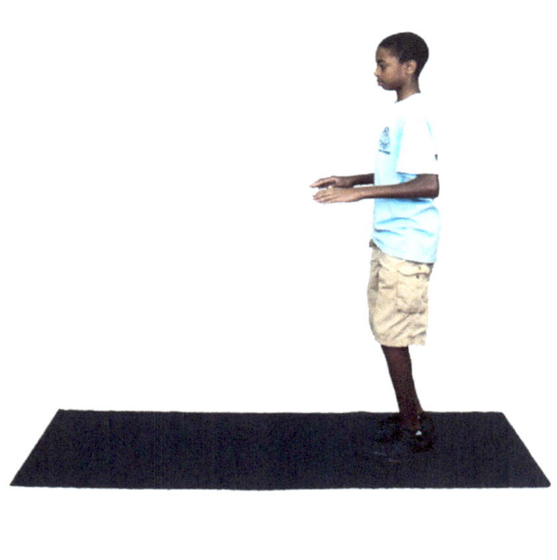

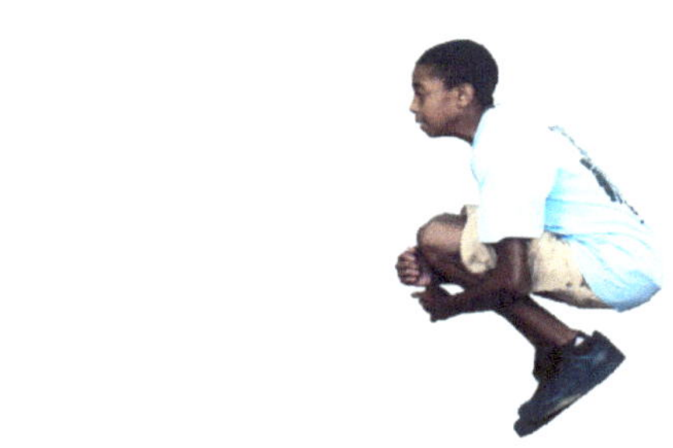

31. TUCK JUMPS, HANDS TO TOES

As if the last exercise was not hard enough, this exercise is even more difficult. Powerful hip flexion, good hamstring range and great timing are required.

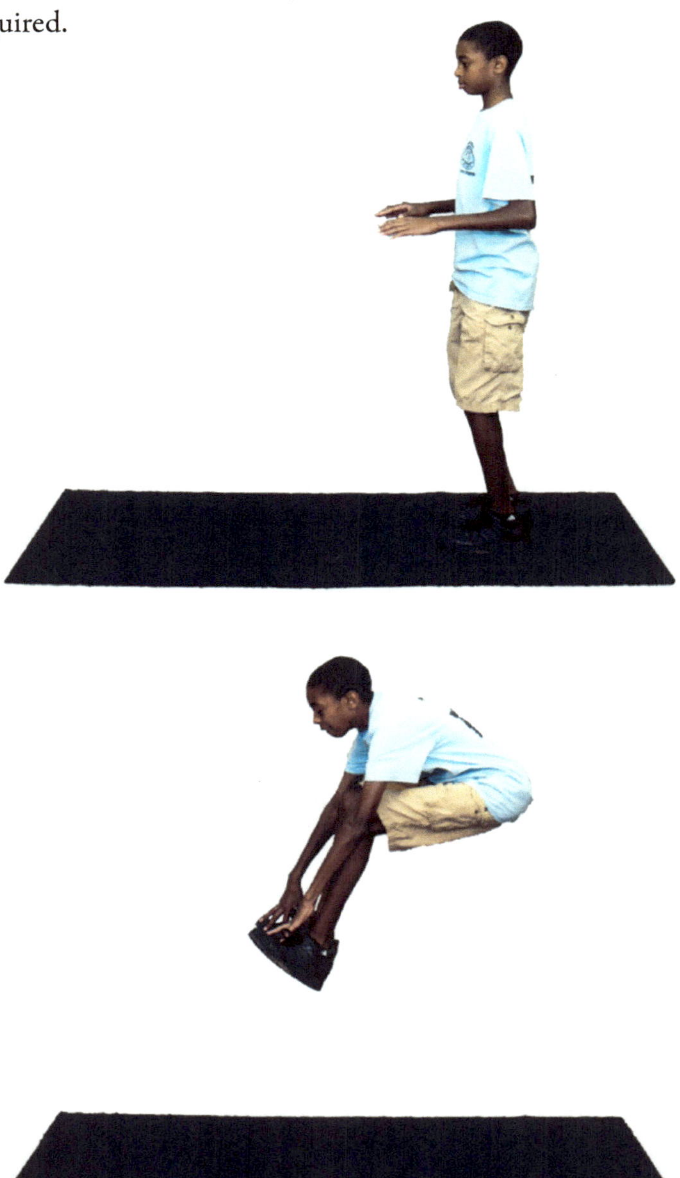

32. BURPEES

I have never known a client who liked burpees. So choose this exercise carefully. This seems to work best for the "hard core" client, specifically the ones who are motivated to excel at a sport. Personally, I like competition for motivation. I challenge my client to a competition of who can do the most repetitions in 30 seconds. I set the timer and have the parent count for the child. I count for myself, and we are off. I almost always get beat. If you want to add an additional challenge to this already difficult task, set a metronome beat to pace a client. See how long you and/or your client can keep pace.

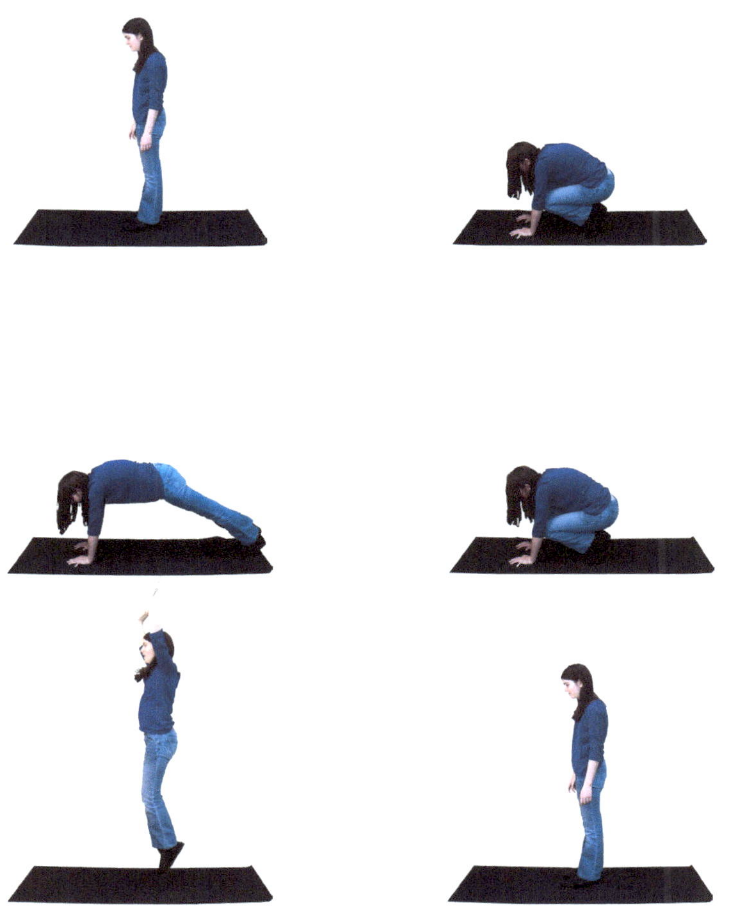

II. HIP EXTENSION

THE HIP EXTENSORS MOVE THE femur away from the pelvis and the lower back or conversely the pelvis and the lower spine away from the femur if the femur is stabilized. This movement is in the sagittal plane. The hip extensors are powerful lower body stabilizers. Weakness or tightness in the hip extensors will affect gait, as well as sitting and standing posture. This chapter includes a wide variety of exercises to improve hip extensor strength.

* * *

1. HIP/KNEE EXTENSION SUPINE ON BALL

I tend to use this exercise with clients who have little idea or capability of pushing with hip and knee extension. If you carefully balance the client-no small task; then a small hip extension push from the client can produce a big and rewarding movement. I often end up taking this kind of client through the movement so she can get the feel of the motion-or as the case often is; so that the client will be motivated by the motion and want to repeat it. The further you have the client on top of the ball, the more gravity-eliminated this movement becomes.

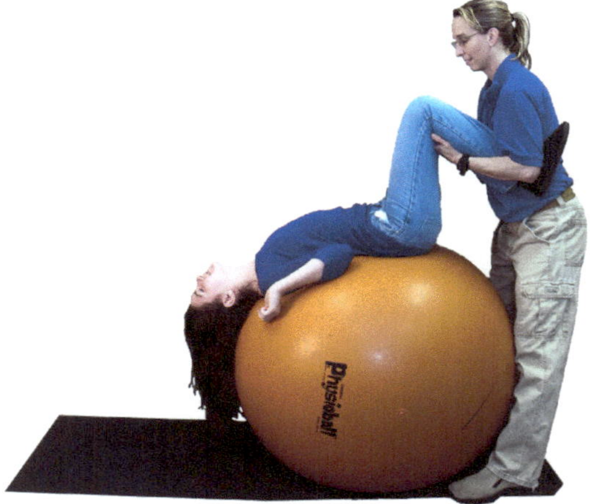

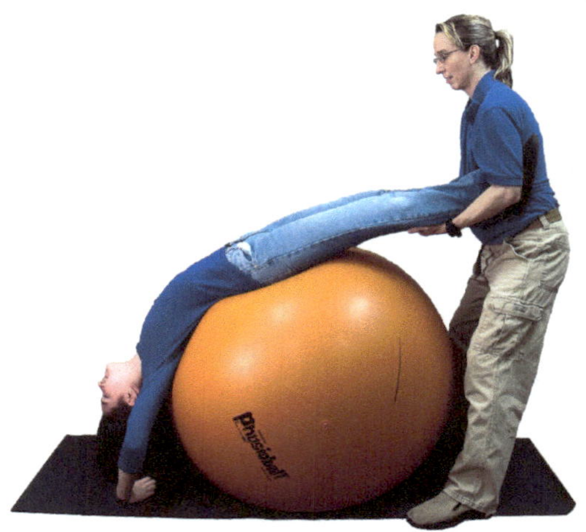

2. BRIDGING

Sometimes I have to block the knees and help the client lift her hips with my hands on her hips/lower back. I have some lower-functioning clients that can only lift their hips in this position if I pretend to start to change their diaper. Other clients like to play the game where the bridge comes up to allow the ball or the car to roll under their hips. The bigger the ball or the car, the harder this is. For some clients I just have them try to clear the floor momentarily, while with others I ask them to hold their hips up for 10 seconds. I have a client now who loves to do bridges on the trampoline. He is nonverbal but he understands that if I help him bridge until we count to 10, then I will bounce him while he lays on his back on the trampoline. He LOVES this and will play the game repeatedly. I document how much assistance the child required, how extended a position is reached and the duration the position was held.

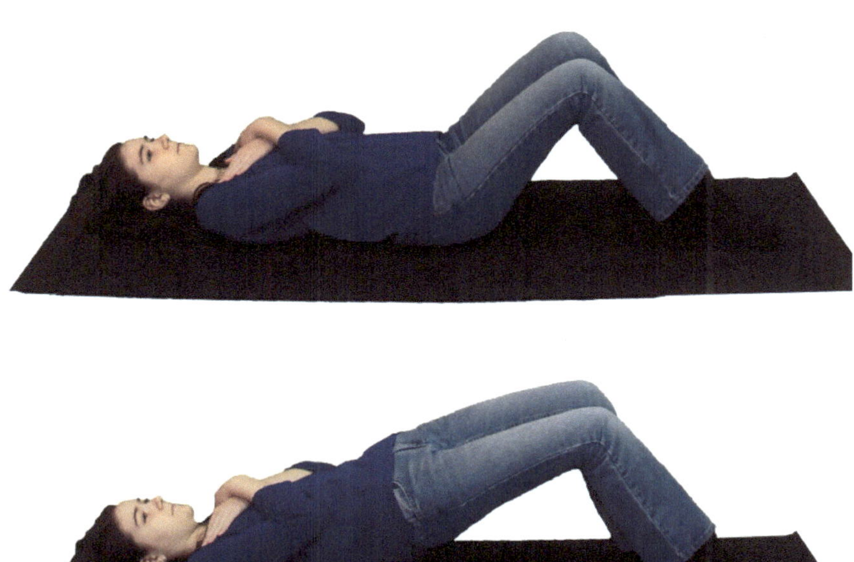

3. BRIDGING WITH ONE LEG CROSSED

This exercise is one step harder than a standard bridge. With the "free" leg crossed across the other knee, it can still help a little bit. This is an activity I might pick for a client with unilateral weakness like hemiplegia. Some clients like to play the game in which the bridge comes up to allow a ball or a car to roll under their hips. The bigger the ball or the car, the harder this is. For some clients I just have them try to clear the floor momentarily and some I ask them to hold their hips up for a specific duration.

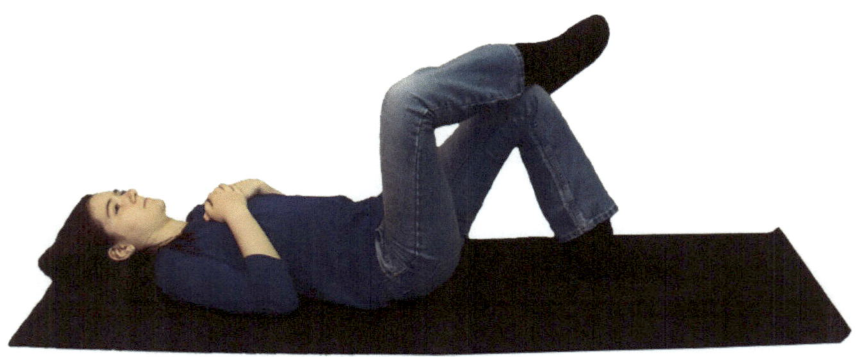

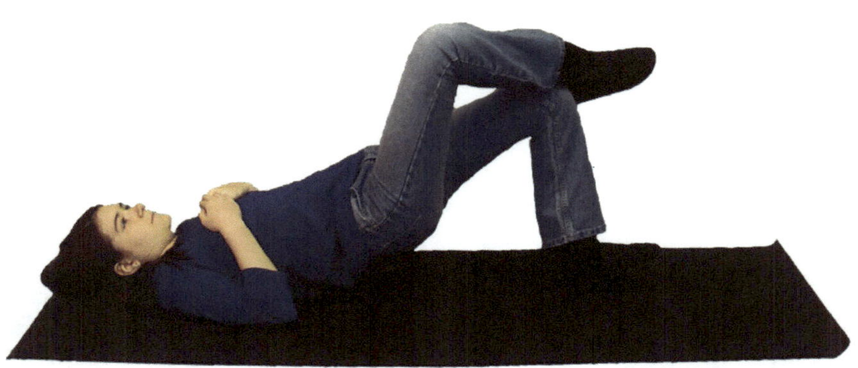

4. BRIDGING ONE LEG UP

This exercise is one step harder than the bridge with one leg crossed. Again, this is an activity for a client with unilateral weakness. This is also good for the game in which the bridge comes up to allow a ball or a car to roll under their hips. The bigger the ball or the car, the harder this is. For some clients I just have them try to clear the floor momentarily. This is harder with a longer isometric hold.

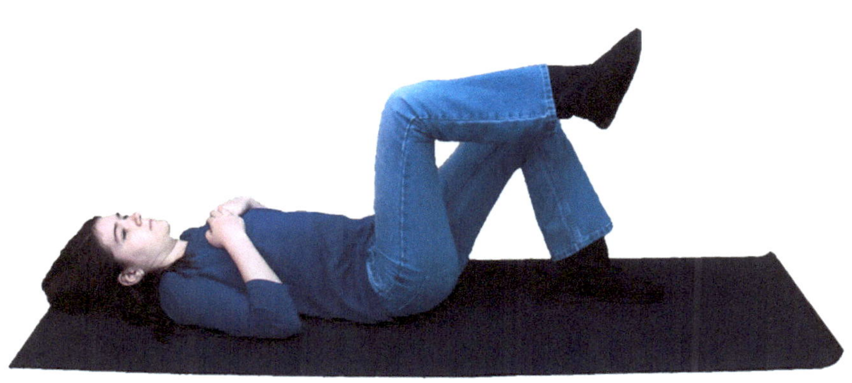

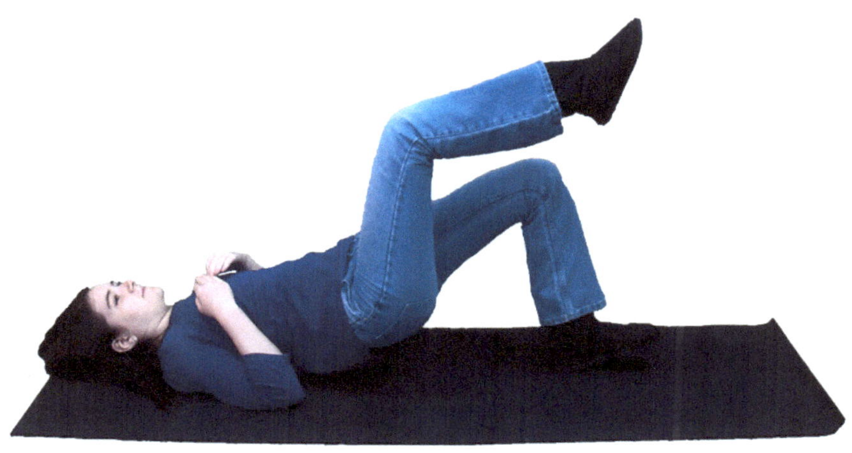

5. STAMP IN BRIDGE

This is a good activity to work on strength and also balance and weight shift for some clients. You can have your client stamp the same foot over and over or alternate legs. I always find my clients do best if I tell them up front how many stamps I am expecting before they can be finished.

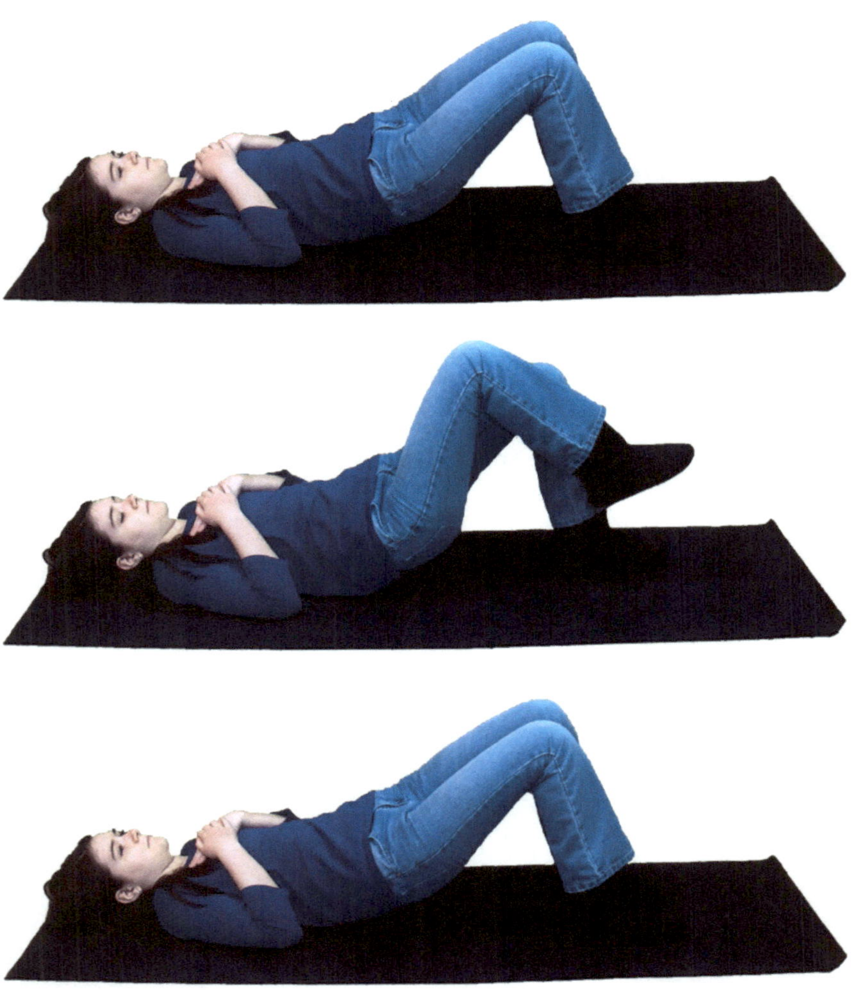

6. BALL BRIDGE WITH KNEES EXTENDED

This emphasizes end range hip extension with knee extension which is often needed in gait. The client can prop her legs on a bench for more stability or on a peanut ball for a little less or on an exercise ball for progressively less stability.

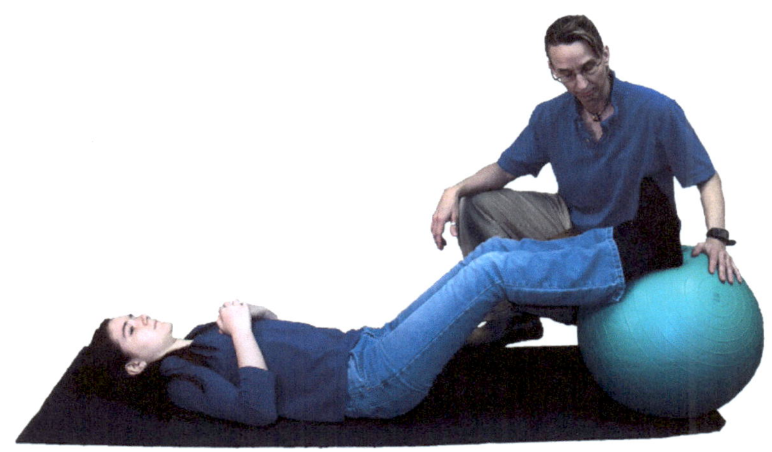

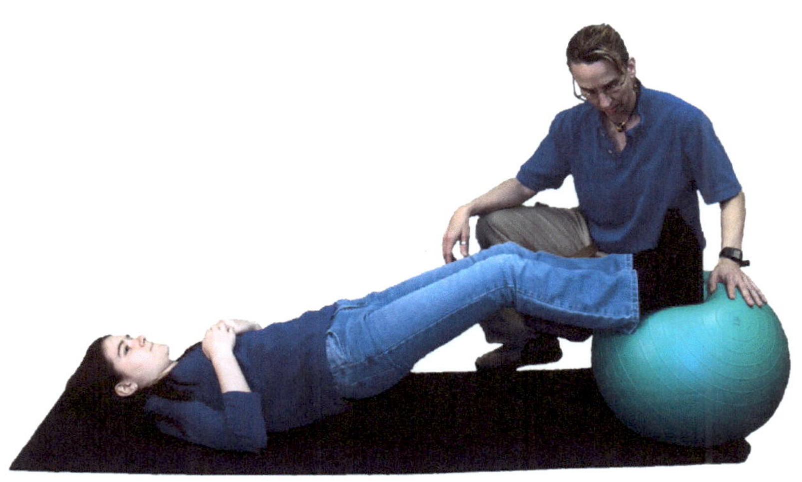

7. TWO LEGS HIP/KNEE EXTENSION SUPINE

I should have called this the human squat press machine! Kids love this activity. I have the child lie back on a bean bag or pillow blocked behind by a wall or large furniture; otherwise kids tend to slide away from me on the floor. If no support is available, I have a parent stabilize the child's shoulders to keep him from sliding. I help the child maximally flex up his hips and knees, then I lean forward putting my upper chest on the child's feet. I adjust my weight on the child according to what he can accept. I apply just enough weight for the child to just barely be successful in pushing me off. I fall dramatically, and oh, how the kids love this exercise! I have no problem getting 8-10 repetitions. I have used this with clients who are minimally to severely physically involved. It works perfectly.

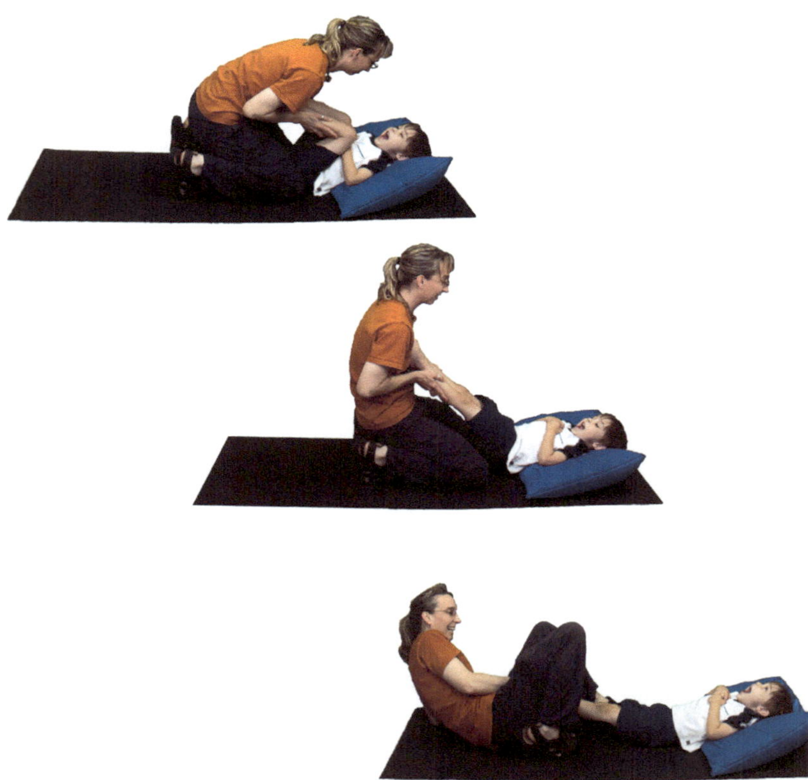

8. ONE LEG HIP/KNEE EXTENSION SUPINE

And this is the one-leg squat press machine! I use this activity when I want to isolate one leg at a time. It is wonderful with children with one-side involvement. Kids love this activity too. The same blocking suggestions apply as on the two leg extension. I tend to block the other leg down relatively straight.

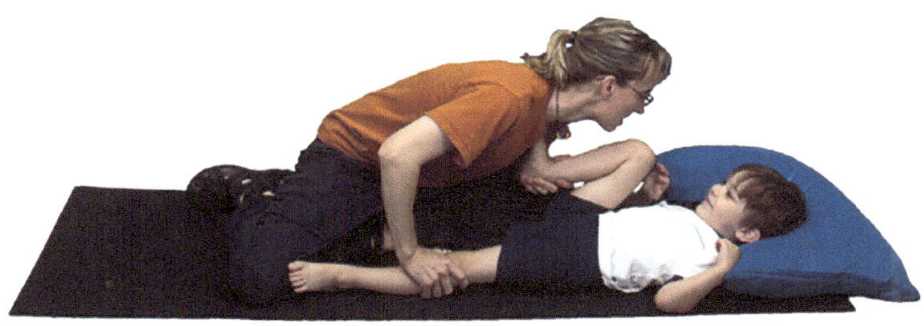

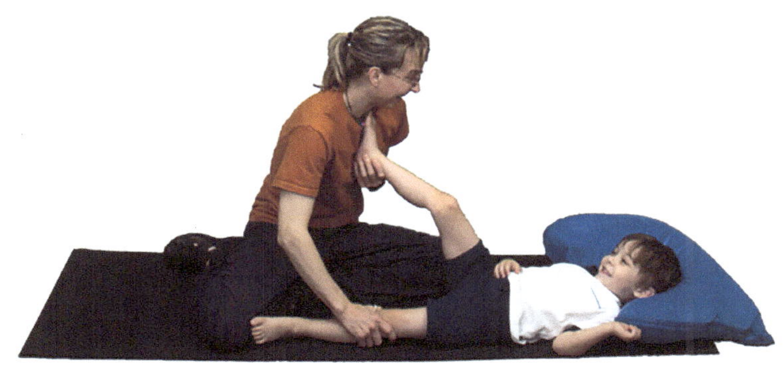

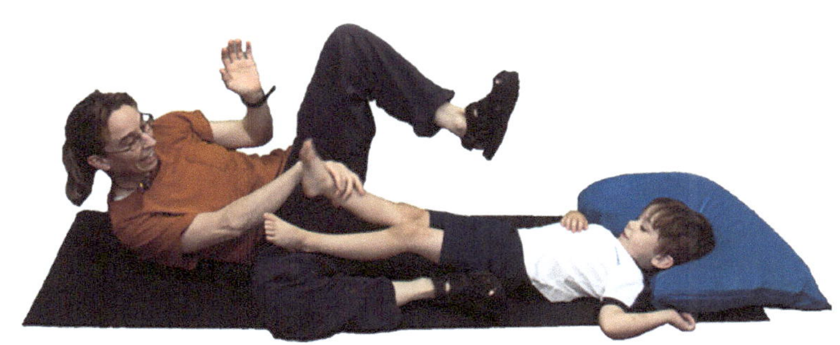

9. ONE LEG ON BENCH BRIDGE

This exercise emphasizes end range hip extension unilaterally. This is great for a client with unilateral weakness or one who needs a greater challenge. I have my client either perform a certain number of repetitions of this and/or hold the end range hip extension with the opposite leg up for certain duration.

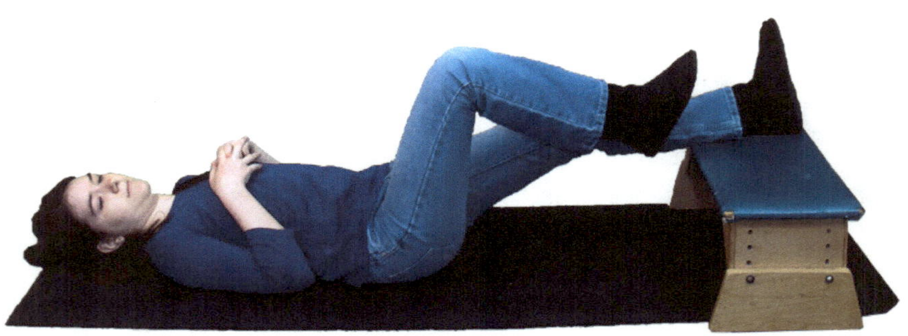

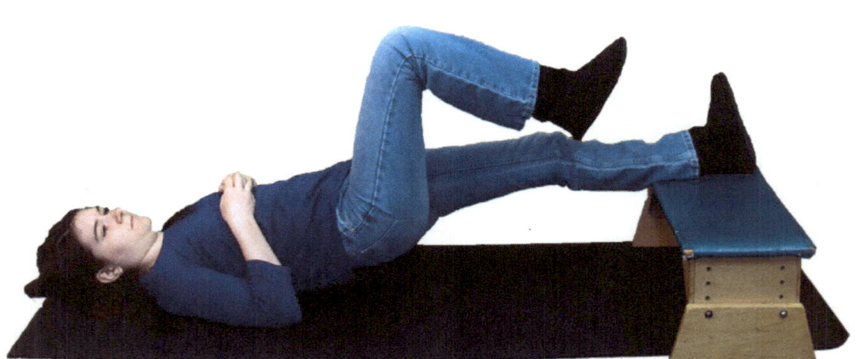

10. ONE LEG BRIDGE, ABDUCTION KICK

So first the client lifts into end range extension with one foot up on the bench. Then she kicks laterally into abduction to knock the cone/block/toy off the bench. This is hard work but most of my kids like knocking things over especially if I act like I am upset about it.

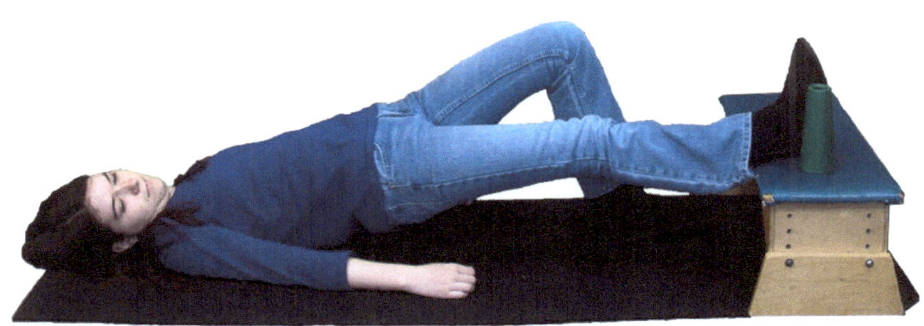

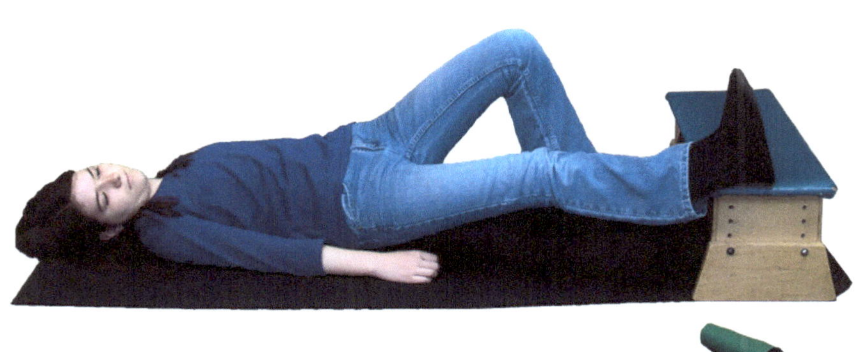

11. LOW TO TALL CRAB

Some of my kids will do this exercise just to do it, but most need a target. I simply hold my hand above the belly button and I tell her to lift her stomach up to my hand.

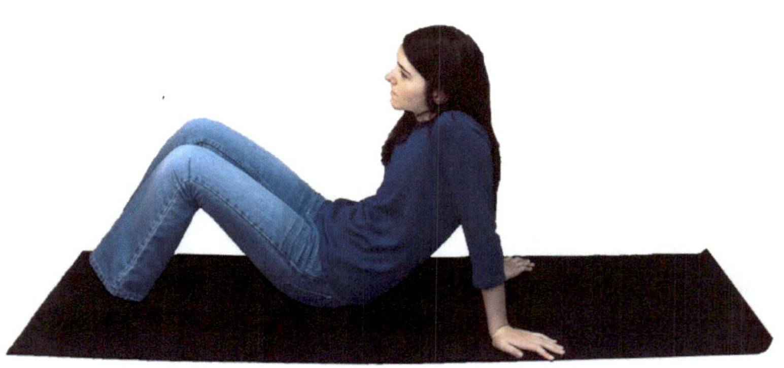

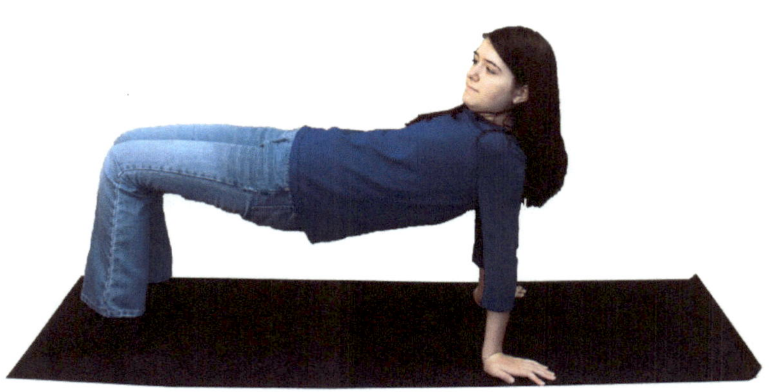

12. BALL ROLLING UNDER CRAB

Some of my kids will work harder if I have a ball or a car that I roll underneath them in crab position. A bigger car or ball requires more hip extension. Having a specified number of cars stacked up waiting to get to the other side makes it a little easier for the kids to tolerate this exercise.

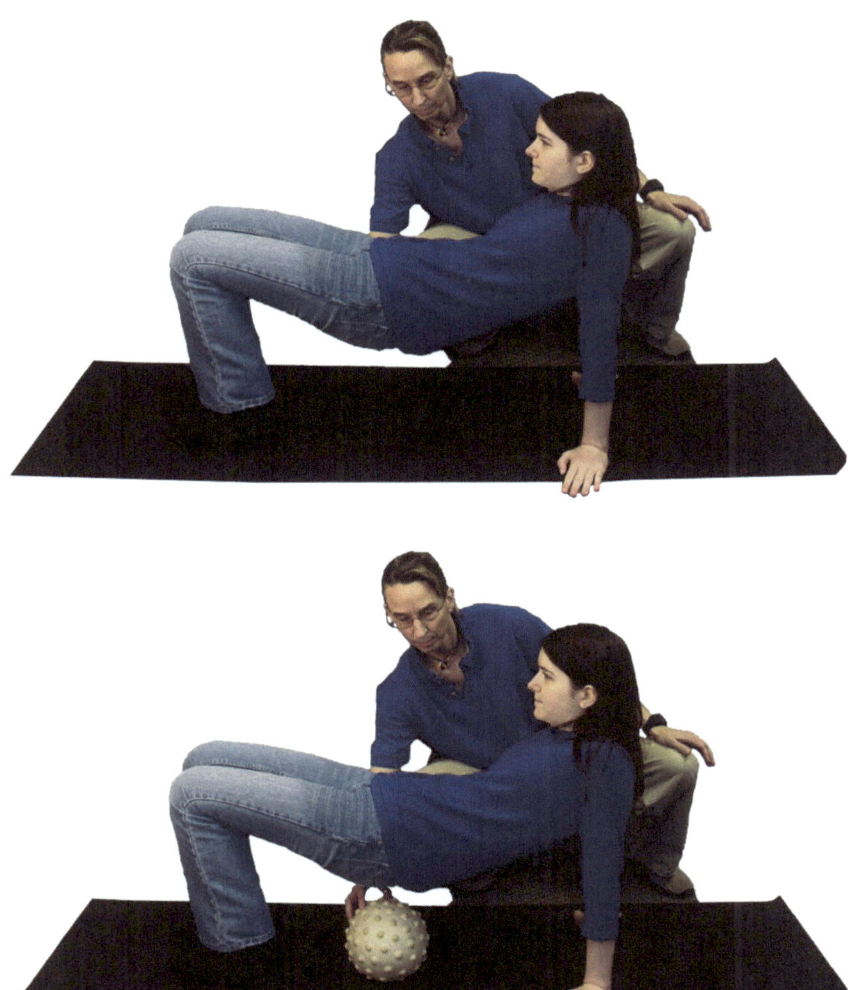

13. KICK IN CRAB

For some clients, the motivation is not a hand target, bridge or a car, but instead them kicking a ball and making me chase it around the room, especially if I playfully moan and groan. I may or may not require the child to be in full hip extension before I roll the ball. This is another activity that is good for unilateral hip weakness or to isolate one side before trying the other side.

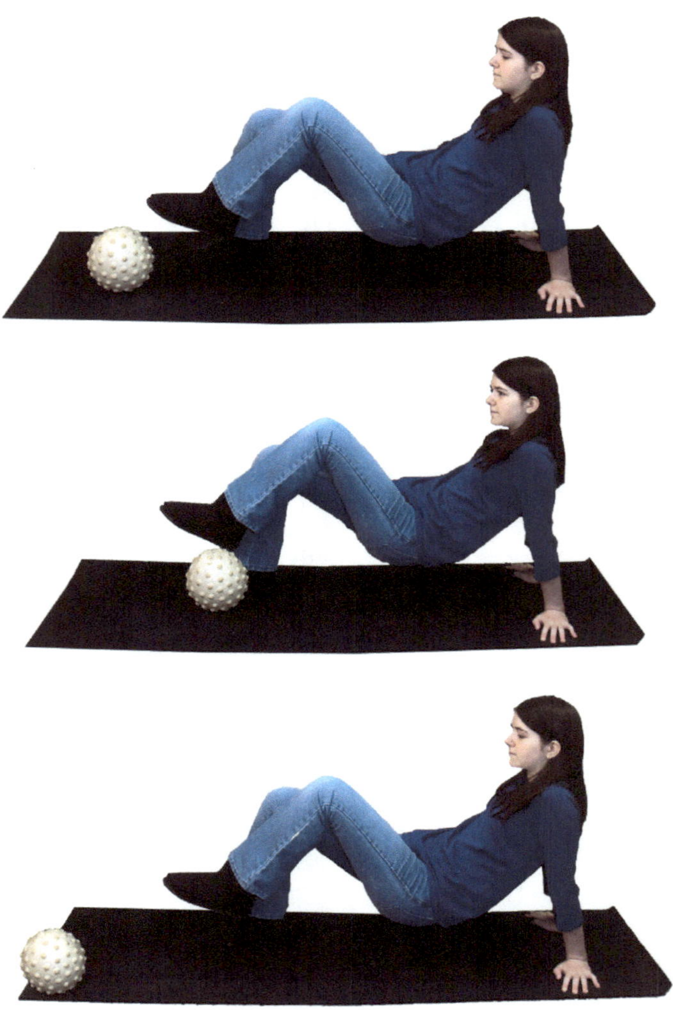

14. CRAB WALK

Oh, the dreaded crab walk! I usually get down on the floor and do it too. If I complain about it, the kids don't seem to mind as much. You can have the child go forward, backward or sideways. I always emphasize keeping the hips off the ground-with more or less success. I may set up races going down the hall. A child is not as miserable crab walking if she is beating her therapist in a hot race. I have also played soccer in this position with my client. Why not get a work out too?

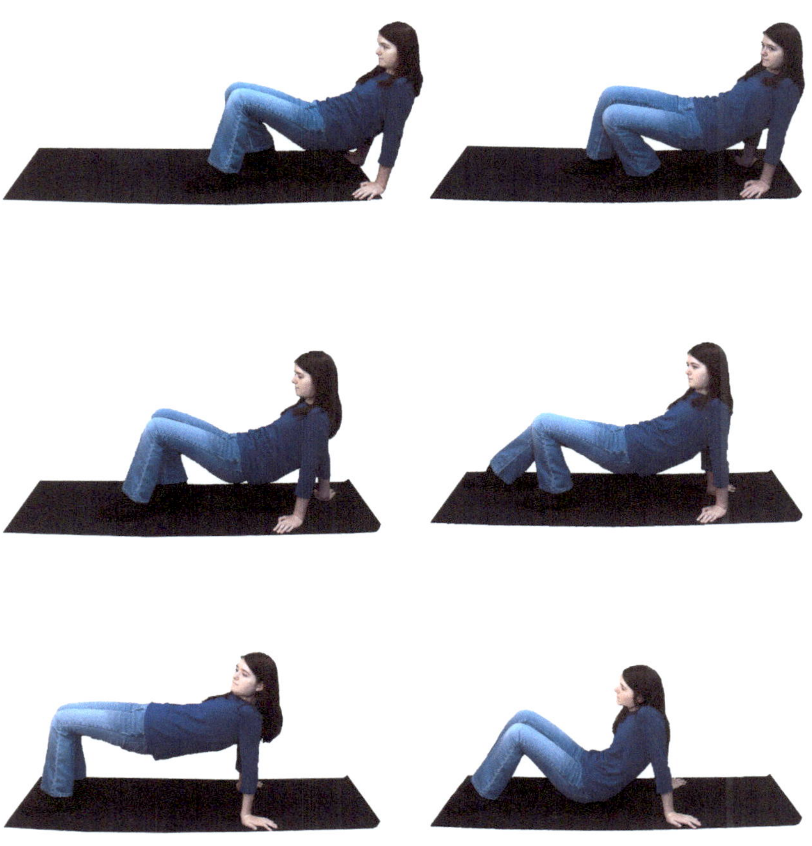

15. INVERTED SUPINE BICYCLE

This is a super hard exercise. The most difficult part actually seems to be the end range abdominals required to get in the start position, and getting the arms in the right position to prop up the hips. Sometimes I have to give up on the lower back being up off the floor.

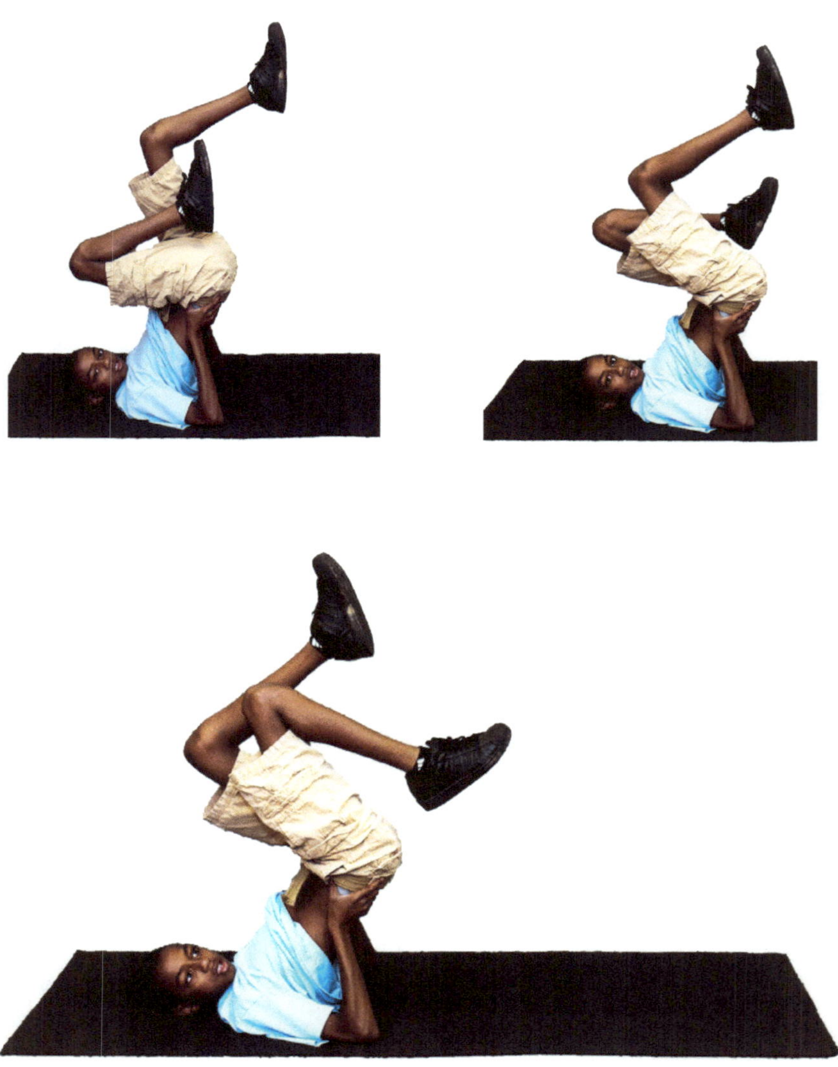

16. QUADRUPED HIP EXTENSION WITH KNEE EXTENSION

This is another boring exercise that is hard to get a kid to perform. I usually have a reward ready at the end. I have seen a variety of short cuts with this exercise. My diplegic kids cheat by flexing their elbows which effectively lowers the front of their bodies and their lower leg goes effectively higher. Brilliant. I have another child who anteriorly tilts her pelvis or sags her back to make it easier to look like she is extending her hips to neutral. You can do this exercise for repetitions or for the duration that the leg is elevated or both. I have a piano that I can put on "organ" function. I have the child extend the leg to hit the piano keyboard that I am holding up. She has to keep the leg up so the organ continues to play for 10 seconds. It is not fun, but it gives her the auditory feedback to know when the leg has dropped and when it has gone high enough.

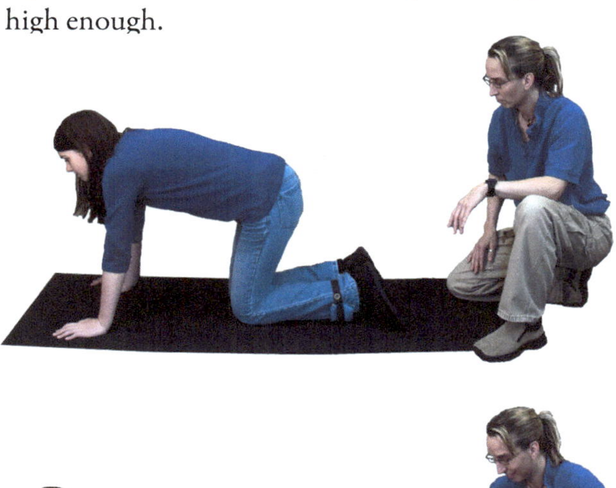

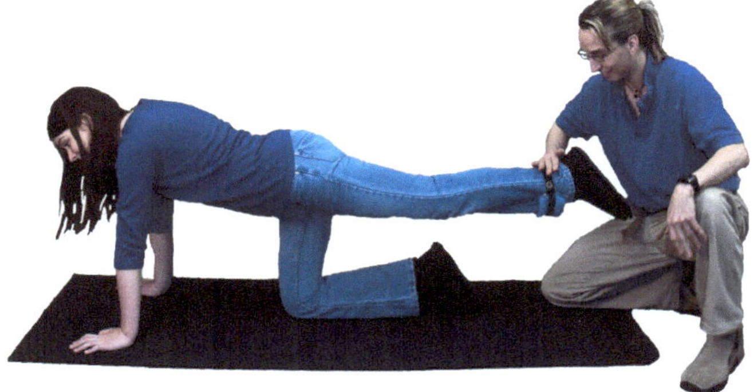

17. QUADRUPED HIP EXTENSION WITH KNEE FLEXION

I constantly try to come up with some enthusiasm for these exercises or some brilliant way to make them fun, but no success with this yet. This knee flexion is super hard for most of my clients with diplegia to hold. The knee flexion helps eliminate the hamstrings from helping but decreases the lever arm to make it easier. I was always miserable doing these in aerobics class. There should be a great reward following this exercise. You can do this exercise for repetitions or for the duration that the leg is elevated or both. I use the piano as described in the previous activity on this exercise as well.

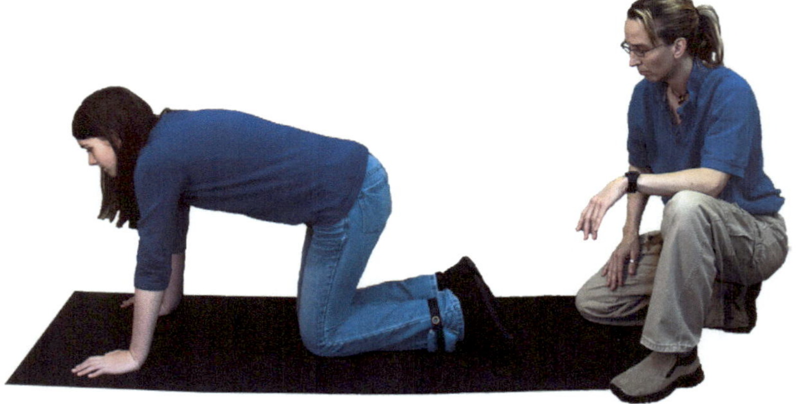

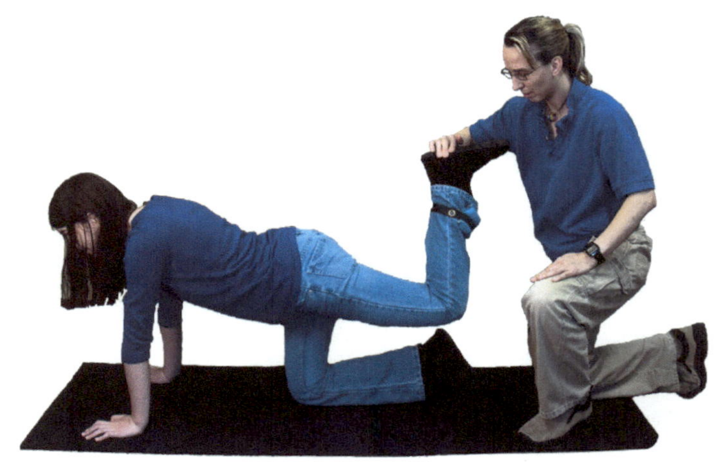

18. HIP EXTENSION BENCH LYING WITH UPPER EXTREMITY SUPPORT

I usually start with my 16" (41 cm) bench and see if this helps the child be successful. If so, I go to the 10" (25 cm) bench, then the 4" (10 cm) bench, then the 2" (5 cm) thick board, and then 1" (2.5 cm) board. With boys, I put down extra padding under their hips to prevent uncomfortable pressure on their private parts. I record the bench height and how long she could keep her legs off the ground.

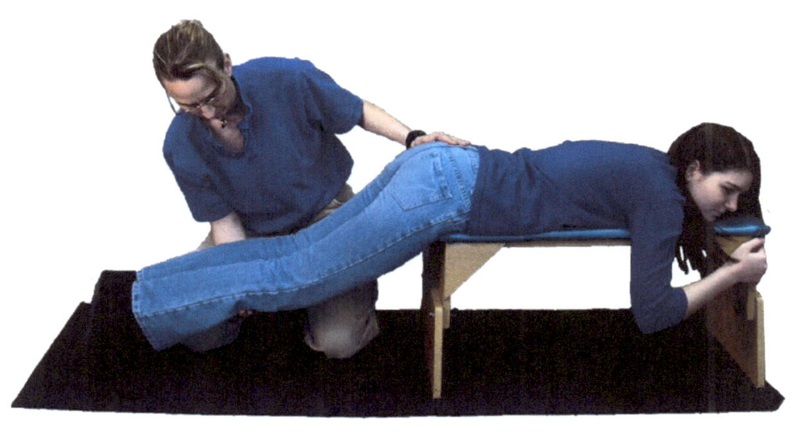

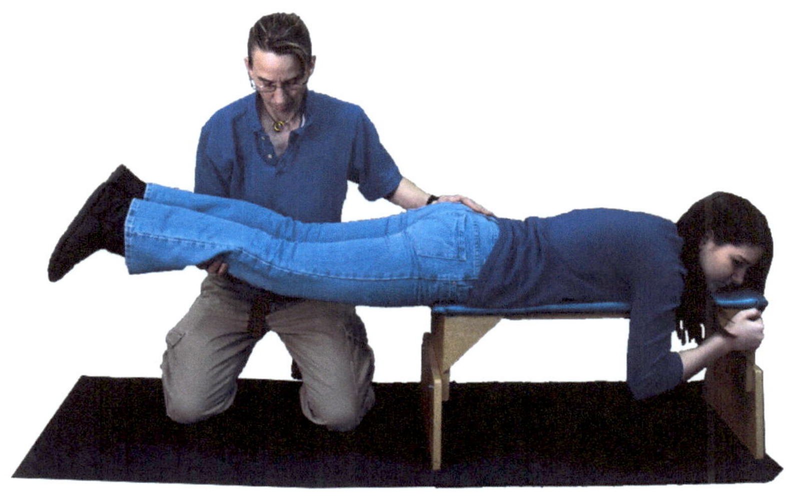

19. HIP EXTENSION BENCH LYING WITH ABDUCTION/ADDUCTION

Sometimes I try having the client abduct and extend her legs in this position to work in opposition to a flexed adducted gait pattern. I try bench heights starting with the easiest and progressing to harder to find the right challenge.

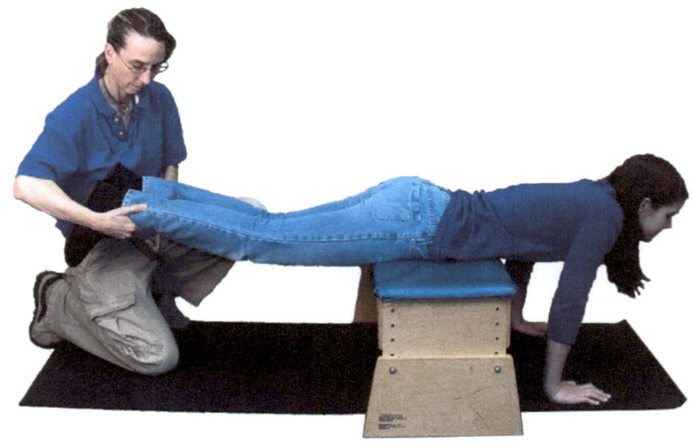

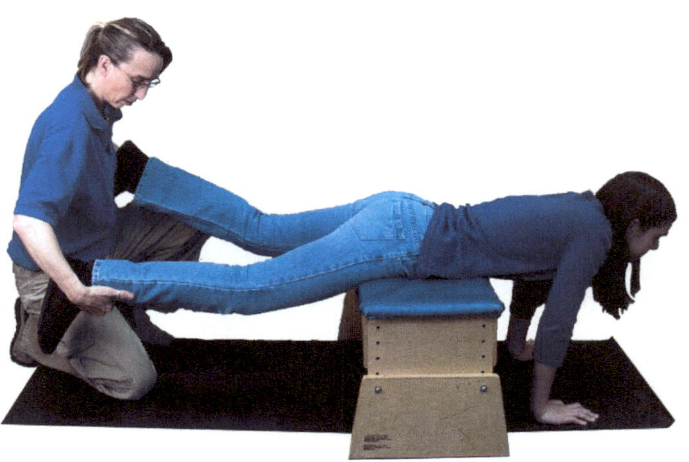

20. HIP EXTENSION PRONE WITH KNEE EXTENSION

This is classic prone hip extension starting from neutral hip extension, thus emphasizing end range hip extension. By having the knee extended both the hip extensors and the hamstrings are active.

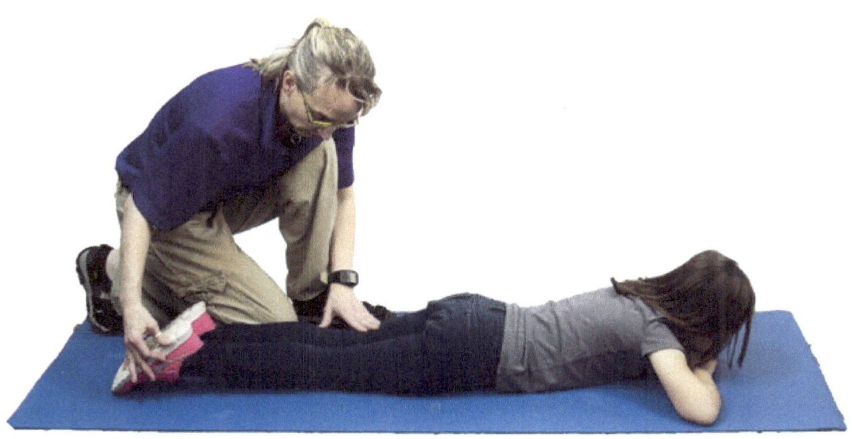

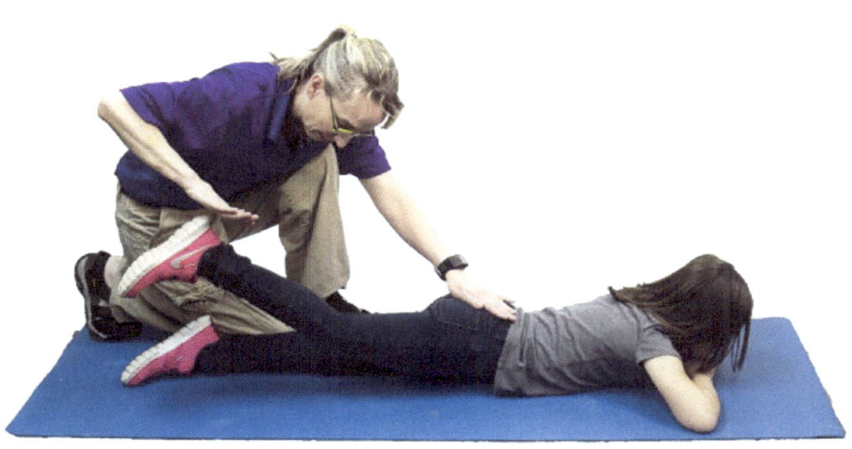

21. HIP EXTENSION PRONE WITH KNEE FLEXION

Again, this is classic hip extension starting from neutral hip extension emphasizing end range hip extension. With the knee flexed, the hamstrings are placed in a disadvantaged position to assist in hip extension.

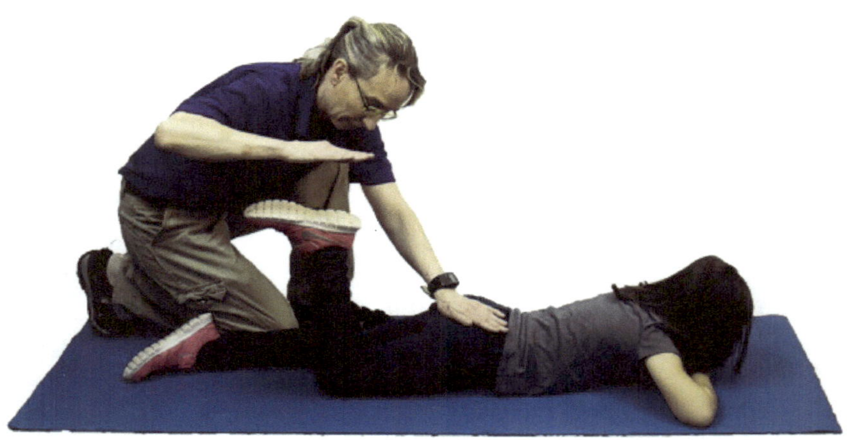

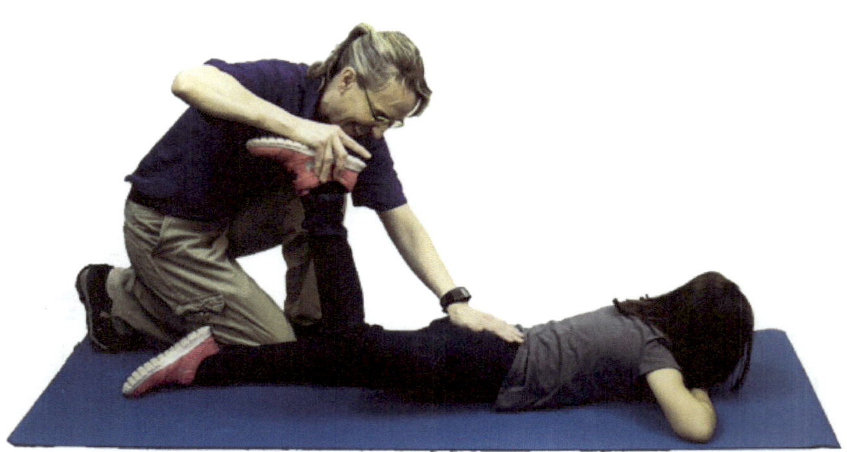

22. BENCH AIRPLANE/SUPERMAN

I work towards progressively lower benches. I also pad the bench for boys for private parts comfort. I document bench height and duration held. I also record arm and leg position, whether bent or straight. I work towards making it to the floor with all extremities extended and arms straight overhead. As the benches get lower, the legs are the extremities that are more likely to hit the ground. So, I keep checking the child's leg height by waving my hand between the floor and her knees to make sure they are clearing the floor.

For whatever reason kids seem to enjoy this activity. I usually do the exercise with them but maybe it is the act of defying gravity that they like. To start I line up the different height benches. When the child is successful with one bench then we all slide down to the next bench. I always have siblings do this exercise at the same time, often starting one bench ahead of the client. I don't start counting until everyone has all of their extremities up.

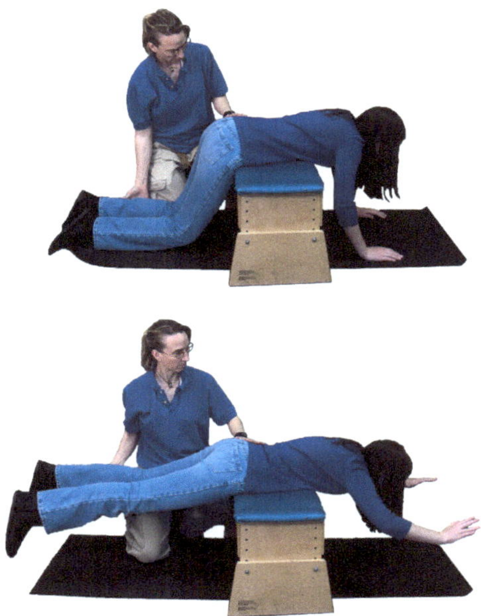

23. LOW TO TALL KNEEL

I start this activity at a bench before a child has the ability to walk. Then I work on it at a wall mirror which eliminates upper extremity help but allows balance assistance. Next I progress to the middle of the room, removing the balance assistance. I may need to give one or two hand held for support, but I prefer to give hip support so the child is not getting upper extremity aid. Several of my children with diplegia lack end range hip extension so they achieve this position with more of a lordosis. Keep an eye out for this substitution.

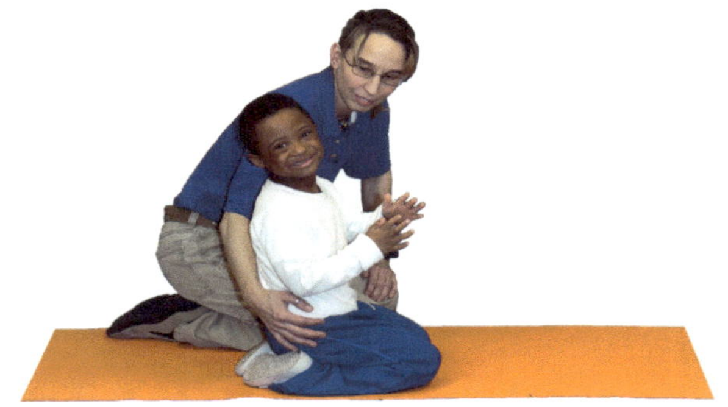

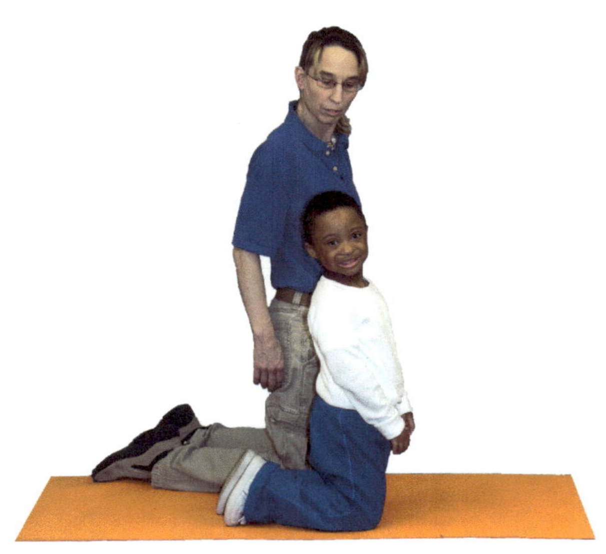

24. KNEE WALK

This is a great exercise for those bunny hoppers. I always use a mat, especially as the kids get bigger. I start with two hands held, then one hand held. As an in-between step to independence, I may have the child knee walk sideways to the wall with one hand on the wall. I document the number of steps taken or the distance knee walked. This is how many of my clients with athetosis and ataxia figure out mobility. I discourage knee walking long term for locomotion.

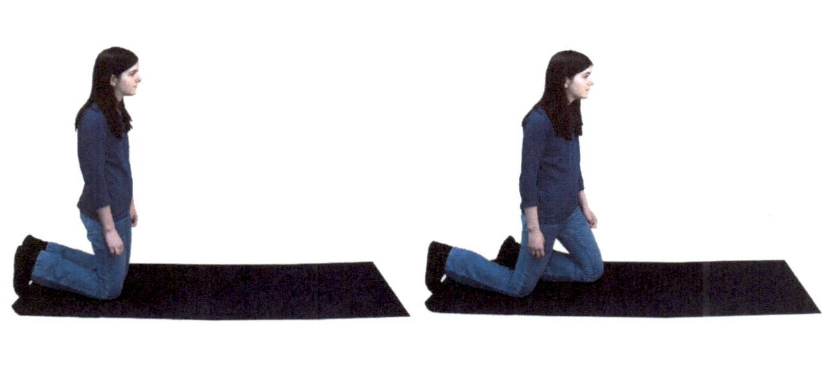

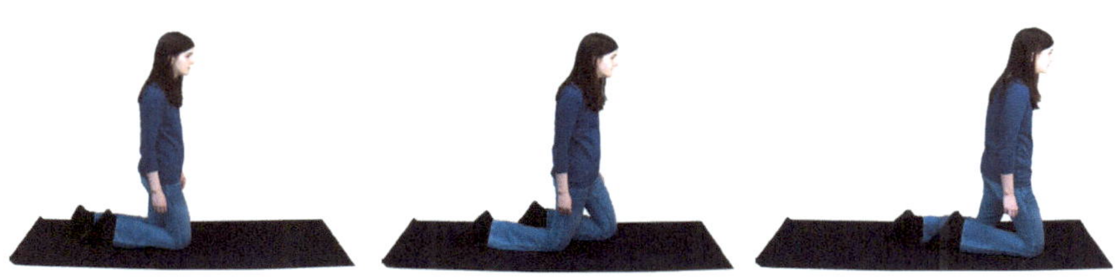

25. LOW TO TALL HALF KNEEL

I usually perform this activity at a bench. I put a puzzle piece or similar item on the floor on the side with the knee down. The child has to go down and back to get the puzzle piece and then he raises up into tall half kneel to put the puzzle piece in the puzzle on the bench. This is an extremely hard activity for my kids with diplegia. I often have to get in low kneel behind my clients with my knees on either side of the client's knee that remains down to give them the balance needed to perform this activity, especially without a bench.

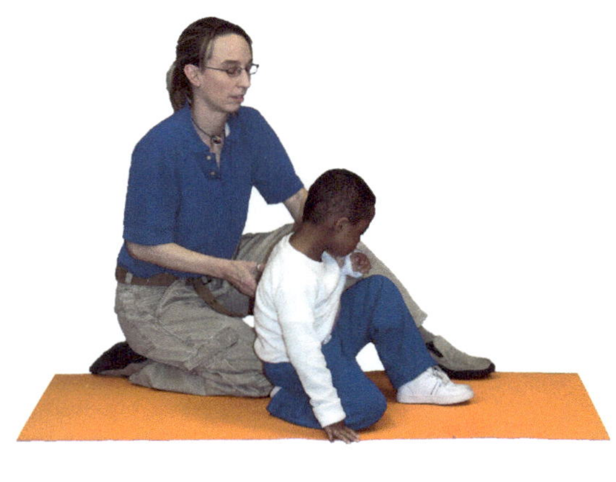

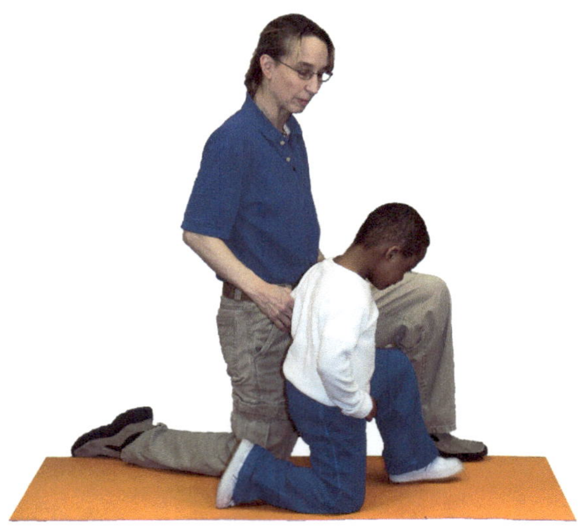

26. KNEEL TO HALF KNEEL WITH TWO POLES

Moving from kneel to half kneel requires hip flexion on one side and maintenance of hip extension on the stationary side. The Kaye Product vertical poles are perfect for this activity. This is one of those exercises that my kids with diplegia need to practice repeatedly.

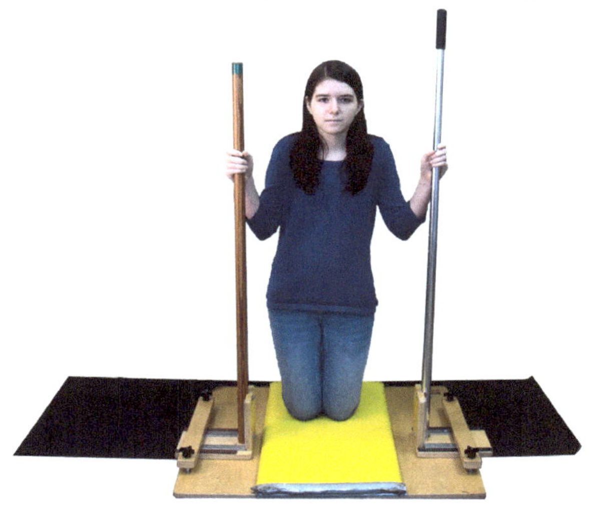

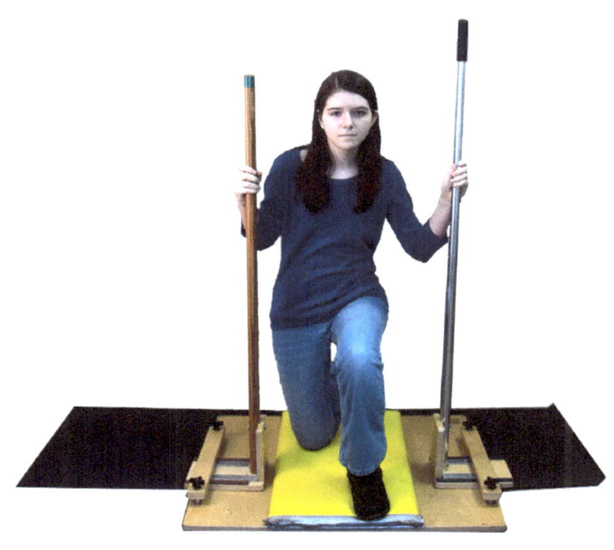

27. KNEEL TO HALF KNEEL ONE HAND HELD

One hand held gives significantly less stable support than the upright poles. My diplegic kids all want to skip from tall kneel up to standing at a support. They need to practice this work on both sides until they can do it in their sleep!

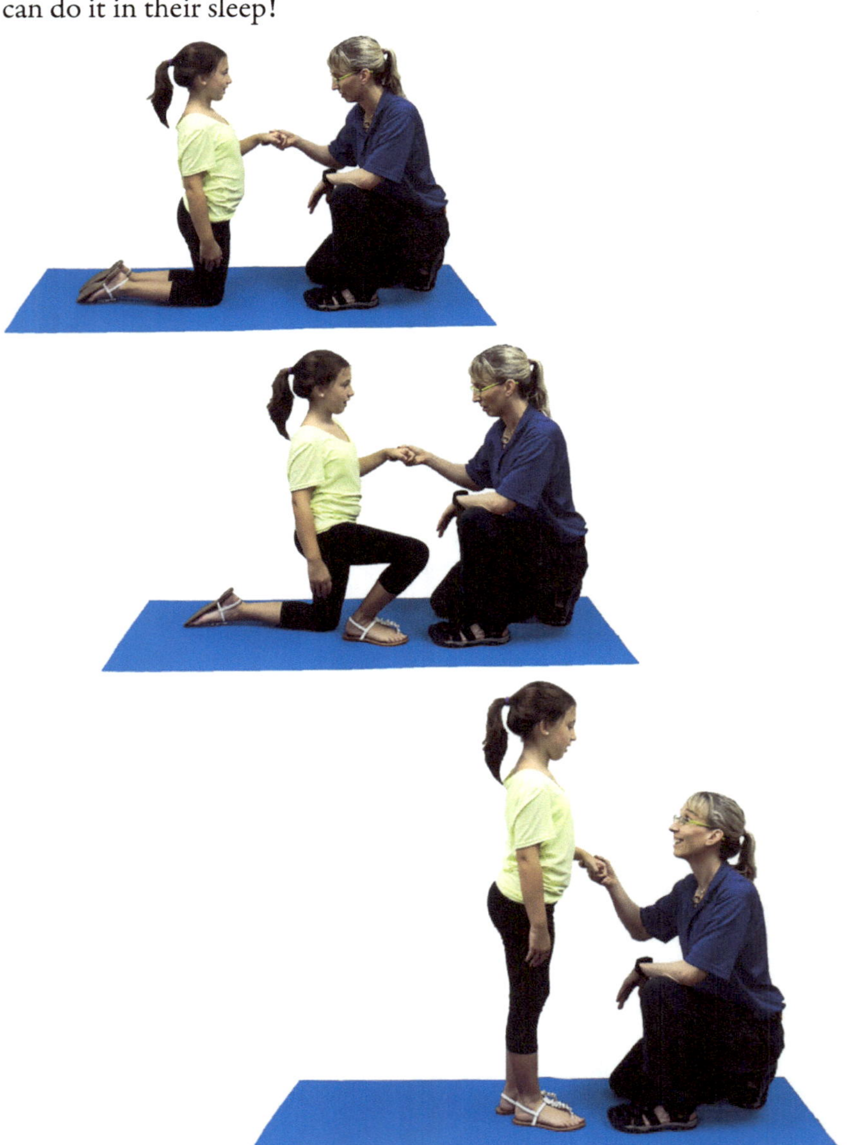

28. HALF KNEEL TOSS

I like work in half kneel. I've had parents read to kids in half kneel. Each time a page is turned, the child has to switch legs. Looking at a story in this position is a less dynamic activity than placing rings on a ring stander. Having to throw a ball back and forth is even harder. Again, the hip extensor on the leg with the knee down is working really hard here. The emphasis on this activity is to have no upper extremity support while engaging in another activity.

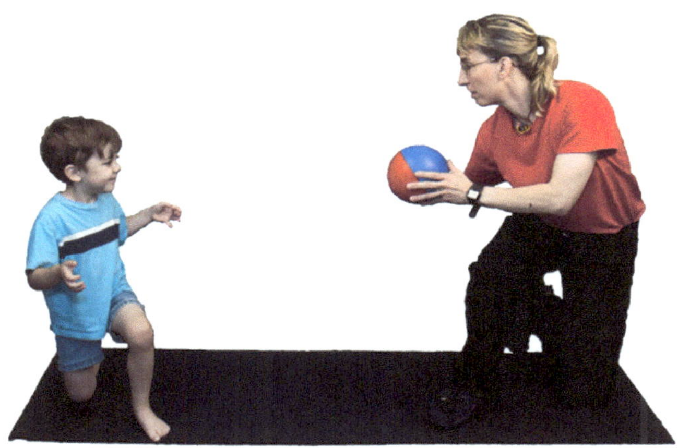

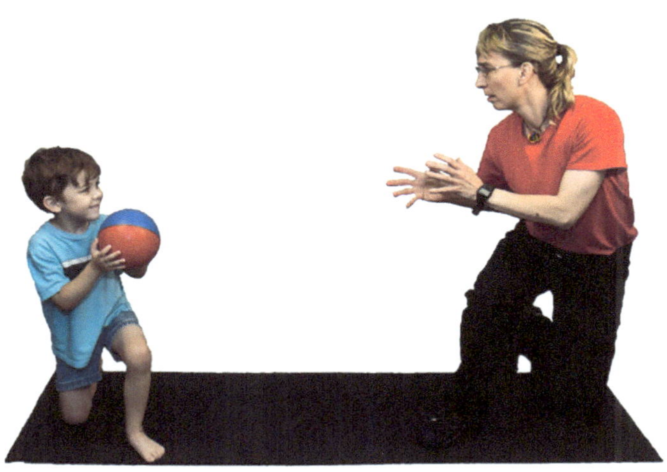

29. TALL KNEEL FRONT PUSH

Being stable in tall kneel requires strong hip extension. I like testing tall kneel balance with a "push." A push from the front requires initially hip flexion and then hip extension to maintain balance. You can push with a series of nudges or with a prolonged push. I often will have my client hold against the push for 10 seconds.

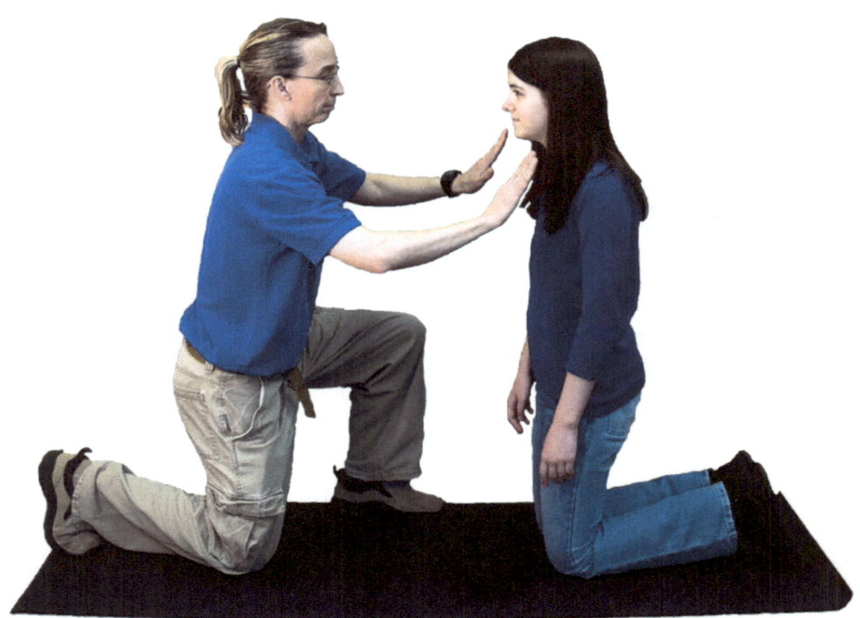

30. TALL KNEEL BACK PUSH

A push from the back requires hip extension to keep the client from toppling forward. I perform this activity similar to how I perform the front push-just from the back. Giving a warning before pushing is always polite.

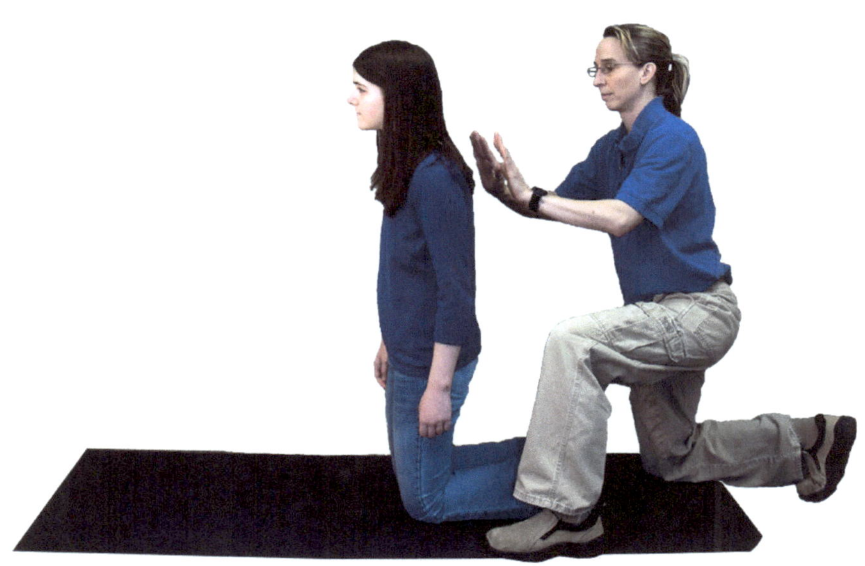

31. HALF KNEEL STAMP

I like this exercise for strengthening both hip flexion and extension. If it is performed without support, the exercise requires significant balance.

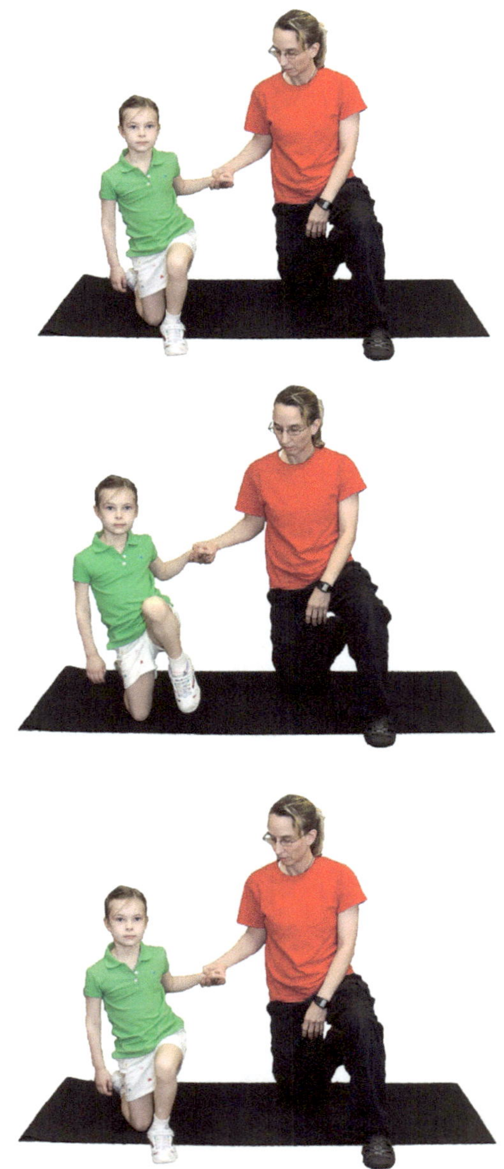

32. HALF KNEEL STAMP

I've always found exercises with toys that make noise make the activity go better. This can be a hard or...a very hard exercise depending on the placement of the toys. Obviously the leg stabilizing and not moving is the one performing hip extension.

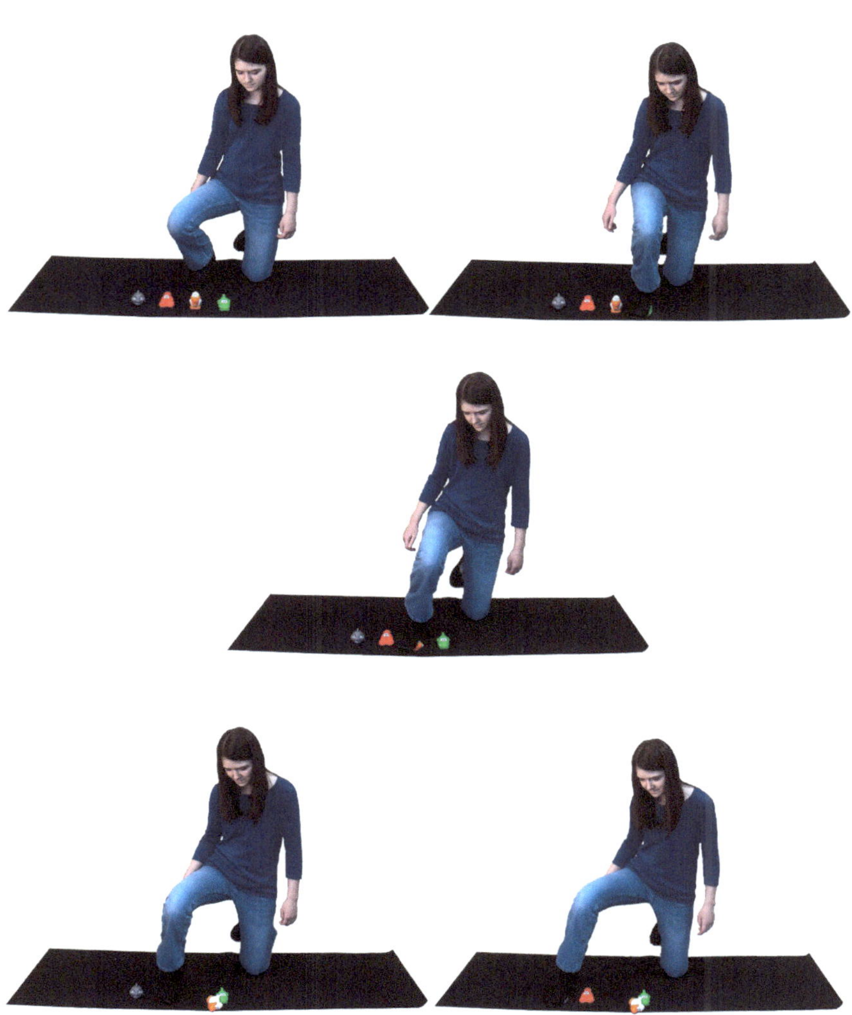

33. BENCH KNEEL TO HALF KNEEL WITH TRAY

Holding a loaded tray prevents my client from using her arms significantly to counter balance as she brings her leg from the behind the bench, to foot up on top of the bench, to foot in front of the bench and back behind again. The stationary leg is getting a strong hip extension work out as she tries to keep stable and balanced.

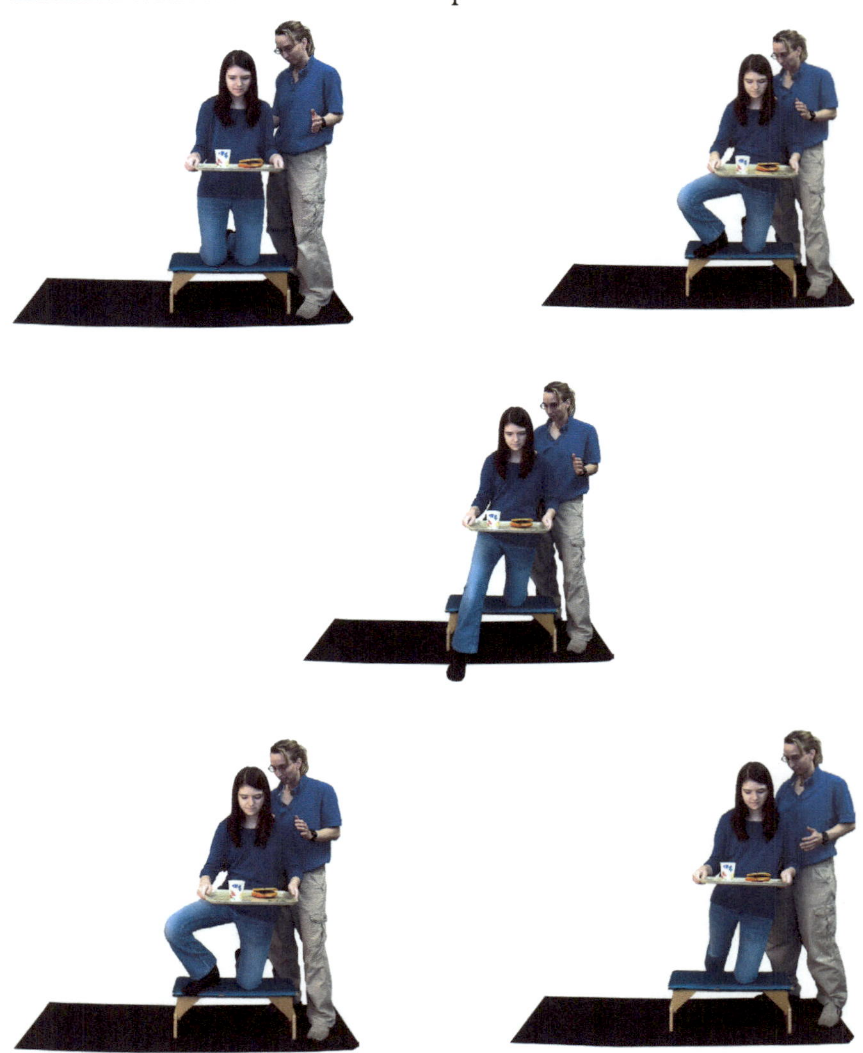

34. KICK CONES IN HALF KNEEL

This can be a hard to very hard difficulty based on the placement of the cones. If the client has to keep her foot up in the air for multiple kicks, then this exercise becomes extremely difficult. I usually let the client put her foot down between each kick. The stationary leg is getting a strong hip extension work out as she tries to keep very stable and balanced for the kick.

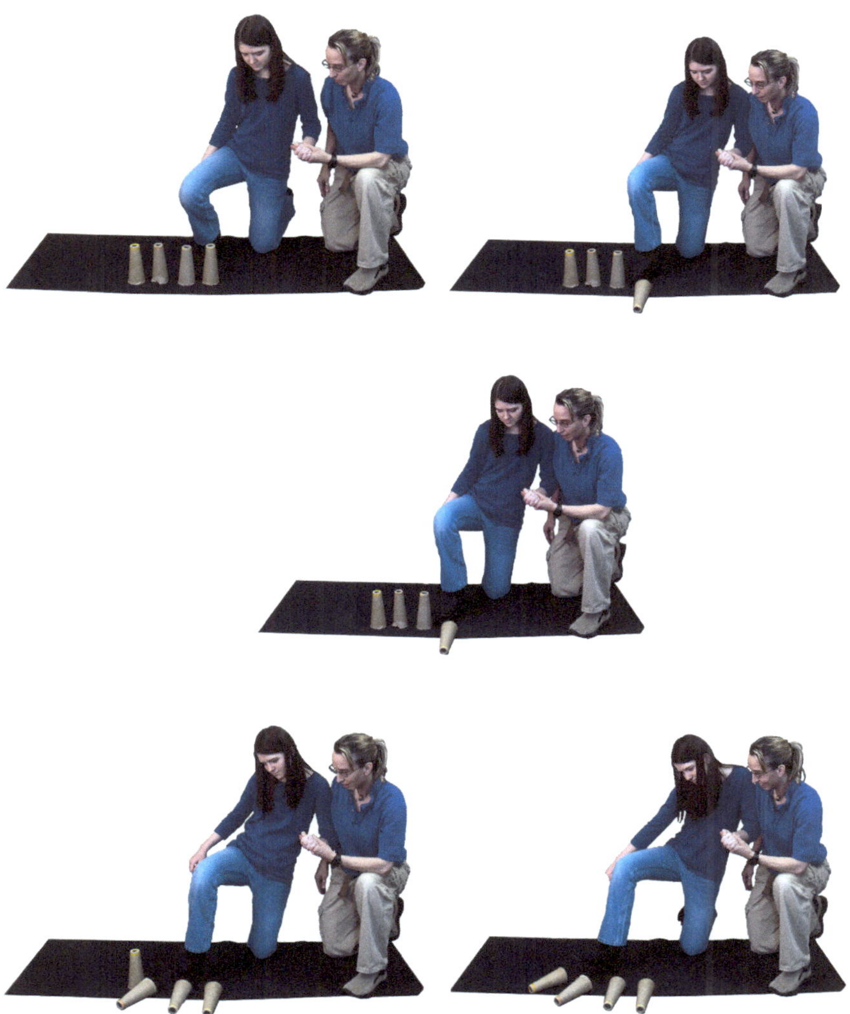

35. STRADDLE SIT TO STAND

I have several kids who pull in their adductors as they move from sitting to standing. Straddling something like a bench or a bolster makes adduction a little easier to block. Usually I have to sit behind the client on the bolster and help keep the knees apart with my hands on their knees.

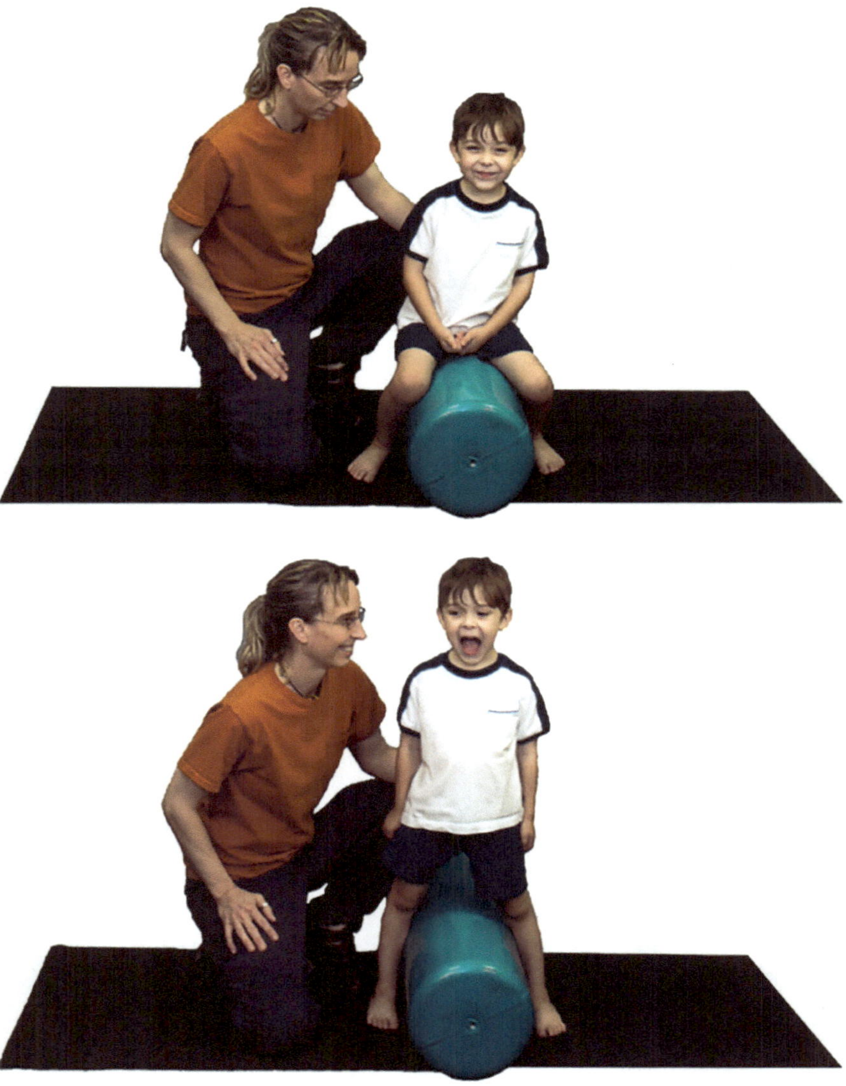

36. SIT TO STAND WITH TWO HANDS HELD

Sit to stand is such a functional daily life skill. The taller the bench the easier this exercise is. This is of course assuming the client's feet are still on the ground. To give the most support, I use two Kaye Products upright poles, two wall grips or two hands held. I have suction cups-wall grips meant for showers. I place them on my mirror in my room. I love them! I can put them where I need-up/down, wider/narrower, or vertical/angled/horizontal. If I am using the poles or the wall grips, I sit behind the client helping at his hips or knees. In the activity pictured, the client is strong enough to stand up with two hands held.

From here I progress to one hand held or two hands on a wall. Then I progress to touch or to no support in the transition from sitting to stand. I pay attention to whether or not the client needs back of knee support by the chair. Some clients can only get up to standing independently if the back of their knees hit the chair. I also like to work on sit to stand when the client is close to being independent by helping only at the knees in the front. I sit on a lower bench in front of the client facing him. I have my hands on his knees, helping the weight shift forward for the sit to stand transfer and then his standing balance.

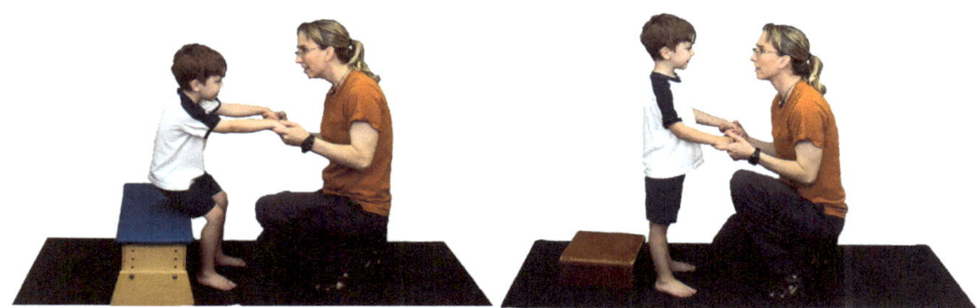

37. LOW SIT TO STAND

This activity is more challenging with a lower bench. Often as a therapist, I find I make one aspect of an activity harder, while making another step easier to compensate. I follow the same progression as described in the previous exercise. I document how much support the child requires and the number of repetitions he can perform.

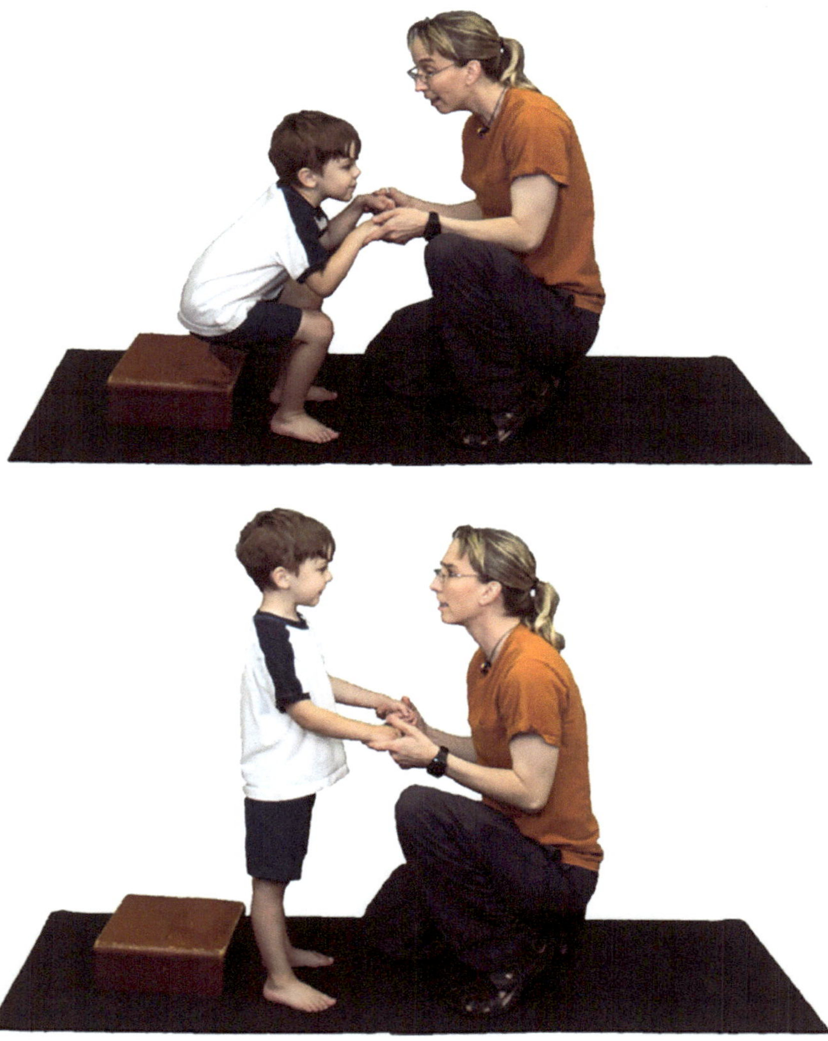

38. SQUAT TO STAND

Squat to stand works hip extensors, quadriceps and plantarflexors concentrically on the way up and eccentrically on the way down. I try to get children to look up as they transition up and down to try to keep an arch in the back. I try to get my client to put her heels down. If she has trouble, I let her stand on a decline or with her heels on a mat and her toes on the floor. Sometimes I assist with one or two hands held. Sometimes I support at the knees from the front or by sitting on a bench behind her holding the knees from the back.

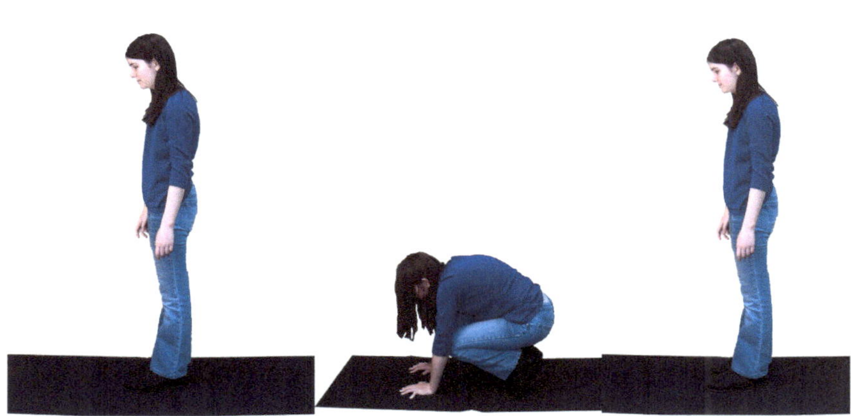

39. TALL BENCH-DON'T SQUEAK!

I have many clients who need to work on midrange control of hip and knee extension. I have the client stand in front of a bench with a squeak toy or piano on it. He is to stoop down and touch the piano or squeak toy-but not squeak it. If his hips or knees bend too much, then he collapses down. Obviously this is much easier if you don't have to go down too low.

I love the Kaye Products adjustable benches that allow you to incrementally modify the bench's height until you find the right height for the perfect challenge for the client. If you don't have an adjustable height bench, you can always progressively make the bench shorter by putting a single thickness mat under the client's feet-not under the bench. You can continue along the same lines by doubling and then tripling the mat to effectively make the bench shorter. I love my clients' reactions when I use sound effects. This exercise is usually fun. Placing the client facing toward a wall mirror helps give him visual feedback about the distance to the squeak toy.

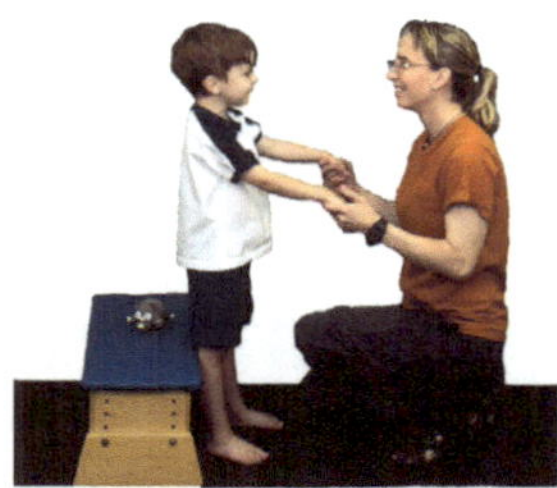
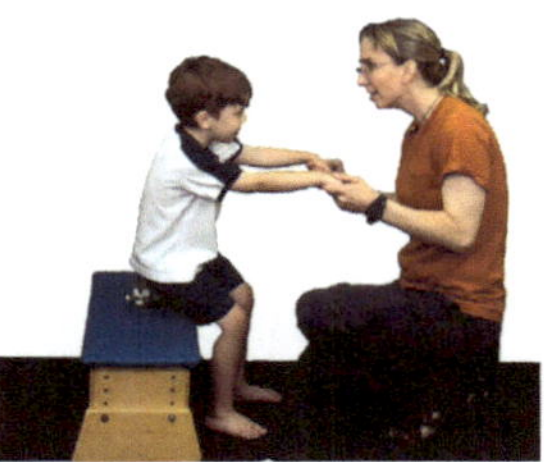
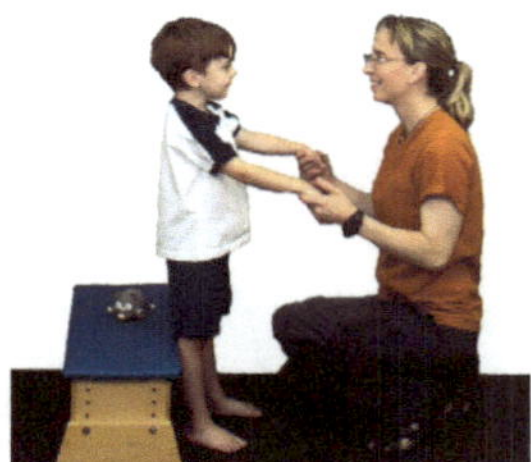

40. LOW BENCH-DON'T SQUEAK!

This is the same as the previous exercise, but one step harder. Simply modifying the bench height even by a small amount can dramatically increase the difficulty.

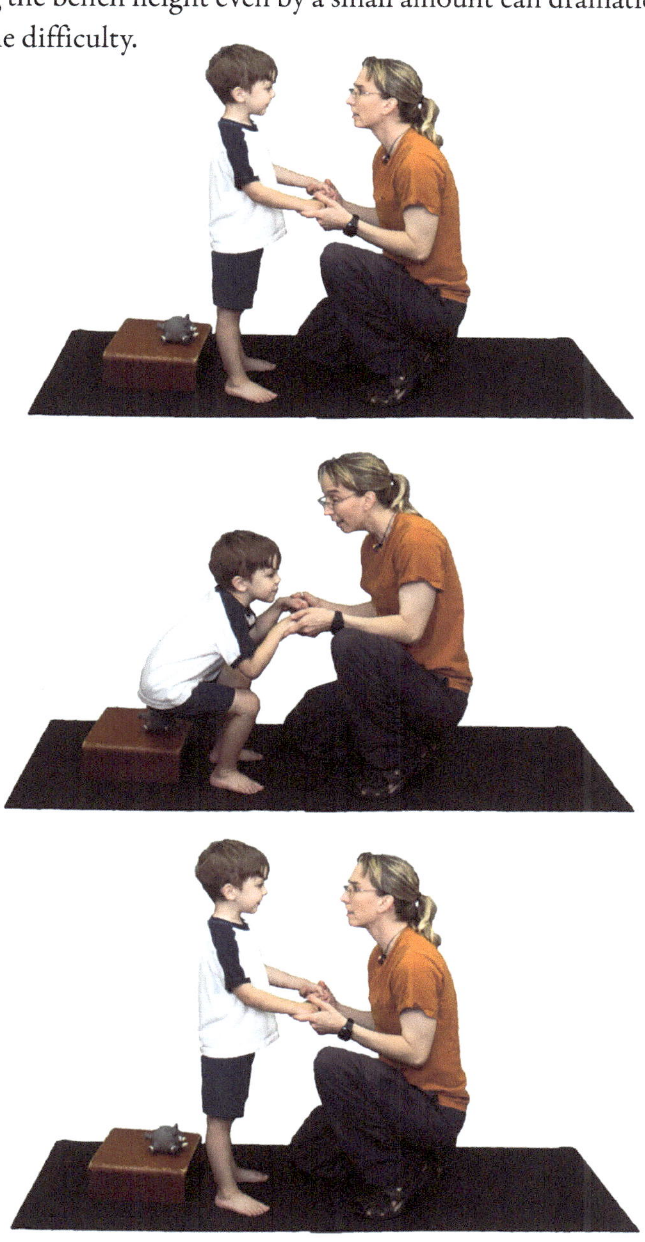

41. HIP HELP HALF KNEEL TO STAND

I work on half kneel to stand at furniture, walls, with one or two upright poles, with one hand held, or with one hand on the wall with my client facing sideways. In the middle of the room I give a variety of support before a child can perform this independently. Makes sure to get the weight shifted forward so the head is over the knee that is up. I facilitate this transition in this picture series with hip support from behind but in reality it is probably more commonly done with knee support from the front when a client is close to performing the transition independently. Several of my kids have learned to do this transition with both hands on the raised knee. Then I fade to only one hand allowed on the raised knee and then completely independently. I am not typically satisfied until a child can perform five to ten repetitions with either leg raised and with hands free.

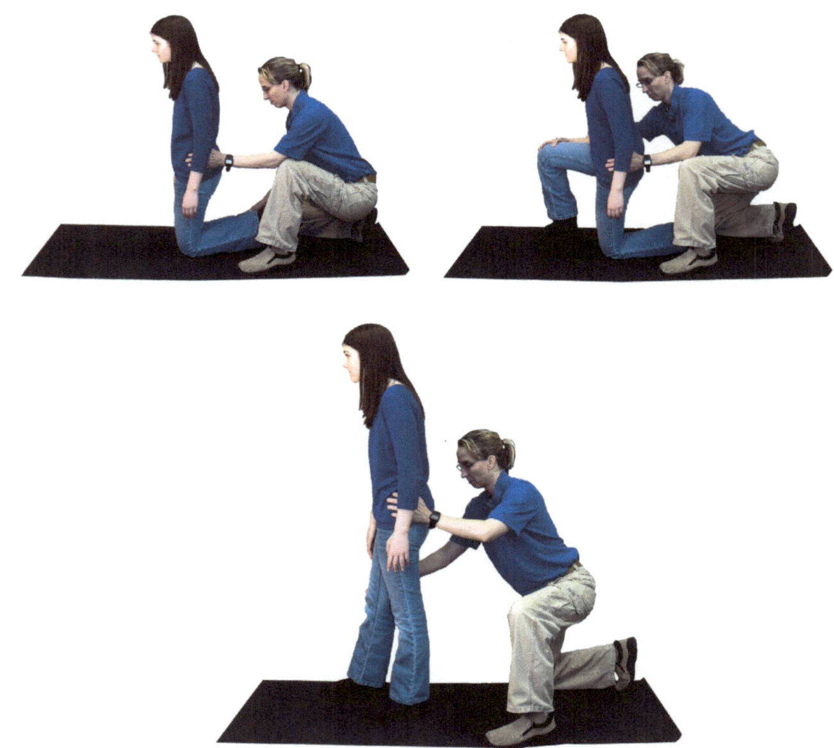

42. KNEEL TO HALF KNEEL TO STAND

Here the client is strong enough to perform this activity with close stand by monitoring/assistance for safety.

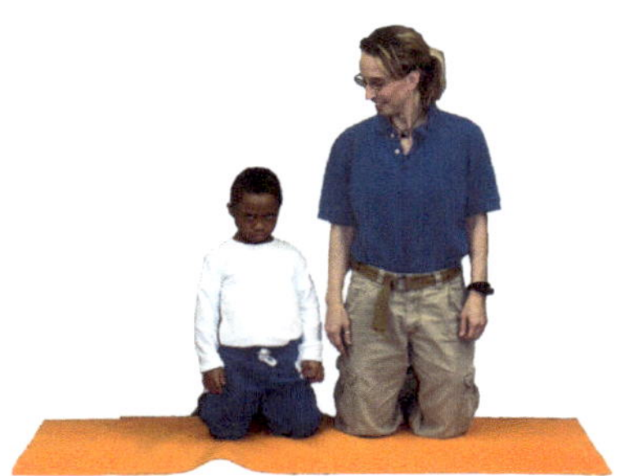

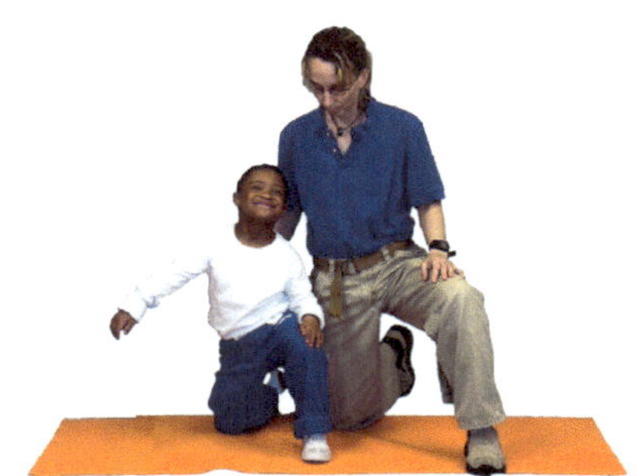

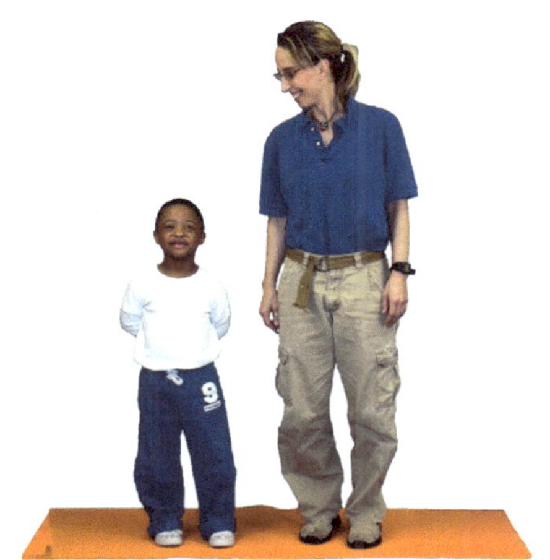

43. STAND TO HALF KNEEL

I love emphasizing both parts of the transition-the half kneel to stand and then the stand to half kneel. Most of my clients figure out the transition to standing with control before they can control standing to half kneel. I frequently have be behind them to help bring back the leg for them to initiate the transition. The movement up to standing emphasizes the concentric muscle contraction and controlling the descent works the same muscle groups eccentrically.

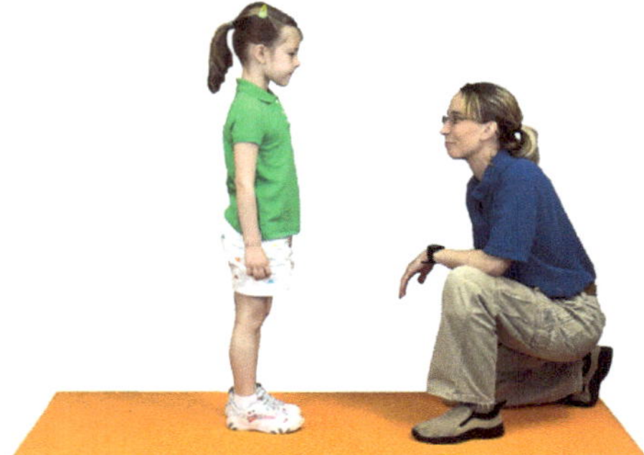

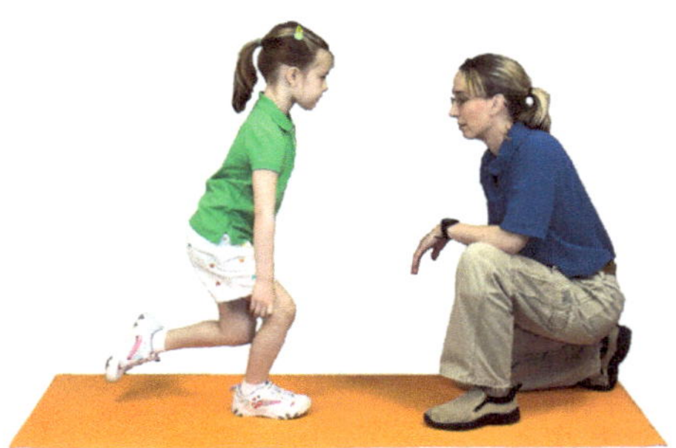

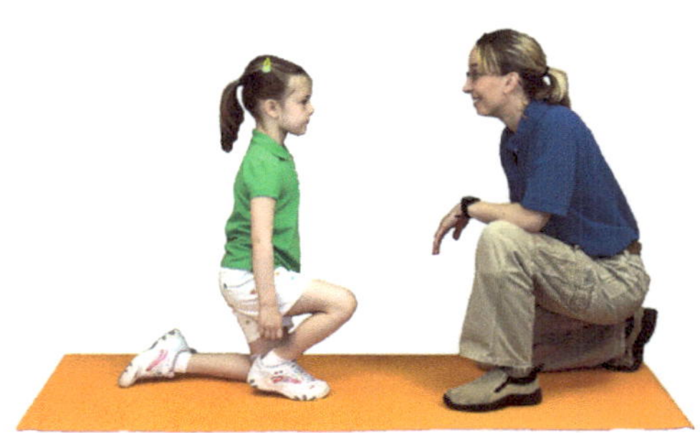

44. KICK BACK STANDING TWO HANDS HELD

If the bench is back a little further, you get hip extension beyond neutral. I usually have my client hold onto the grips placed on my wall mirror instead of holding my hands. For the ease of the photo, I held my model's hands. If you use the wall grips, a wall bar or furniture for your client to hold on to, then you have your hands free to help the child with the movement. My children with diplegia have such a hard time with this exercise. It is easier for them to rotate their trunk posteriorly than to extend their hip in neutral. It is not uncommon that I will have the mother block the child's hips, while I assist in the movement of kicking backward with hip extension.

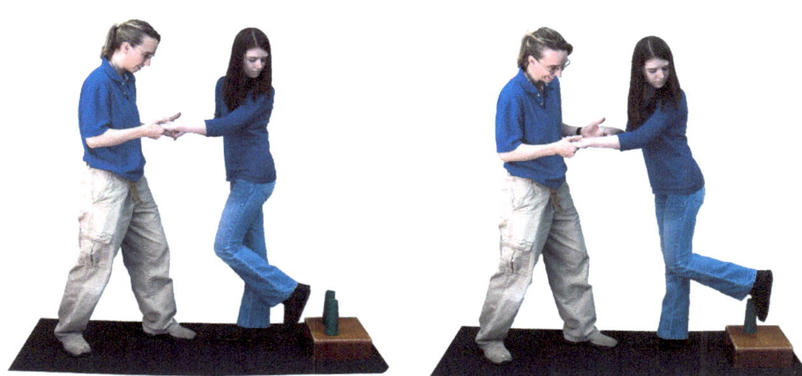

45. MODIFIED BEAR HIP EXTENSION WITH KNEE EXTENSION

I call this modified bear because it is the bear position modified by use of the bench. I like this exercise because my client is stable, and I can help her perform the movement. This exercise is tricky because she can't see the target easily. Here I am simply using my hand as a target. I typically rely on sound effects like a "ding" when my client has gotten to the right height. I may "ding" or a make a sneeze sound or go through a gamut of strange sounds that might keep my client engaged enough to continue. Many of my clients with neurological impairments have difficulty getting one leg significantly separated from the other leg. So this activity with one leg flexed while one leg is extended is quite difficult. It is also hard to make this activity fun, so have a reward planned after this one.

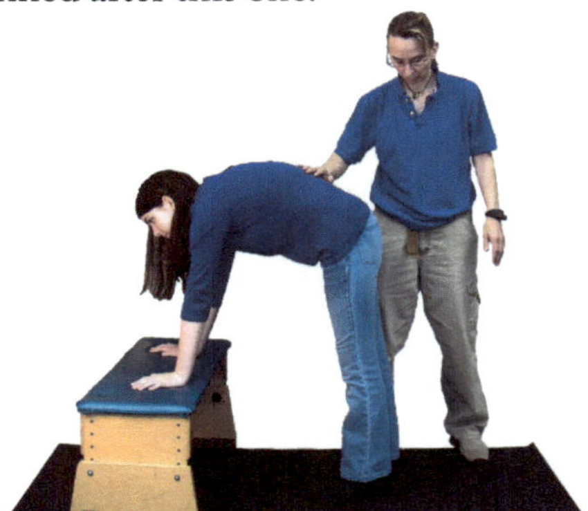

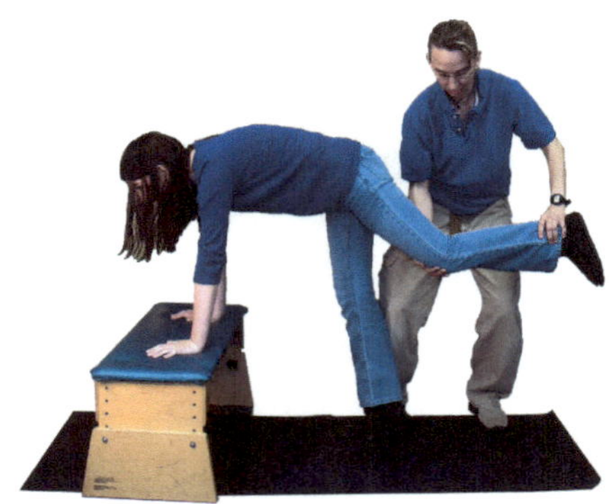

46. MODIFIED BEAR HIP EXTENSION WITH KNEE FLEXION

The flexed knee is often just as hard to assume as the hip extension is for my neurologically involved clients, due to weak hamstrings at close to 90 degree knee flexion. Clearly the flexed knee encourages the hip extension to be generated without as much assistance from the hamstrings.

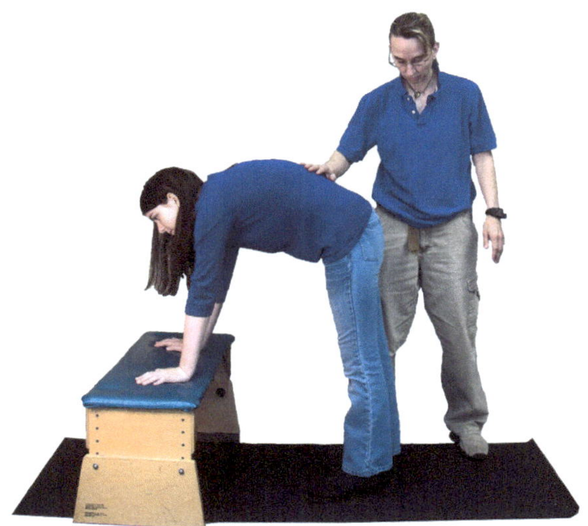

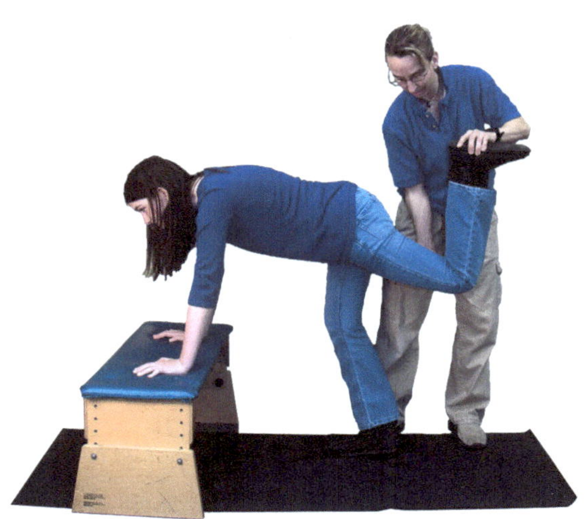

47. MODIFIED BEAR BENCH KICK

Having a target on the bench makes it easier for my client to know where the target is. There is a certain satisfaction gotten from knocking something over that makes this activity a little more desirable for my clients than the previous two exercises. In this picture I wish I had put the bench further back to obtain more hip extension; however, the closer bench encourages more knee flexion to clear the edge of the bench. This activity does not require as much pelvic disassociation as the previous two activities so it may be easier for your neurologically involved clients.

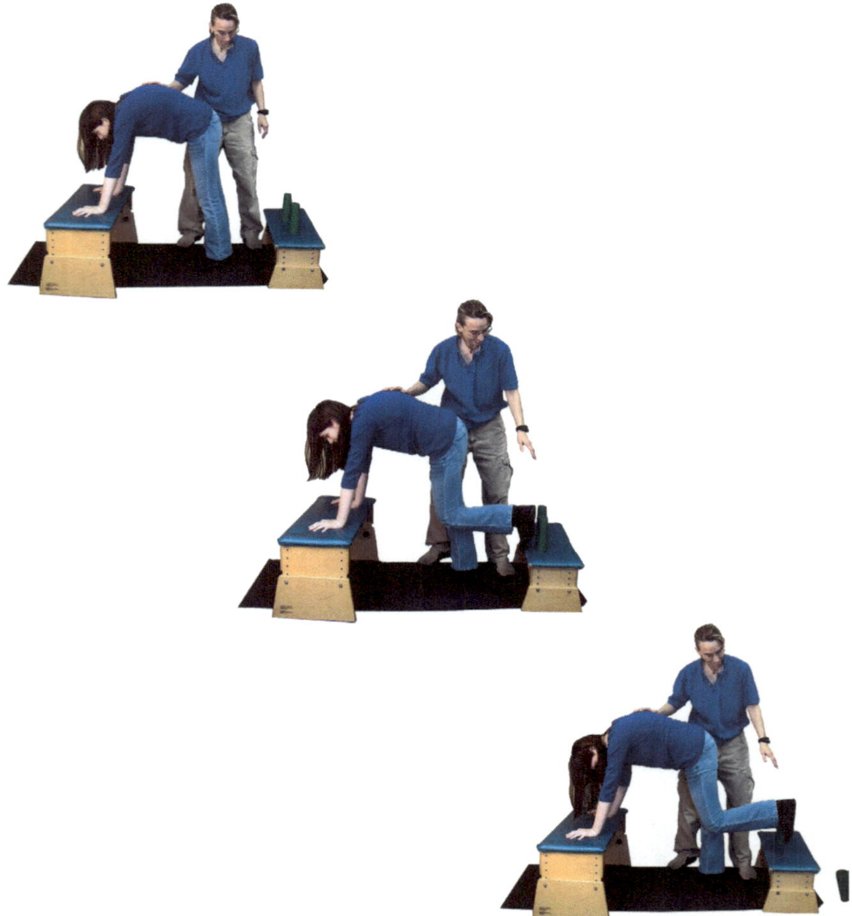

48. HIP EXTENSION STANDING

The way I typically do this exercise is with my client holding onto the grips placed with suction cups on my wall mirror. She could also have held onto furniture or a bar placed on the wall. You can vary the resistance with the choice of elastic band strengths. My children with diplegia have such a hard time with this exercise. Again you may need the mother to block the child's hips to access more isolated hip extension. I also have done this exercise with a bungee pulley attached with velcro straps at the child's ankle. This exercise is usually performed with active assistive. Watch for your client to flex forward at the hip to eliminate having to extend beyond neutral hip extension.

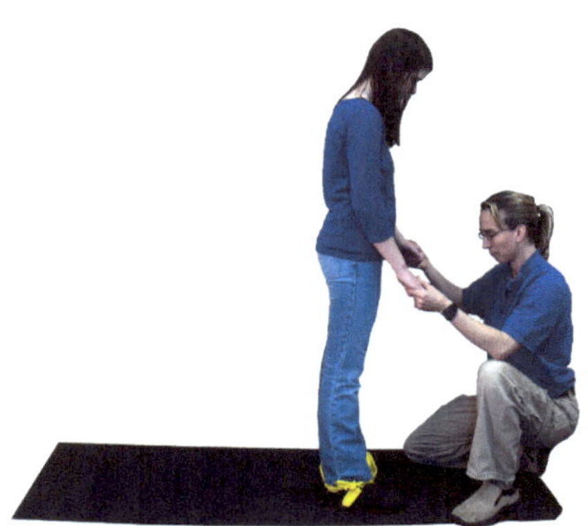

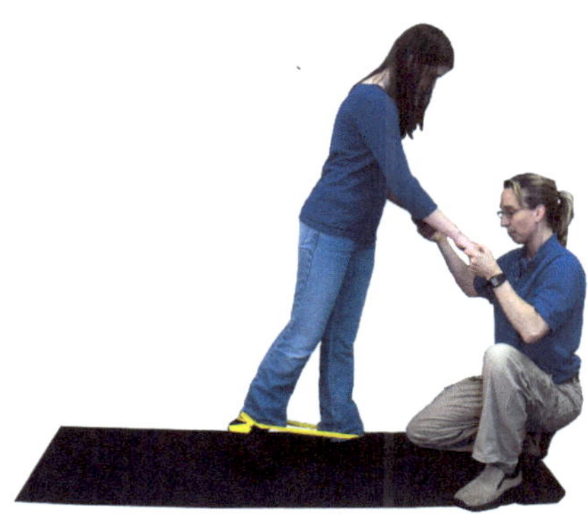

49. RESISTED BACKWARD WALKING

This is another great exercise! I also perform this exercise sitting on a scooterboard facing my client. I set it up similar to this picture here, but I have the client drag me along on the scooterboard as she walks backward. I like having the elastic bands above the knee to isolate hip extension.

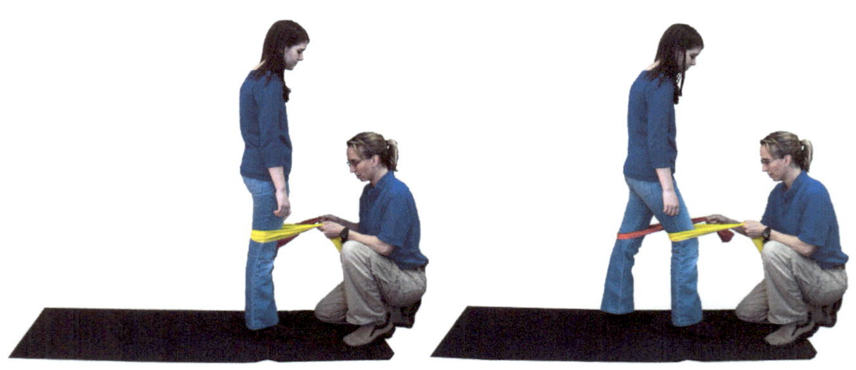

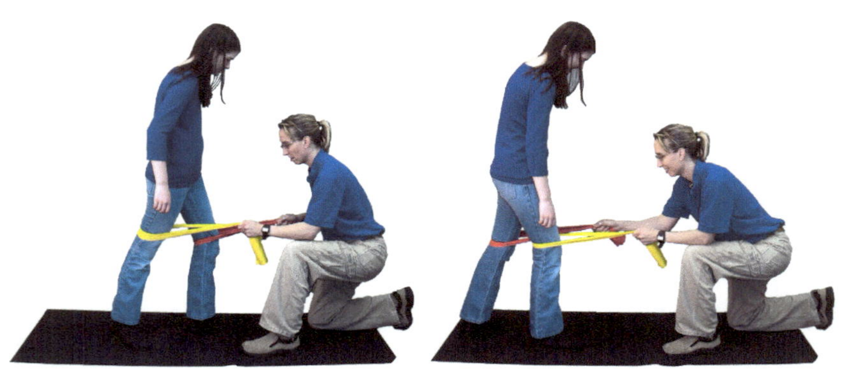

50. PUSH YOU ON THE ROLLING CHAIR

I am the one that loves this activity because I finally get to go for the ride! I sit on a rolling desk chair or stool. They can be hard for the child to simultaneously push and steer, but a challenge can be a good thing. Remember that pushing on hard floors like wood, vinyl or tile are much easier than carpet. If there is a sibling in the room, I usually let him or her take the ride. A parent is fun to push too, but often help by pulling some with his/her legs. Kids love when I return the favor and push them for an equal distance. I usually start off giving the child a ride and then I take my turn.

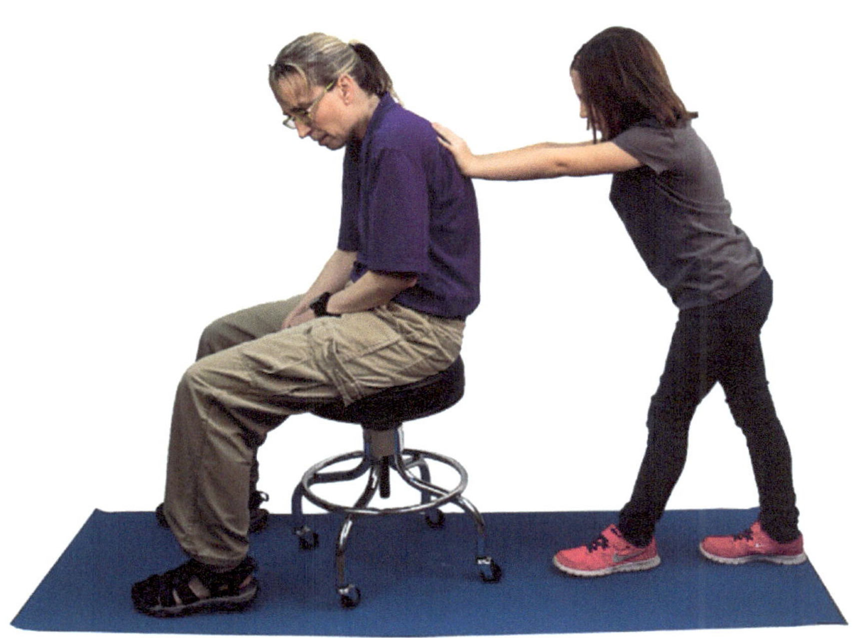

51. YOU PUSH ME ON THE SCOOTERBOARD

My comments from the previous activity still apply. I often will motivate the child by putting stacked blocks at the finish line. The person riding knocks down the blocks dramatically and with flare. This adds to the fun.

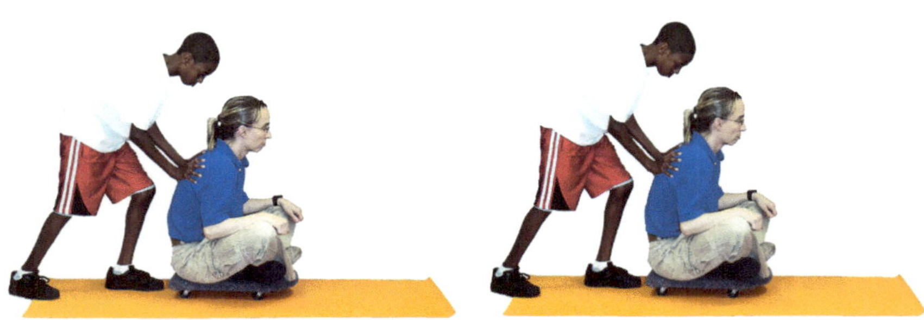

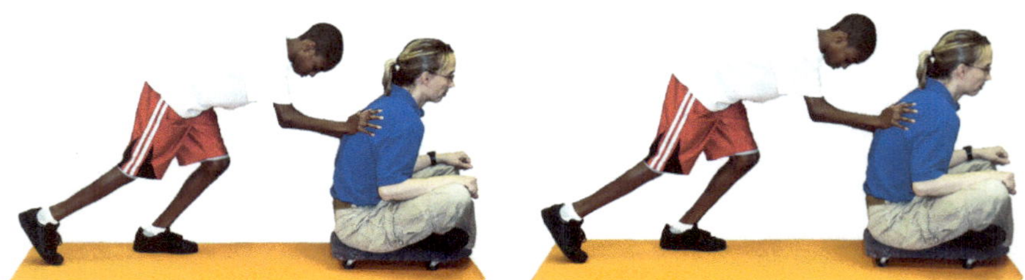

52. WALL SITS

I know, I know, collective groan from all the children I have ever made do this exercise. It is a tough one and there had better be something really fun afterward. Sometimes I go for repetitions up and down and in other cases I ask the child to go down and hold the wall sit for one to ten seconds. Miserable perhaps, but a great strengthening exercise. I do the exercise along with the child if I think he won't fall down without my assistance. If I think the child might collapse, I sit on the floor in front of the child facing him. I put up my index fingers and ask the child to dip down until he touches his knees to my finger tips. This seems to work best as it gives the child a target. It also puts me in position to catch the child by blocking his descent at his knees. I have a child with a myopathy who can only control the first ten degrees of a wall sit. He collapses if he tries a lower dip. So we work the range he can safely control. Since he is bigger, I put a 10 inch bench waiting under him between his feet and the wall to catch him if he falls.

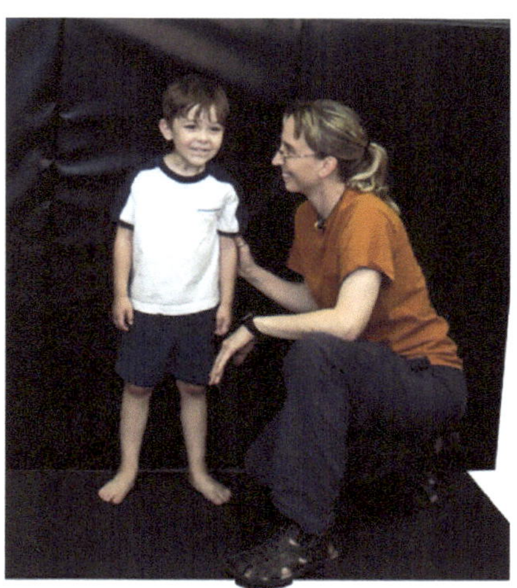

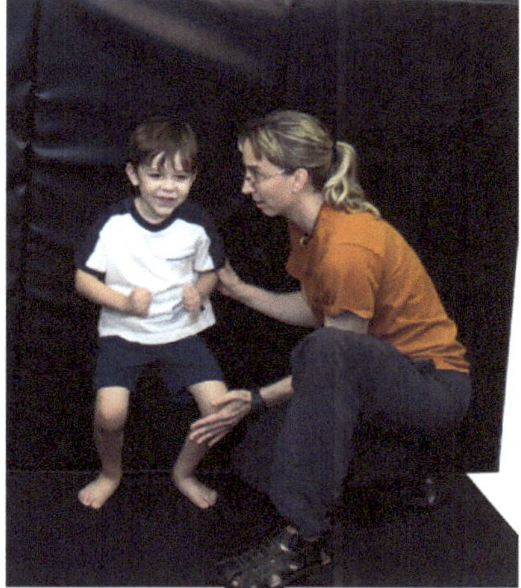

53. WALL TALLS

For the crouch walkers I do almost the reverse of a classic wall sit. I let the child stand with his back to the wall with his typical knee/hip flexion. I sit on the floor in front of him facing the child. I put my index fingers on his knees and I say, "Stand up taller, straightening your hips and knees to get your knees off of my fingers." As the child extends his hips/knees, I reposition my fingers to touching his knees again and repeat. At the child's end range, I may have the child keep his knees off my fingers and time how long he is successful.

In another variation of this exercise that I use with a child with quadriplegic cerebral palsy who has difficulty getting end range knee/hip extension in stance, I stand the child with his back on the wall. I hold his hands and lift the child to a less crouched position pushing with my knees through his knees until we find the tallest he can stand with assistance. I have a helper Velcro a box to the wall touching the top of the child's head with convenient pre-placed Velcro strips I have on the wall. Then I unblock the child's knees but still hold the hands, and the child immediately sinks. His head is no longer touching the Velcro box. I ask the child to push with his legs so he is tall enough again to touch his head to the box, either momentarily for a certain number of repetitions or for a specified duration.

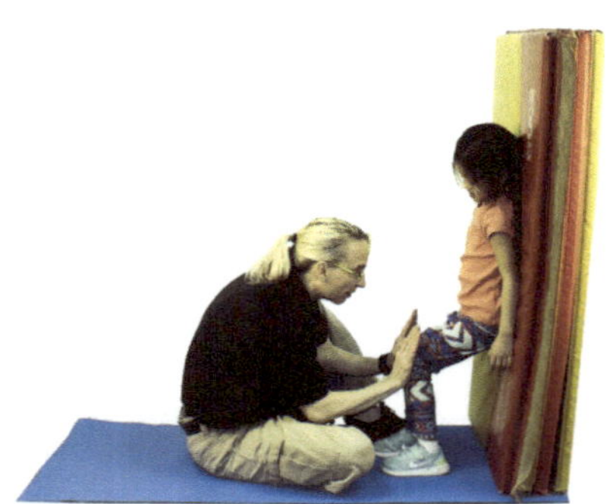

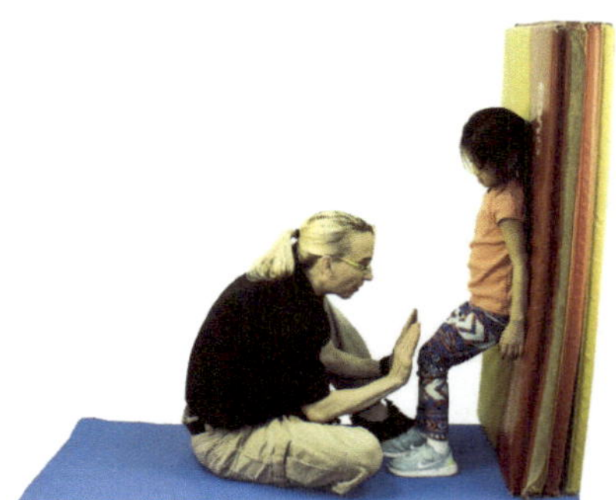

54. LUNGES

Clients have to be fairly physically adept to perform this exercise. I usually mark on my carpet with Velcro lines where I want my client to start, to step out to, and to step back to in one big step. I start with small distances and work further out with success. I always try to get the child to put the knee of the non-stepping leg down to the floor. I have done these with and without hand weights with my clients.

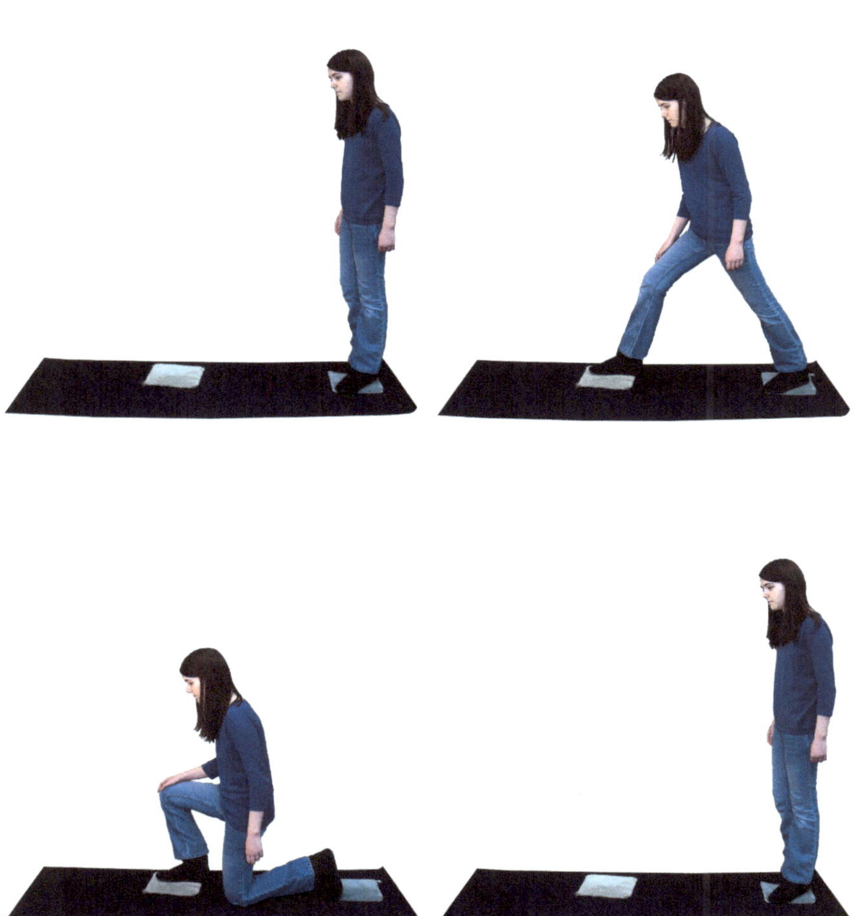

55. ONE FOOT UP SIDE PICK UP

This exercise is particularly good for clients with hemiplegia. By putting one foot up on a bench, the client is immediately more likely to put more weight on the foot on the floor. But I have seen more than a few kids try to figure this exercise out without putting more weight on the foot on the floor. With these kids, I often support the knee on the down leg to guide the weight shift over to pick up the object. The higher the bench the foot is on, the more the weight is shifted to the down leg. Some clients need trunk support, a hand held, or a bench in front of them to stabilize on to complete this activity. This is where toys with pieces are wonderful.

I may put a puzzle with ten pieces on a bench in front of the child for him to hold onto. I put puzzle pieces down below-on floor or on a lower bench for the child to pick up. Then he stands up to put the piece in the puzzle on the bench in front of the child. I may initially not put the toy all the way on the ground. I may not even put one foot up relative to the other. I measure progress by how close to the floor I can hold/place the toy and the child still manage to pick it up and return to upright. Any child who can cruise is ready to start working on this game, albeit with a bench/furniture in front of him. If the child is stronger and has more balance, then I do it without out the bench in front like in this picture.

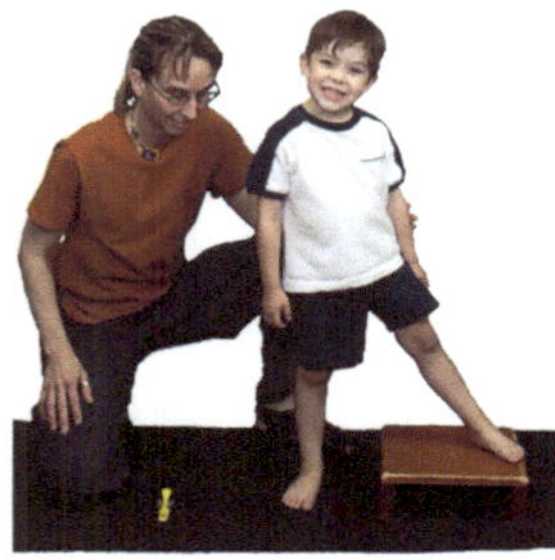
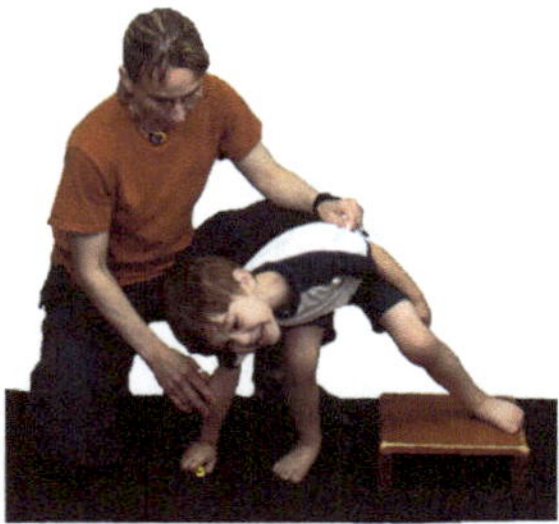
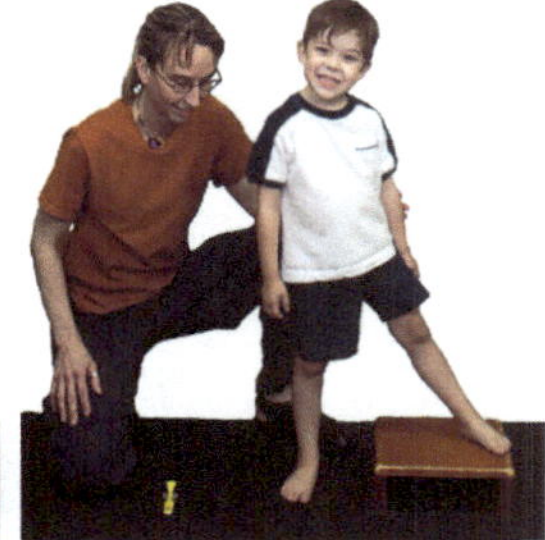

56. PICK UP IN FRONT WITH FOOT UP IN BACK

This activity is tough and doesn't win me any points with the kids. This is harder with a taller bench in back. I usually don't place the back foot up any higher than the kid's knee. I usually have to remind the child that I only want the toe of the foot in back on the bench-not the whole foot flat. I love this activity because it works on balance as well as hip and knee extensors and plantarflexors. You get eccentric muscle contractions on the way down, and concentric on the way up. Toys with pieces are the key. Here the child is picking up an oreo cookie shape puzzle pieces. I see more flexion at the three joints when the toy is placed further out relative to the child's foot.

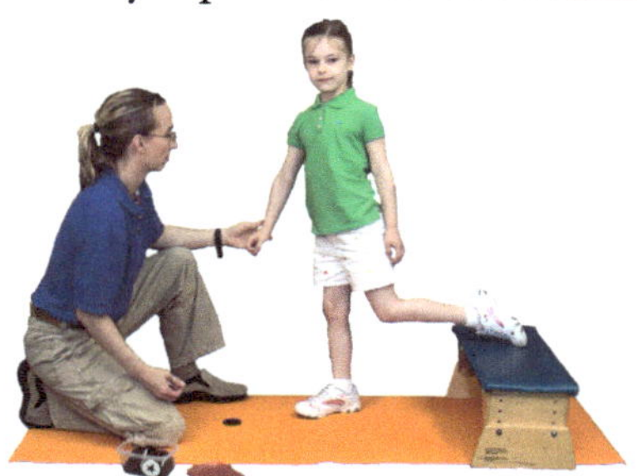

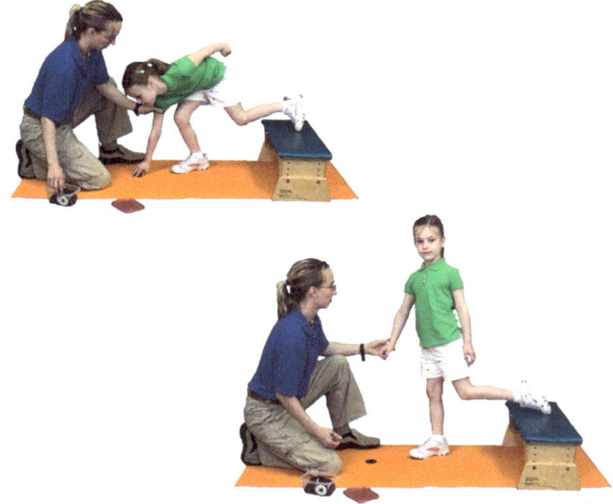

57. PICK UP IN FRONT WITH FOOT ON SLANT IN BACK

This activity is similar to the exercise in which the child picks up a toy with one foot back on the bench. This can be easier or harder depending on how steep the slant is. I typically use a mat leaning against a wall. This activity is easier with a lower incline and harder with a steeper incline. It usually takes me a few reps to determine the correct slant, and then I try to get ten repetitions.

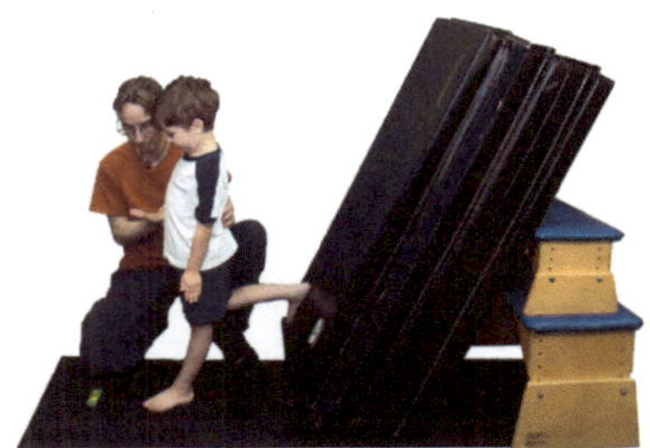

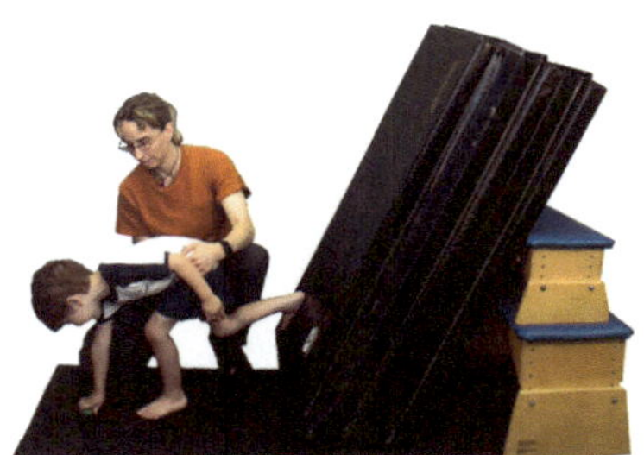

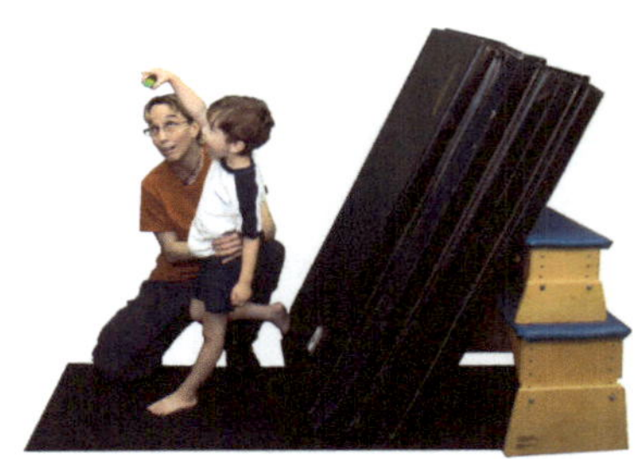

58. ONE LEG PICK UP WITH UNSTABILIZED POLE

I love this exercise! Most of the time I do this exercise with clients with the pole stabilized in the Kaye Product pole frame, but I have performed this exercise with an unstabilized pole. For the most advanced clients I still use the pole, but I don't let my client hold onto it. More hip extension strength is required when the ring is put further forward. When clients are having a hard time, I tend to help the free leg as I demonstrate in this photo series. Kids seem to like this exercise. In the photo I am using rings that children dive for in a pool, but a lot of my kids like to use as jewelry bracelets. They are fun because if you spin and drop the bracelet correctly on the pole, it will spin in a most satisfying way before falling. If the client needs a little more stability then I have the child lift the leg closest to the pole for a wider base of support. For a little more of a challenge, I have the child lift the foot furthest from the pole.

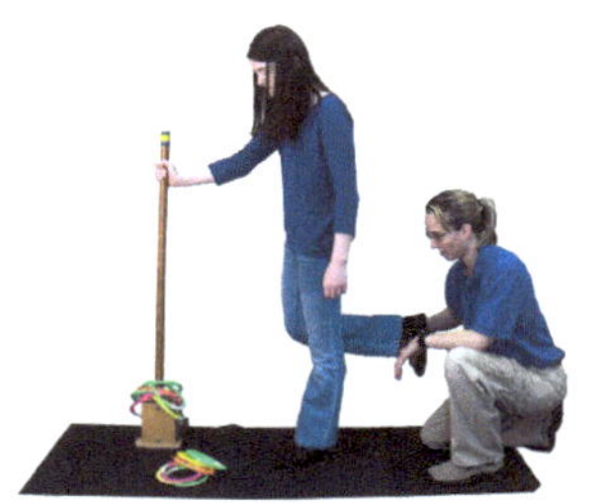

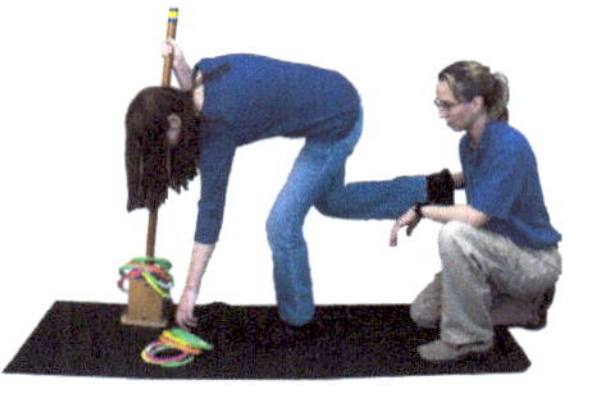

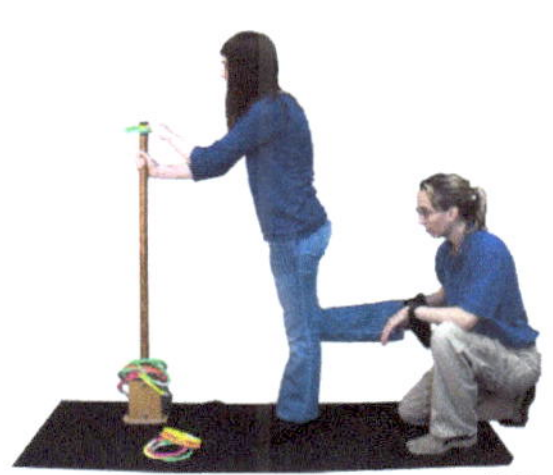

59. ONE LEG PICK UP BELOW

This would be a way to progress the one leg pick up and to encourage more hip extension by having the client pick up an object lower than the level she is standing on. I have had a few higher level clients with hemiplegia who could perform this activity with hands free but the majority can't get to this level without additional assistance.

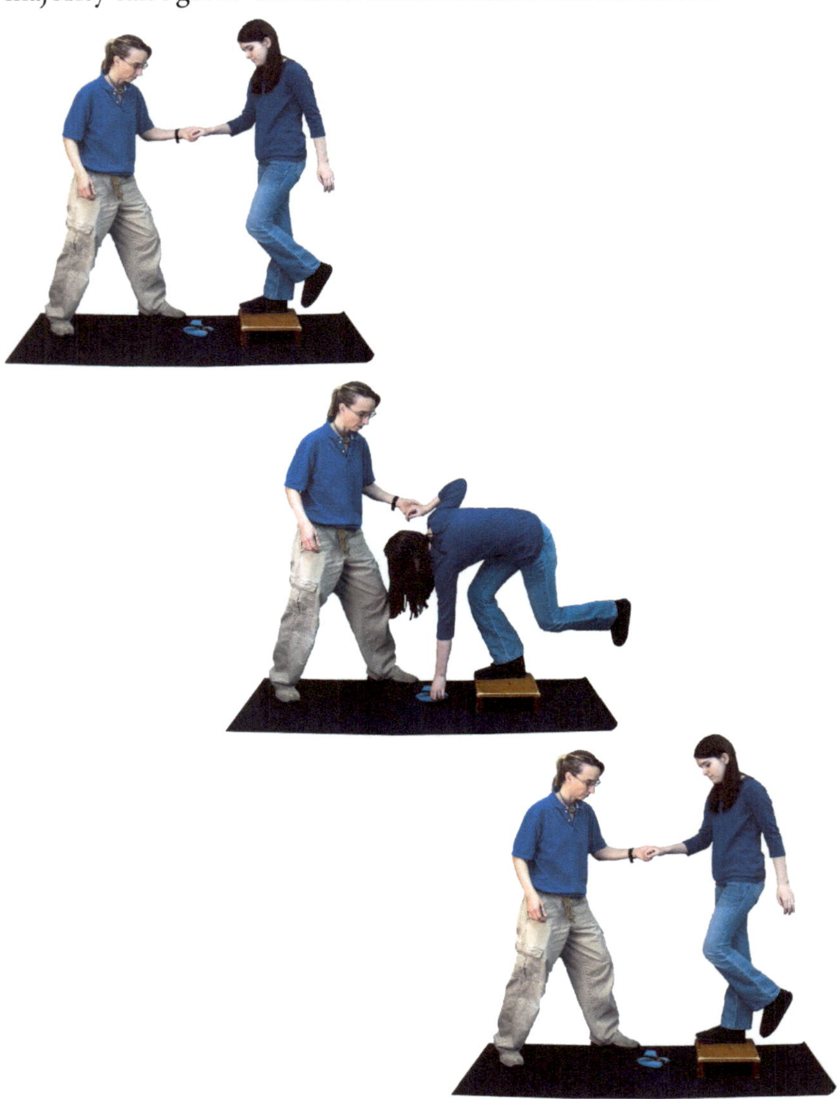

60. LAME DOGS

I can usually get children to do this one time and then they remember how hard it was after that. In this exercise your client hops along on her hands and one back leg like a dog who has a hurt back leg. Since legs are longer than arms, the child has to bend the weight bearing leg which sets her up for quadriceps and hip extensors to help out. This is really difficult. For encouragement, I always do the exercise along with my clients. We have a long hall at work, so we lame dog down the hall and take a rest and lame dog back.

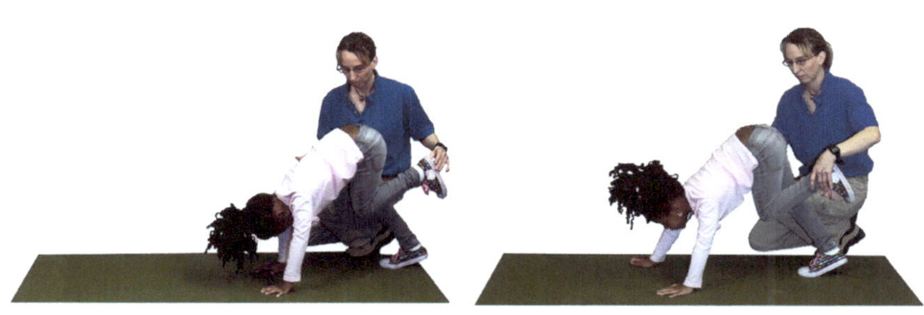

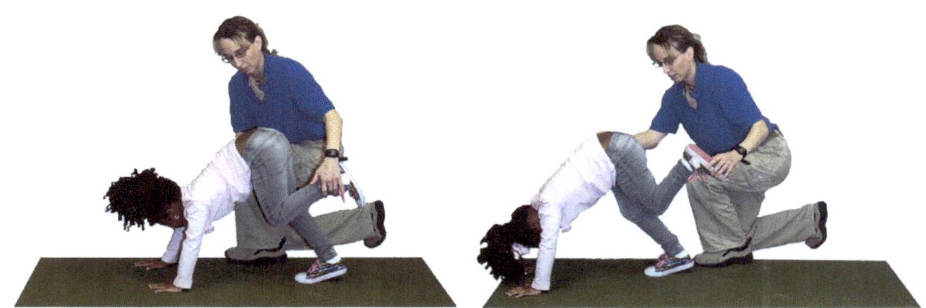

61. DIP KICKS WITH TWO POLE SUPPORT

I love this exercise, and I am always amazed that kids tolerate this activity so well. The picture on the next page illustrates the way I typically perform this exercise. I have also used one railing and a hand held or the inside of a door frame, but upright poles are perfect because a child of any height can hold the pole at the right height for them. I start with two poles and then work to one pole. When I use just one, I place the pole on the side of the stance leg if the child needs a narrower base of support. I put the pole on the kicking leg side if the child needs a wider base of support for success.

For a greater challenge I progress to one hand on a wall. A taller bench makes this harder as well. Technically this activity is more difficult with a greater height differential between the bench on which the child is standing and the height of the toy that the child is kicking. So my first line of offense is to make the toy lower relative to the bench the child is standing on. If that is not enough, then I make the bench higher.

I should note that at first a child tries to simply plantarflex the kicking foot to knock over the toy. You will have to put the toy low enough that the child has to flex her hip/knee. If a child has an ankle foot orthosis with a plantarflexion stop then you won't need to make the toy as low.

To make this activity more difficult, I put the bench close to the wall but I only ask the child to use it if she loses control. I could also resort to the dreaded double, triple, quadruple, etc.; dip kicks. This means I hold the toy and the child must repeatedly dip down to kick the toy before putting her foot back on the bench. This is hard. It never hurts to have a spot on this activity. Because I am usually down low placing the toy to be kicked and not in a great position to spot the child in case there is a loss of balance, I will often have a parent stand nearby to spot.

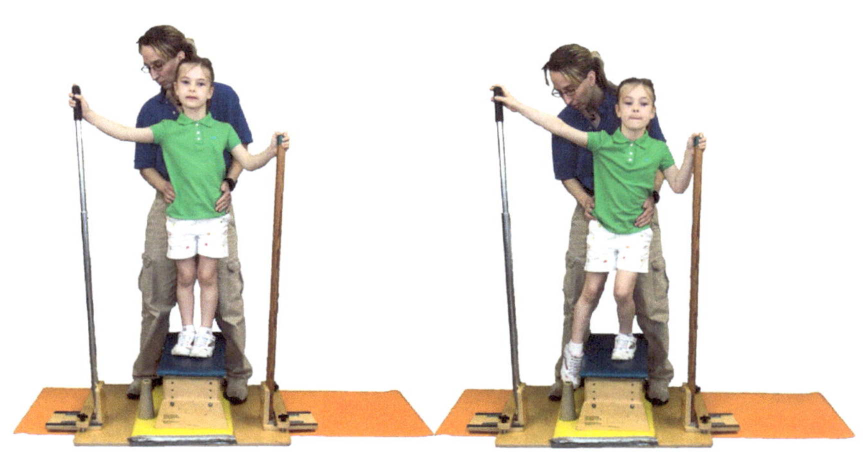

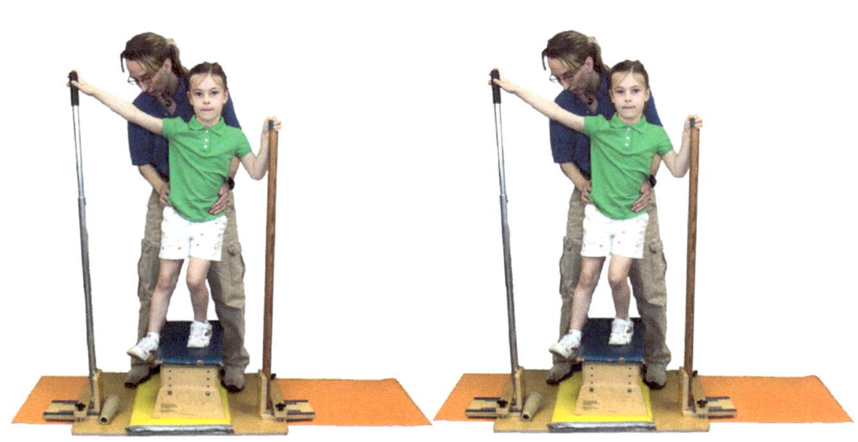

62. DIP KICKS WITH ONE POLE SUPPORT

This is one of my favorite exercises. While in the pictures on the right I am stabilizing the pole only with my foot, I typically stabilize the pole with the Kaye Products Upright Pole frame.

I also modify the difficulty of this activity by changing the distance the client has to dip to kick the object. I can make the bench higher or the block lower. I have some foam blocks/animals that I like to use. The client should kick over the object but not touch the floor. I also like using stacked cones/cups because I can make the distance that she has to dip down harder simply by removing one cone/cup from the stack. Here my client is tall, so I switched from the cones to my foam animals because I can get significantly lower with those than I can with the cups. I could also have put my client on a taller bench. It is not uncommon for my clients to lose their balance on this activity. If I don't have a second person to spot for safety then I would rather use lower objects to increase the dip distance than use a taller bench.

If I find the perfect support level then I can modify the difficulty by having her dip down repeatedly touching the object two to ten times before returning to the resting position on the bench. In this case I have to hold the object to keep it from being kicked away. Take care as I have had my hand smushed by the client when he or she lost eccentric control and collapsed down onto it. Ouch! I usually rig this game up by challenging my client with a taunt that goes something like this, "Oh, you kicked it one time. I bet you can't get it twice. Oh you got it twice. How about three times?" and so on.

Even with clients with one side better at this activity such as clients with hemiplegia, I will often let the client perform a few repetitions on their less/uninvolved side first to get the feel of the movement, and to document how low the client can go with the less/uninvolved side.

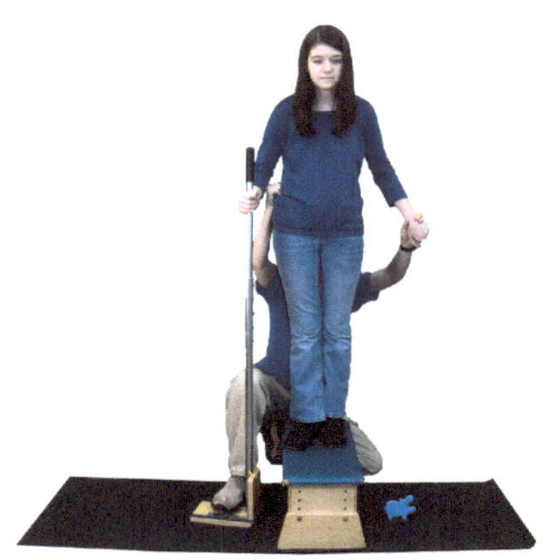

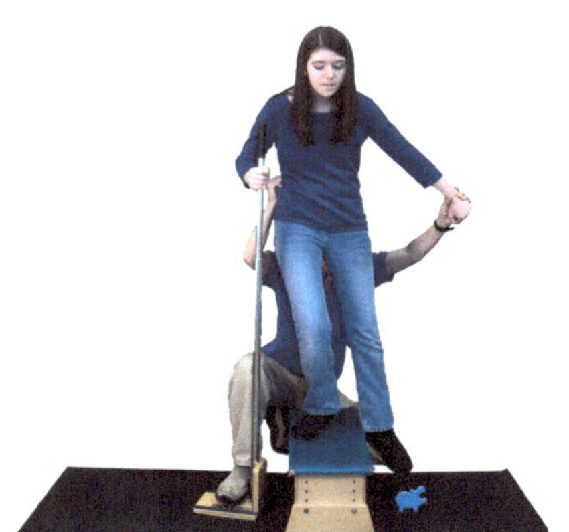

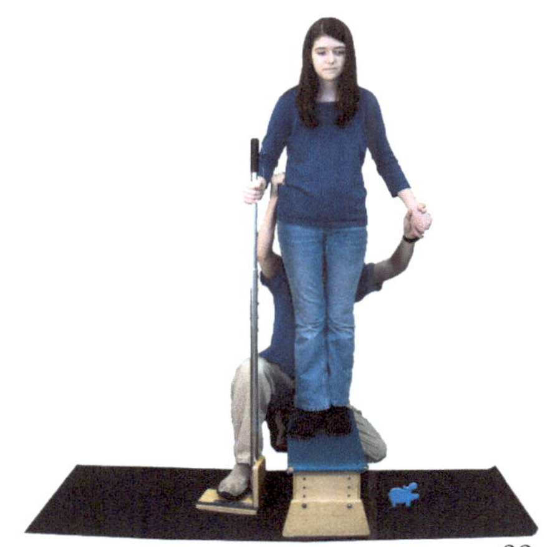

63. SQUAT JUMPS

This is a fatigue-inducing activity, but my clients don't seem to mind. Often kids don't go into a full squat before the jump. I either verbally cue, "All the way down." or provide assistance at the hips to go all the way down. I do this exercise with the child when I can so we can have all the "fun" together. I have a few children who are unable to assume a full squat so I will either let them sit on a low bench like a four inch (10 cm) bench to be able to jump up from or I let them hold onto grips on a wall and jump from a squat from there.

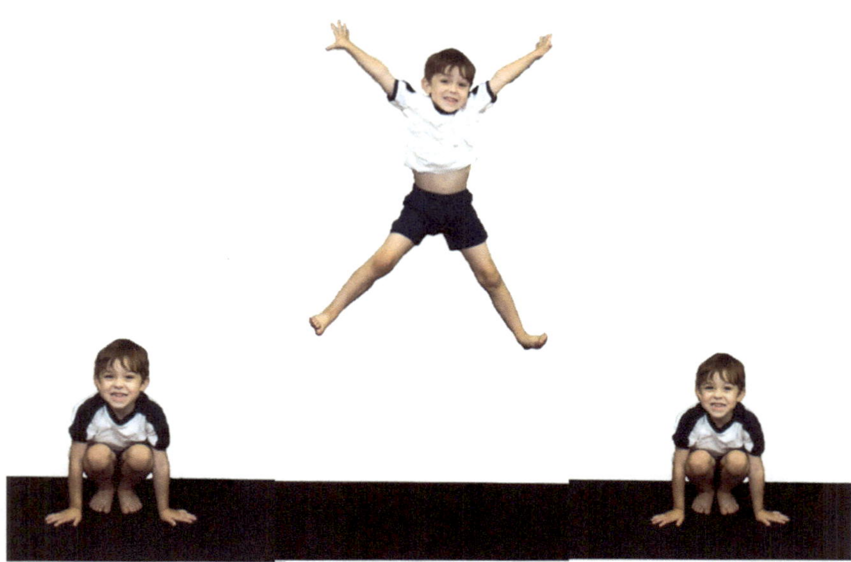

64. SKIP STEPS UP STAIRS

My kids are usually so proud to get to this exercise. They think it is cool. I either let a child hold two rails, one rail or try it independently. I strongly prefer to do this exercise on a real set of stairs. We have 20 steps between floors at work so I can get 10 reps by going just one flight.

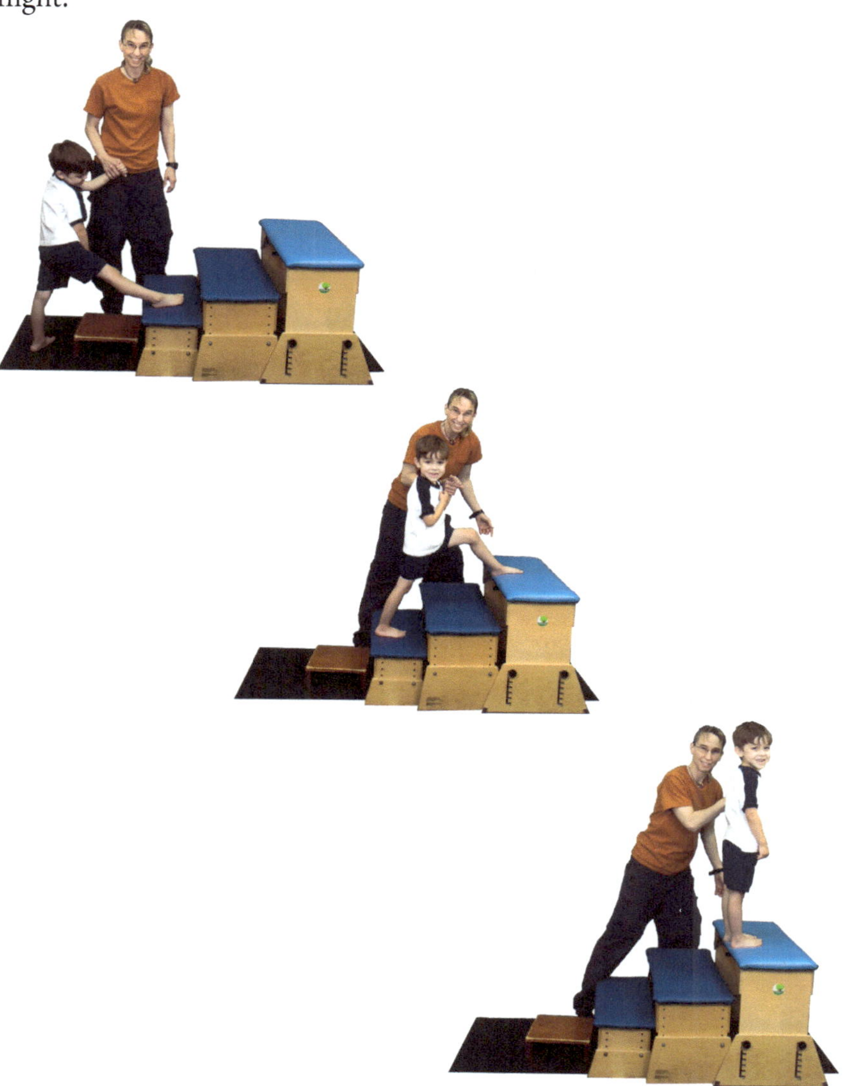

65. HOP UP STAIRS

This is really hard and falls into the category of exercises that kids think are cool the first time they try it. I try not to do this exercise if I don't think the child is ready. It is really easy not to jump high enough and clobber your shin on the next step-never a popular result. I start out with two hands on the rail (one on each side), and then one hand, after which some kids are good enough to try this with no hands on the railing. Since this height is extreme, kids usually recruit help at the ankle, knee and hip. It is a great lower body work out.

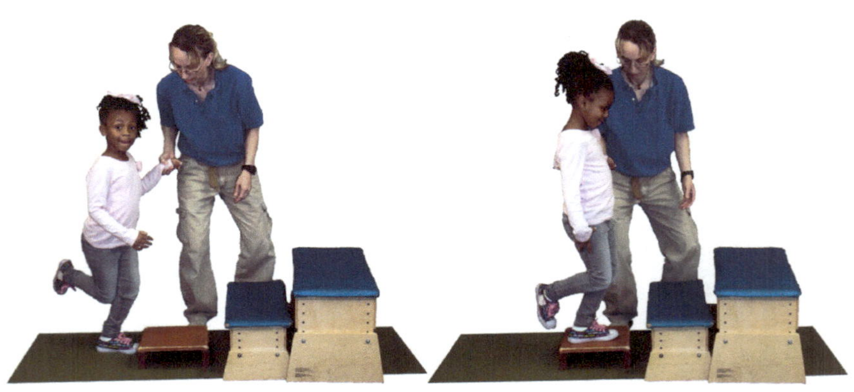

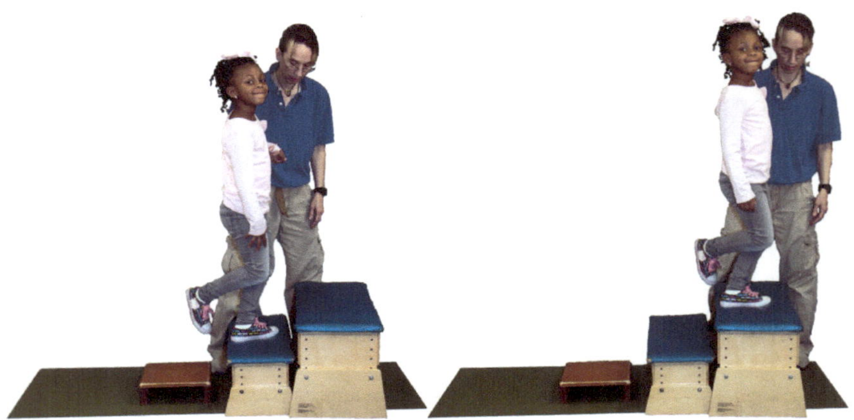

66. BURPEES

Unlike squat jumps that I can pass off like frog jumps, no one seems to like Burpees. So I better have a good reward waiting at the completion of this activity. I do this activity with them if I can for encouragment.

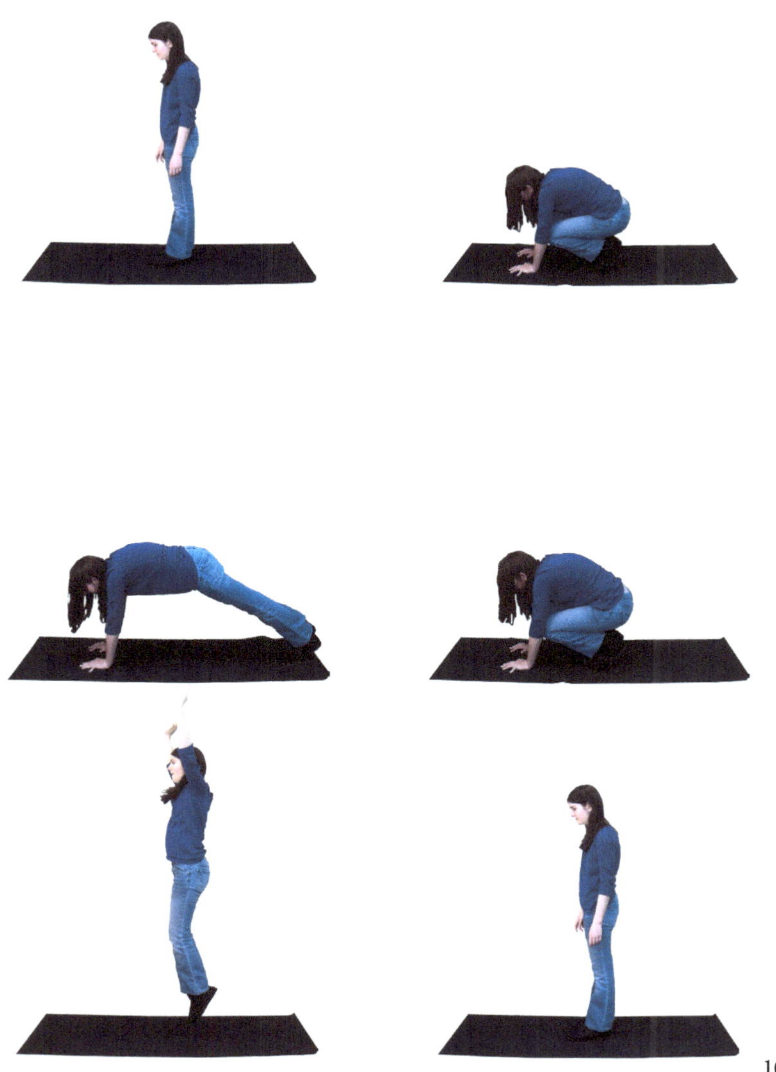

67. MOUNTAIN CLIMBERS

I love how mountain climbers encourage hip extension range of motion on one leg with the other leg flexed. I do these exercises with my clients. Sometimes I use chalk or Velcro lines down on the carpet to show the child where I want her feet to go up to. Some children are simply unable to get in this position. A well placed bench for the child to prop on with her hands really helps. Higher benches provide more support than lower benches.

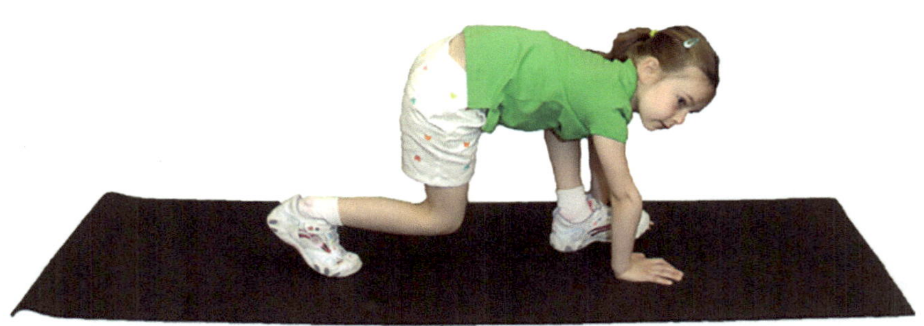

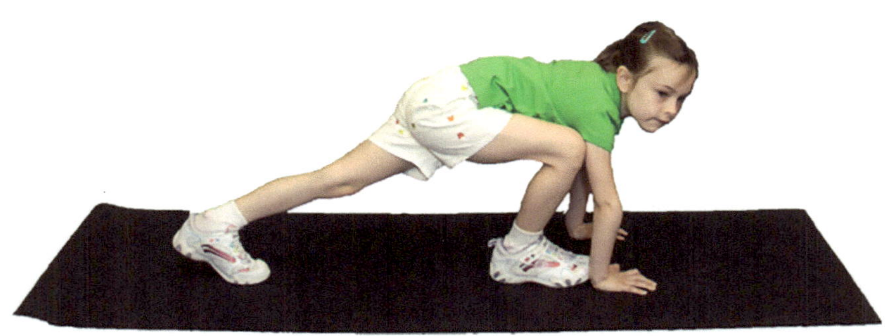

PEDIATRIC PHYSICAL THERAPY STRENGTHENING EXERCISES FOR THE HIPS

III. HIP ABDUCTION

THE HIP ABDUCTORS MOVE THE femur laterally away from neutral or midline or conversely the pelvis away from the femur if the femur is stabilized. Both movements are in the frontal plane. The hip abductors are powerful lower body stabilizers. Weakness or tightness in the hip abductors will affect gait and particularly skill at standing on one foot. This chapter includes a wide variety of exercises to improve hip abduction strength.

* * *

1. SUPINE ABDUCTION, ONE LEG IN SLING

Sometimes a client is so weak in abduction that she is unable to overcome the friction of the surface to move her leg into abduction even in gravity eliminated supine. In this case, I may try a couple of options. I can simply hold under the ball of her foot and I compensate for the friction to help the client move her leg. Sometimes, I put a slick sock on the client and put her foot on a slippery surface to minimize the friction to allow her to move her foot more independently. The other option is to put the client's leg in a suspended sling. This allows her to move her leg with the most minimal effort. I try to support the leg comfortably in the sling and raise it off the supporting surface as little as possible. A target such as my hand or a block to knock over often seems to help.

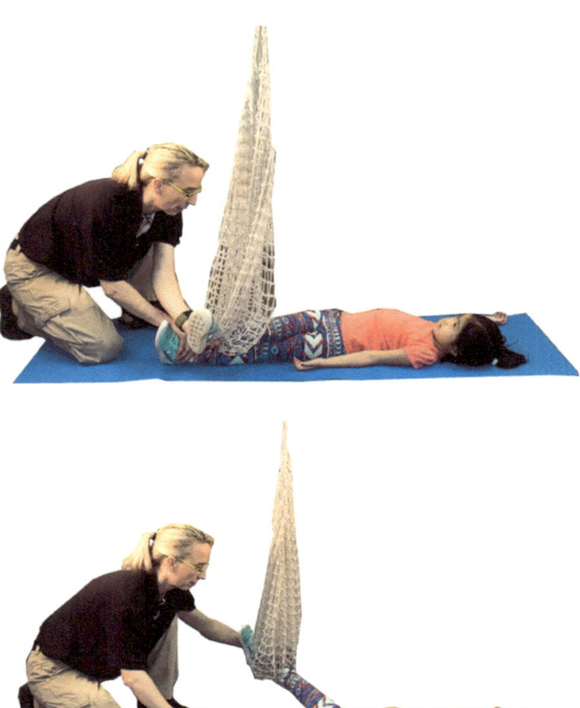

2. SUPINE ABDUCTION WITH ELASTIC BAND ASSIST

If you don't have a suspended sling handy, elastic bands are useful. You can support the client's leg with the elastic band or the client can support her leg at the heel. The elastic band gives proprioceptive feedback through the leg and allows the client to assist abduction with her upper extremities.

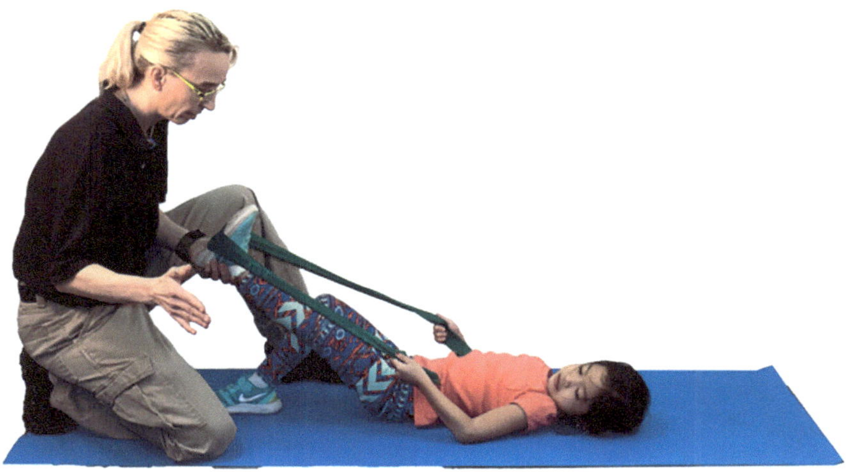

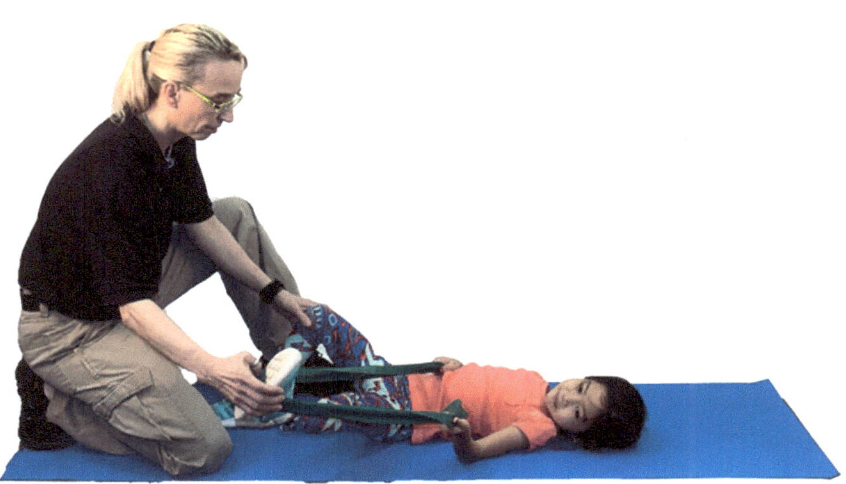

3. SUPINE UNILATERAL ABDUCTION

What kid can resist knocking down blocks? This is always a popular activity. If needed I will prop the child's head up with a pillow so he can see better. I can resist or assist the movement of abduction according to the need of the child. I often find that in part of the range I am resisting and part I am assisting. I usually resist manually, but I can also add ankle weights or elastic bands or tubing wrapped around both legs. When I place the block wider, this acivity is harder. I recently found sliders used in the gym that would be perfect for making the leg slide along the ground, if the floor is hard like vinyl or hardwood. This activity works well on a hard floor if I put a little baby powder on the floor and the child's shoe on a piece of paper. If I want to minimize but not eliminate the resistance, then I may put his leg on a scooterboard.

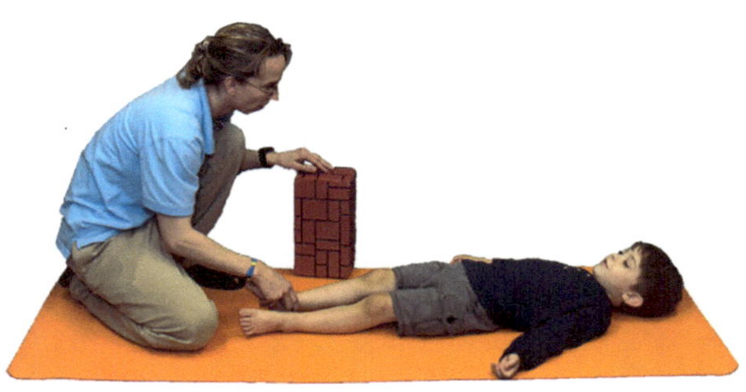

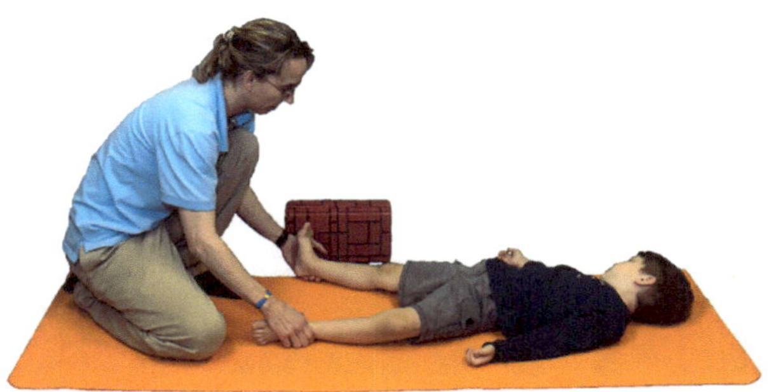

4. SUPINE BILATERAL ABDUCTION

This is the same activity as the unilateral one, except now I am requesting abduction of both legs-either simultaneously or sequentially. As before if needed I will prop the child's head up on a pillow. I resist or assist the movement of abduction accordingly. I often find bilateral abduction to be harder for a child than unilateral. It is often difficult for the child to move both legs simulaneously.

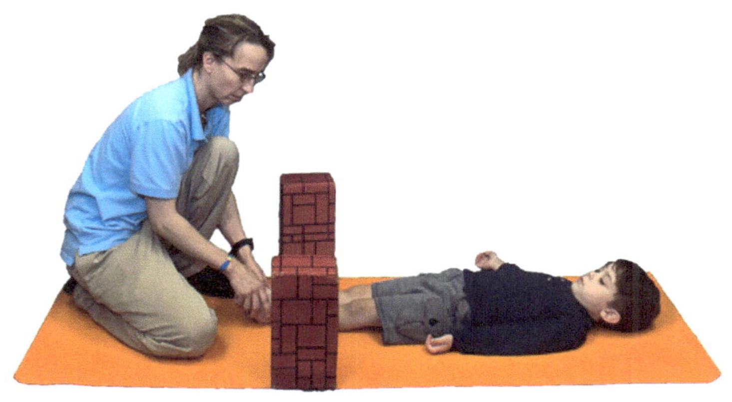

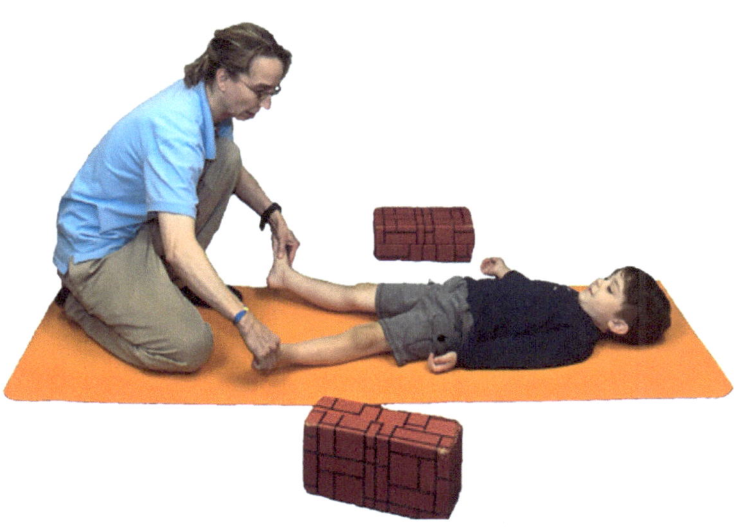

5. HOOKLYING HEEL TOUCH

In supine, the client has to laterally flex far enough to touch his heel when he lies hooklying. This means that more than just core work has to activate. Abductors and adductors are assisting according to the leg and the direction my client is going. This is a fantastic exercise for my clients with diplegia and hemiplegia, but also good for those with proximal weakness. This exercise is easiest on slick floors, harder on mats, and quite difficult on carpeting.

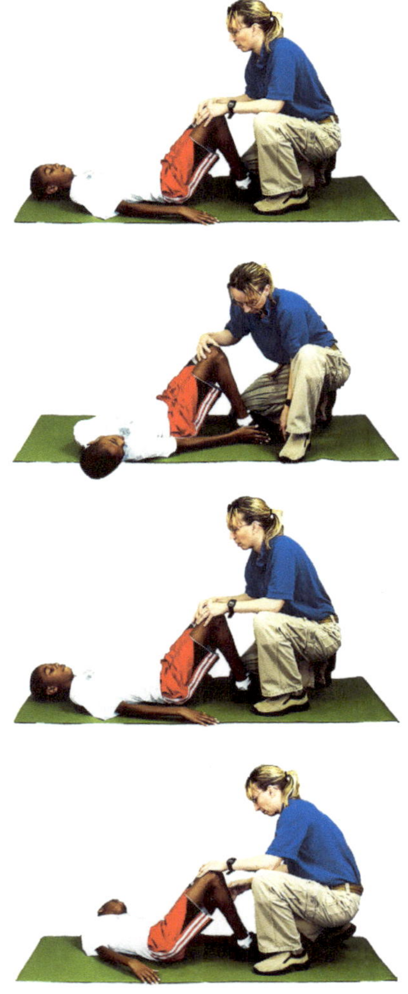

6. HOOKLYING DINNER PLATES

I have the client lie down in hooklying or bridge. I have her lift one lower leg keeping the thighs at least initially level. Then I have the client make dinner plate sized circles with her foot. While doing this she keeps the other thigh as still as possible. This works the proximal hip stabilizers and is much more difficult than it looks.

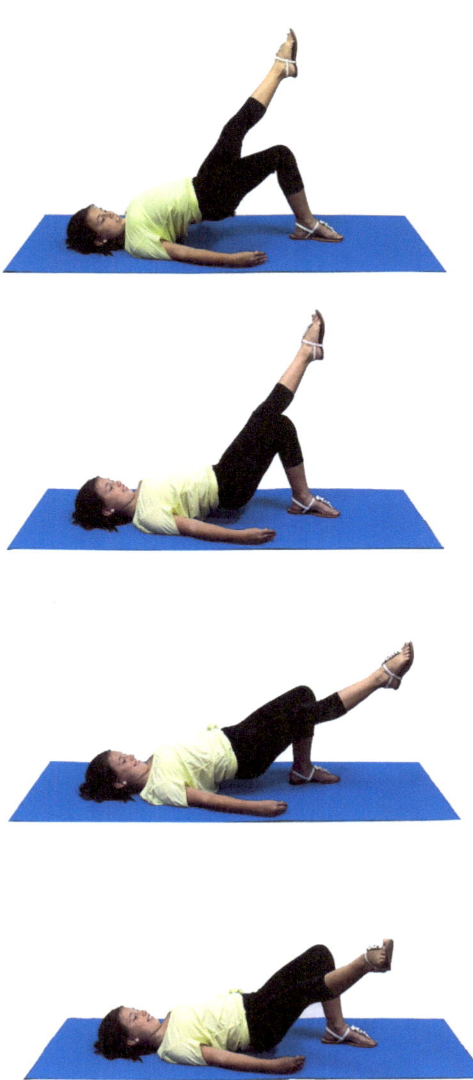

7. ONE LEG BENCH BRIDGE ABDUCTION KICK

First the client lifts into end range hip extension with one foot up on the bench. Then she kicks laterally into abduction to knock off the cone/block/toy off the bench. This is hard work but most of my kids like knocking things over especially if I act like I am upset about it. In a variation, both feet are on the bench before kicking out.

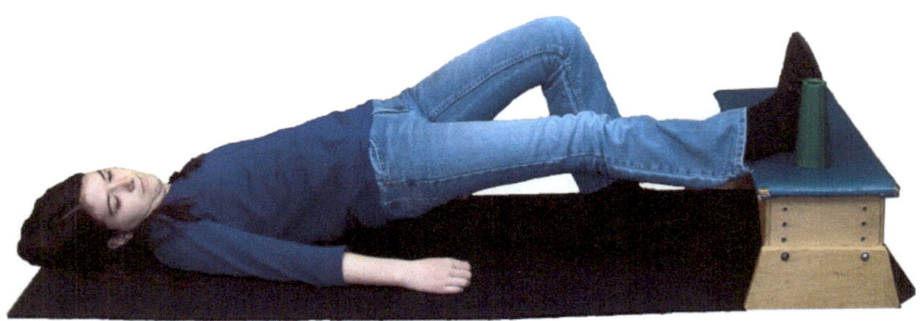

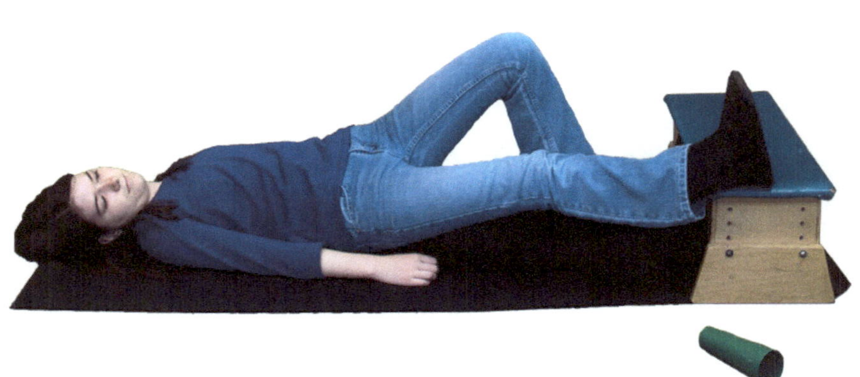

8. ABDUCTION SIDE LYING WITH KNEE EXTENSION

I try side lying in the middle of the floor only with my most reliable clients or with the ones who are too heavy to move. Typically, I put my client side lying with his back to the wall to encourage a straight plane of movement into abduction. Often a client who is trying to abduct their leg will substitute with knee flexion, external rotation or hip flexion. A wall makes these substitutions more apparent. I am strict about making sure the child keeps his hips and back flat against the wall. I frequently have to verbally cue the child to think about leading with his heel in abduction. Frequently the child will turn his leg into external rotation and go toe first. I often put my hand up above the child's foot as a target for him to hit as he raises his leg. Obviously a higher target is harder. I may place a weight on the child's lower thigh or manually resist or assist abduction. This activity lends itself easily to repetitions or holding the leg in abduction. I may tell the child to abduct his leg for a ten count as I try to push the abducted leg down to meet the lower leg for eccentric muscle contractions. I push as hard as I can still allowing the child to win.

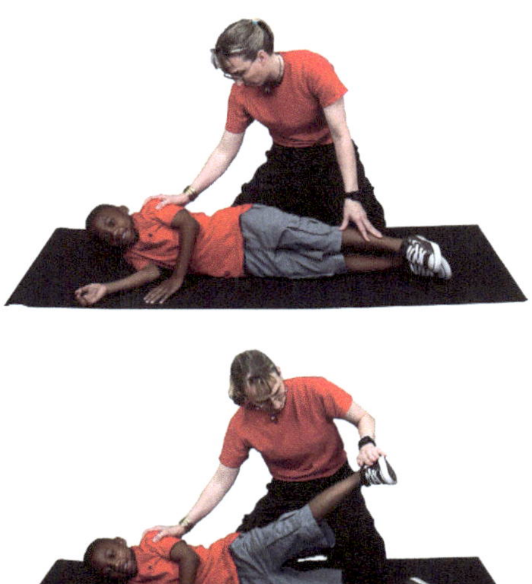

9. ABDUCTION SIDE LYING WITH KNEE FLEXION

This is a hard exercise and it takes a very cooperative and/or motivated client-preferably both-to perform this accurately. Sometimes I do this exercise with the child lying on his side facing a wall with only a little space between him and the wall. I tell him to abduct his leg with his knee bent but keep his knee off the wall. So many of my children get hip flexion when they try to abduct their hip. You can have the child perform this activity with no resistance or manual resistance, with Velcro soft weights at the thigh. I document the number of repetitions and whether I used weights in the daily note.

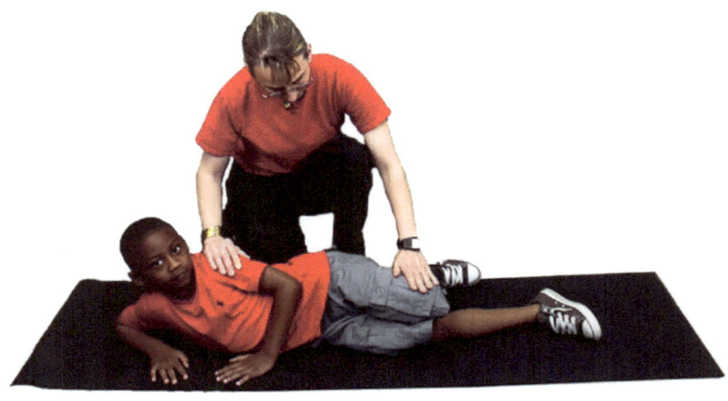

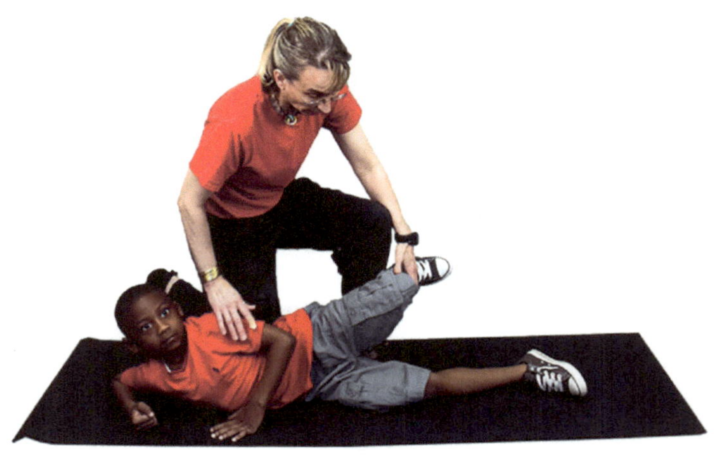

10. PRONE HIP ABDUCTION WITH EXTENSION

Sometimes I try having the client abduct and adduct her legs in this position to encourage abduction with progressive hip extension. I usually start with my 16" (40 cm) bench and work progressively lower. As always I use extra padding for male clients. I document for the record how low the client could go and how many times the client could move her legs out and in.

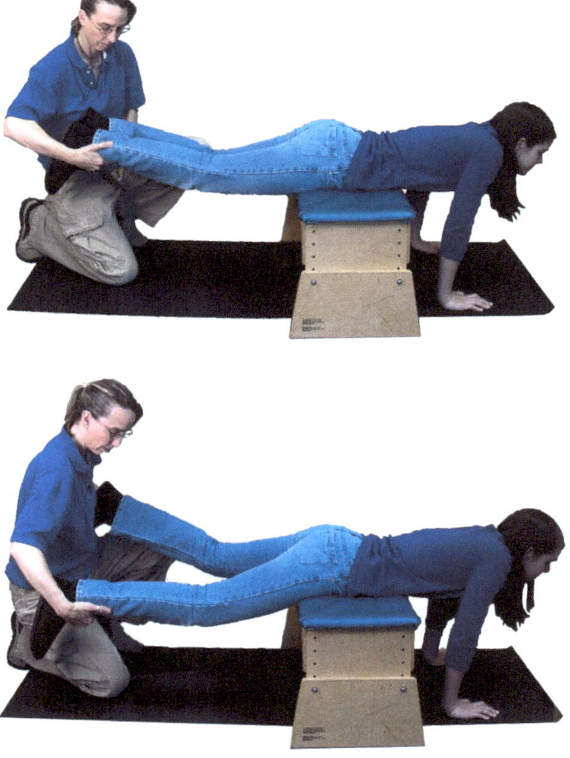

11. STRAIGHT ARM SIDE PLANKS ON WALL

This is the easiest way to start side planks. I am using the mats here as a wall. Make sure the client keeps her body moving only in the frontal plane. The elbow should stay straight.

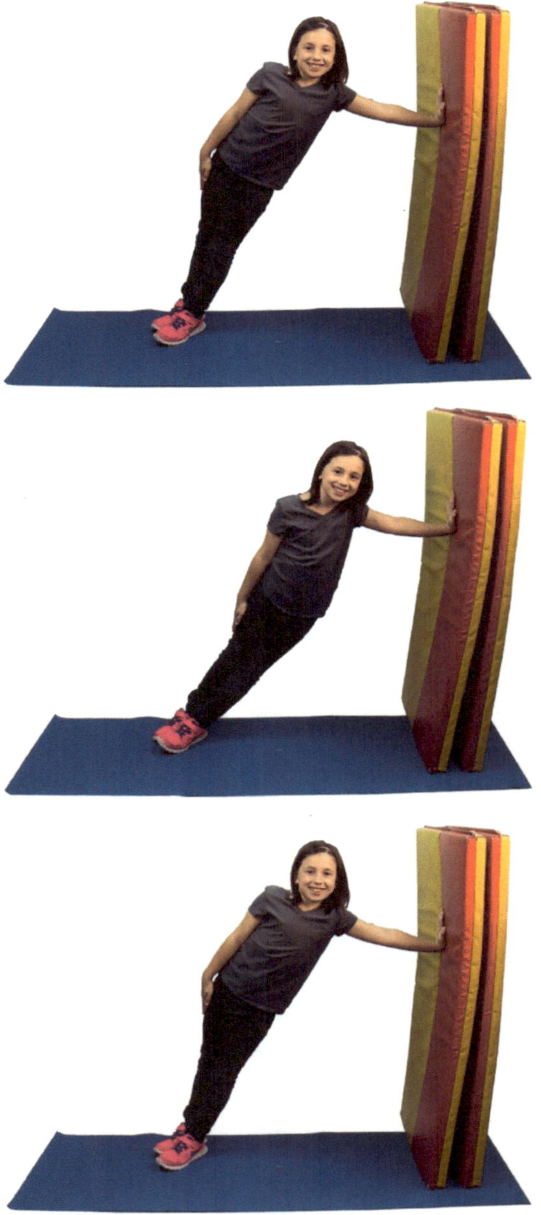

12. STRAIGHT ARM SIDE PLANKS ON BENCH

After the client masters the wall side planks I work slowly progressively lower. Instead of going straight to the floor I used benches to achieve an intermediate level of difficulty.

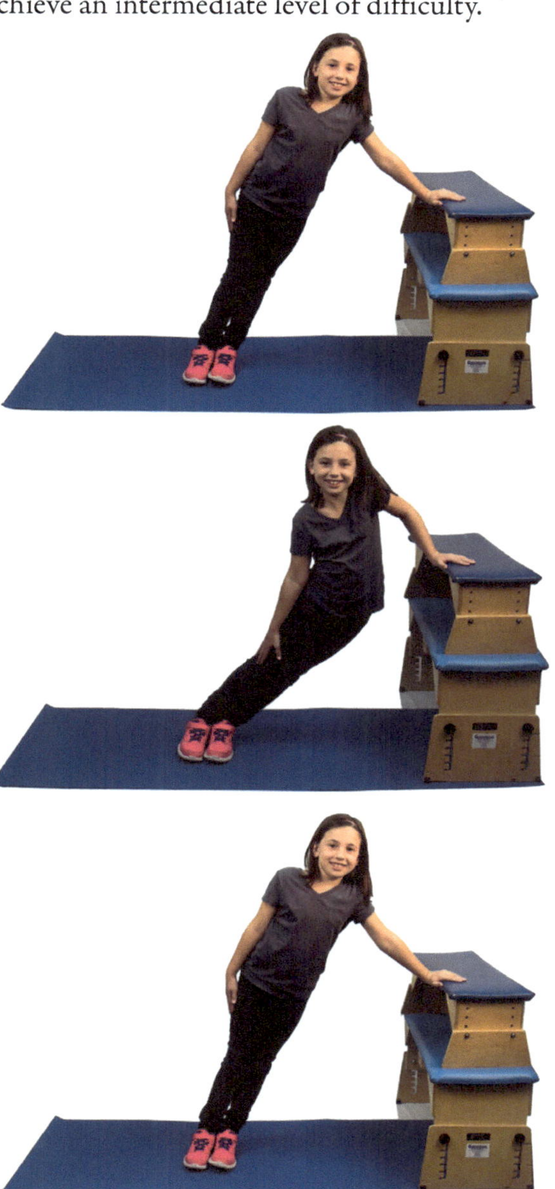

13. FOREARM KNEE SIDE PLANKS

These can be performed from the forearm or on a straight arm. The movement is very small if your client is on forearms and knees. Watch to make sure your client doesn't roll forward and up, instead of straight up. Put your client's back to a wall to discourage substitutions.

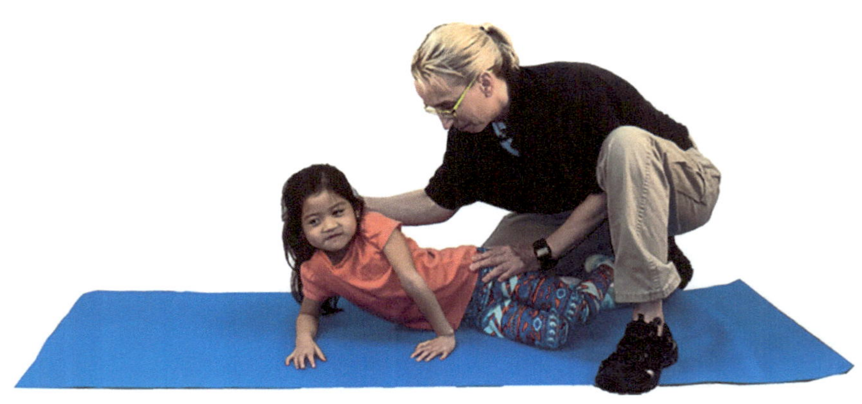

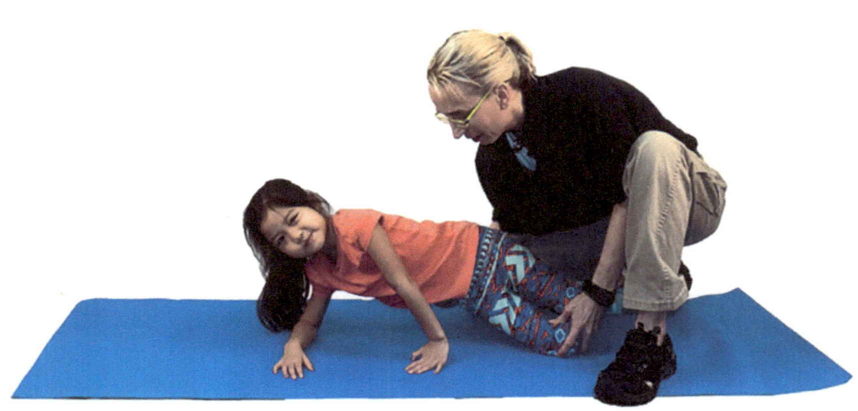

14. STRAIGHT ARM KNEE PLANKS

These knee planks allow for a little more movement. This is harder shoulder work but the client is not as low down against gravity. If a client cannot perform the forearm knee planks, I'll try the straight arms ones and vice versa.

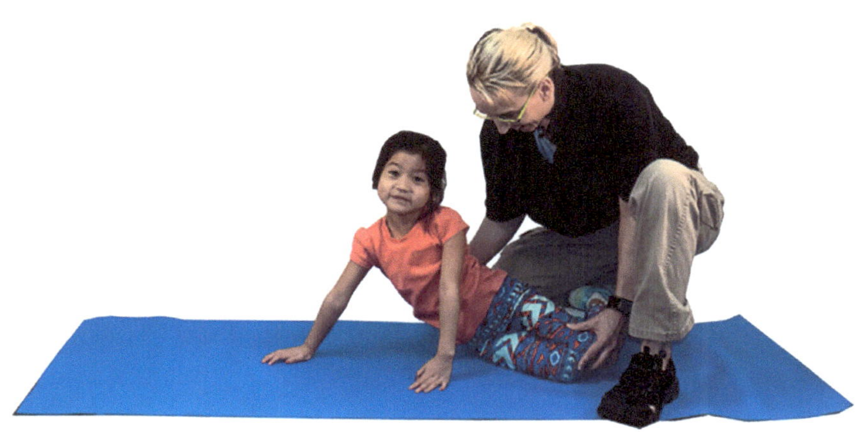

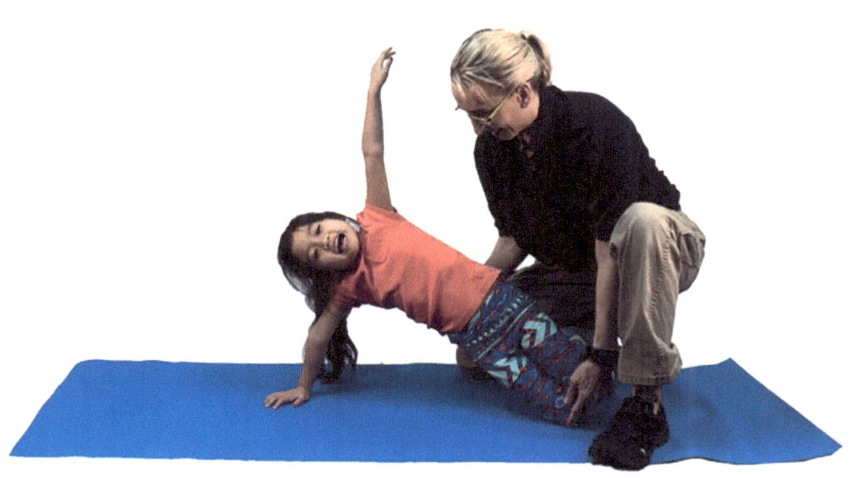

15. FOREARM SIDE PLANK

Oh my goodness, this is a tough exercise! I only have one client who is exercise obsessed that really likes this one. It is another great general body strengthener. This requires trunk activation in general, abdominal and back as well as abduction/adduction depending on the leg. This exercise is marginally easier on a forearm than on a straight arm. For my clients who will tolerate it, I love it for those trying to hold off scoliosis surgery or who persistently shorten one side. On the floor I often see the client kind of roll forward instead of lifting his hips straight up toward the ceiling. When this is the case, I have him start lying down with his back to the wall. I ask him to lift his hips up straight along the wall. It is then visually obvious to everyone when he rolls forward instead.

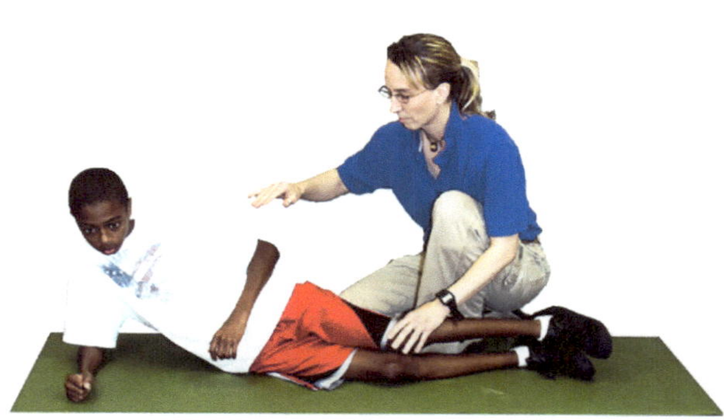

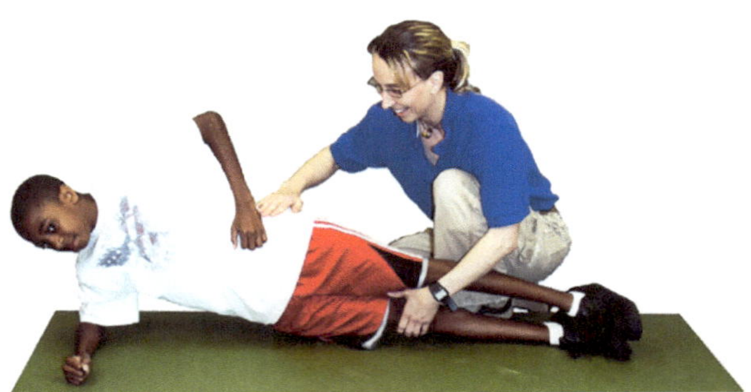

16. STRAIGHT ARM PLANK

This exercise is marginally easier on a forearm than on a straight arm. The floor is really hard. So this requires more shoulder strength, but makes the client move through a greater range, getting more abduction. However, with the client angled higher off of the floor, he is not fighting gravity as much as on his elbow.

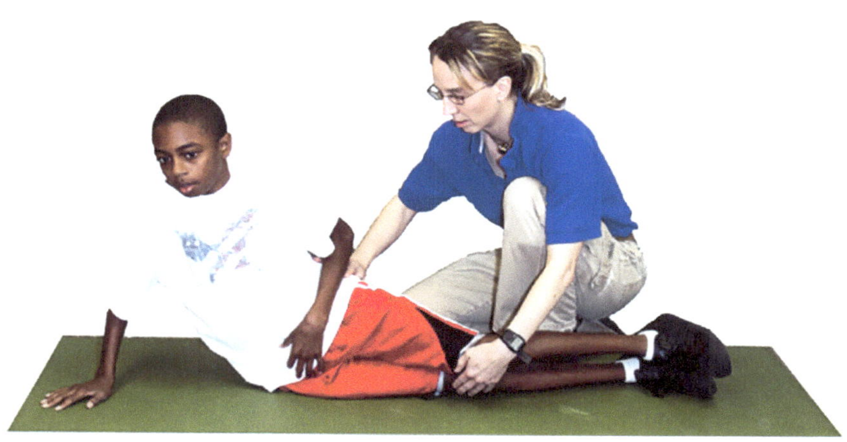

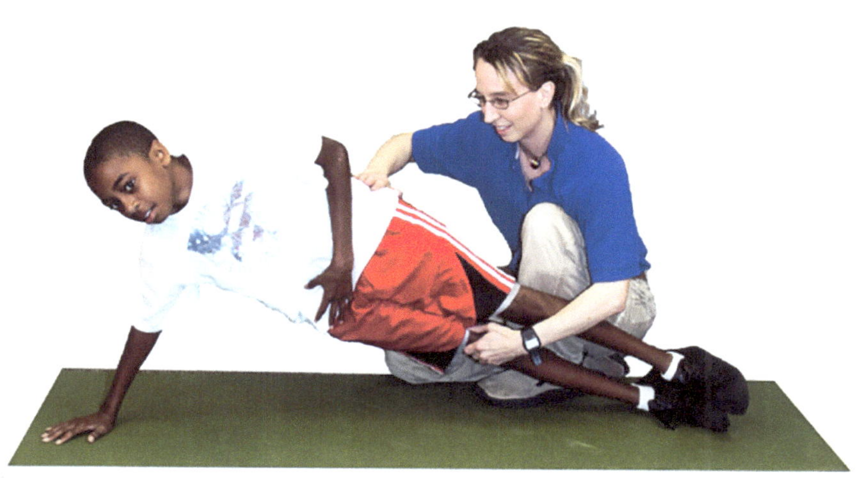

17. SIDESIT PROGRESSIVELY NARROW

When a child sits side sit with his knee spread as wide as possible, the pelvis is fairly level. As you have the child put his knees closer together the pelvis becomes more tilted. When the knees are completely on top of each other in side sit, the pelvis is very angled. The position is more challenging when the pelvis is more angled. This exercise requires lateral flexion, internal/external rotation and hip abduction/adduction strength depending on the leg referenced. I have a child typically start with his knees very wide and progress the difficulty until the child can no longer hold or sustain the position.

I also do this with the child sitting on a trampoline, rockerboard, ball or even a platform swing so I can bounce/rock/swing the child ten times to make it more dynamic. If I am performing the activity on a dynamic surface, I determine what level of leg overlap is challenging, and I make sure the child can hold the position for ten seconds. If the child is successful with small bounces/rocks/swings, I progress the medium, large and then extreme. Kids love this.

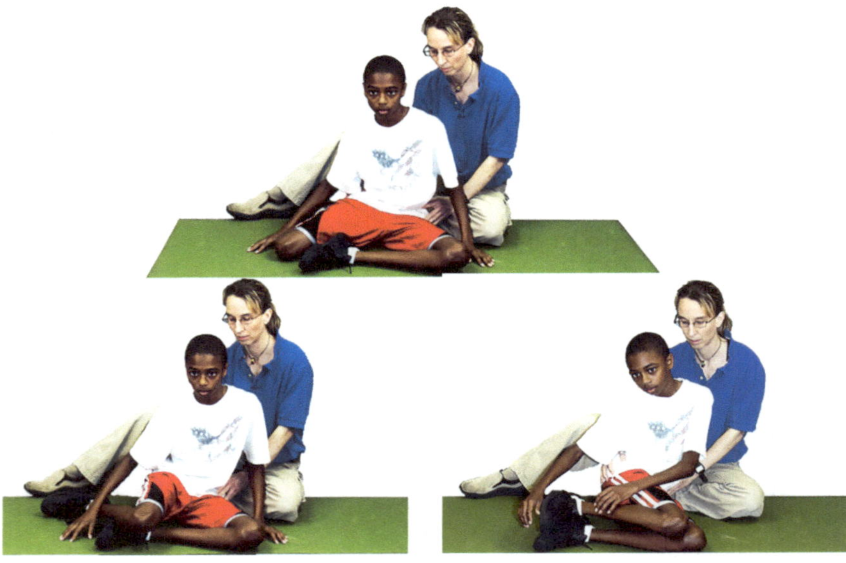

18. SIDESIT TO TALL KNEEL

Often this is a very difficult transition for my clients. It requires lateral flexion, hip internal/external rotation, and hip adduction/abduction depending on the leg. To make it easier, I may use a four inch (ten cm) bench down for the client to sit down to from tall kneel. If he is successful with the bench, I have him sit down to a doubled and then single thickness pillow. If still successful, I progress him to the floor as shown here. This exercise is quite hard in general, but if you need to challenge your client more, have him cross his arms on his chest.

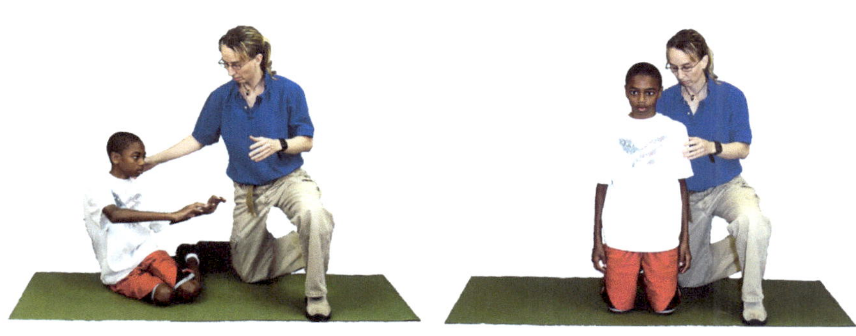

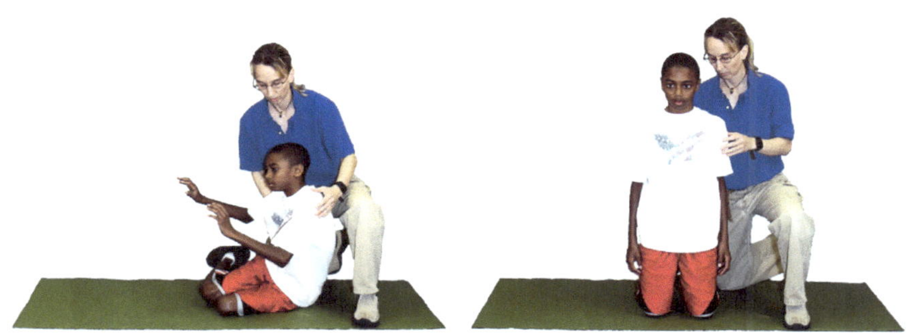

19. SIDEWAYS KNEE WALK

This picture shows this model knee walking sideways holding my hand, but I rarely do sideways knee walking this way. I usually put the mat down next to a wall and have the child knee walk sideways facing the wall with two hands on the wall/mirror. Sideways walking looking at the mirror is usually a good option as children always seem to like to look at themselves. It is worth cleaning the mirror later. Unless I am targeting only one leg, I have the client go both to the right and left. Having a mat down makes this activity more comfortable on the knees.

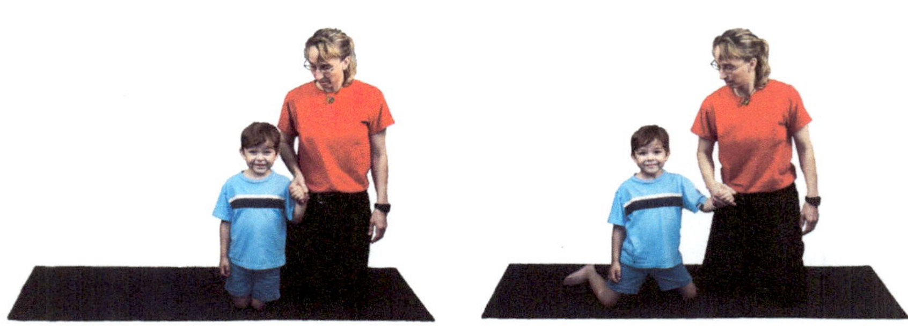

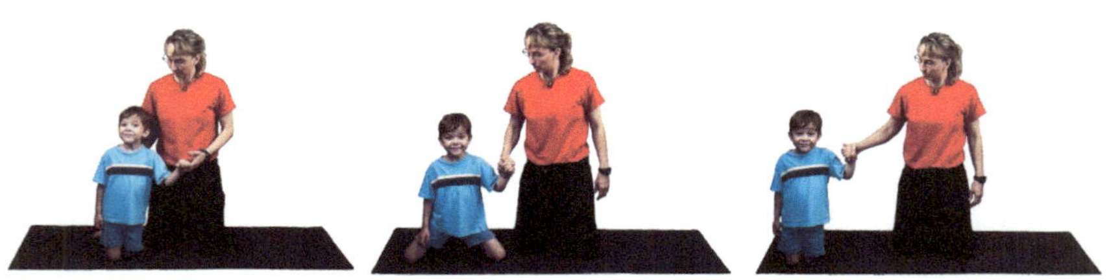

20. RESISTED HALF KNEEL

I often see the limiting factor for clients being able to hold half kneel on the floor is weakness in abduction and external rotation. The knee that is in the up position in half kneel falls into internal rotation and the client ends up back in kneel. In order to make sure I get abduction in this exercise, I make sure I push on the lateral aspect of the knee that is up along with the hip. You elicit active abduction on both legs. You can push in pulses or sustained resistance. For someone who is not as strong, I start with ten pulses and progress to a ten second press. I document the style and intensity of the push.

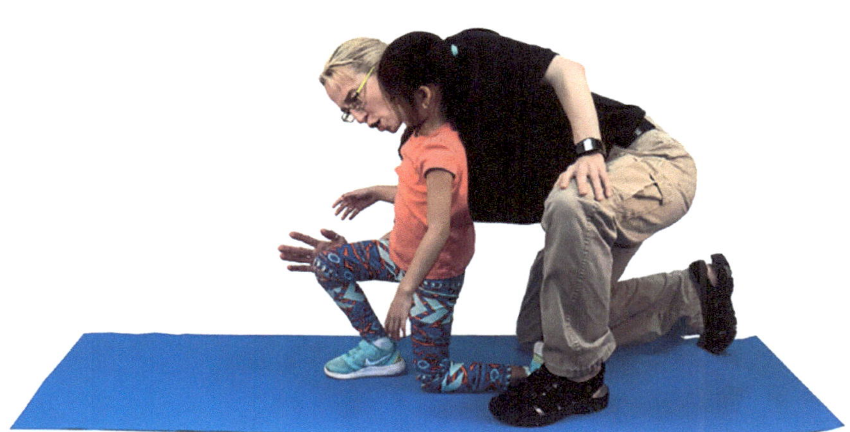

21. BENCH KNEEL TO HALF KNEEL

Because of the nature of moving from kneel to half kneel on a bench, the child must abduct and actually externally rotate the leg to get the foot planted out and beside the knee.

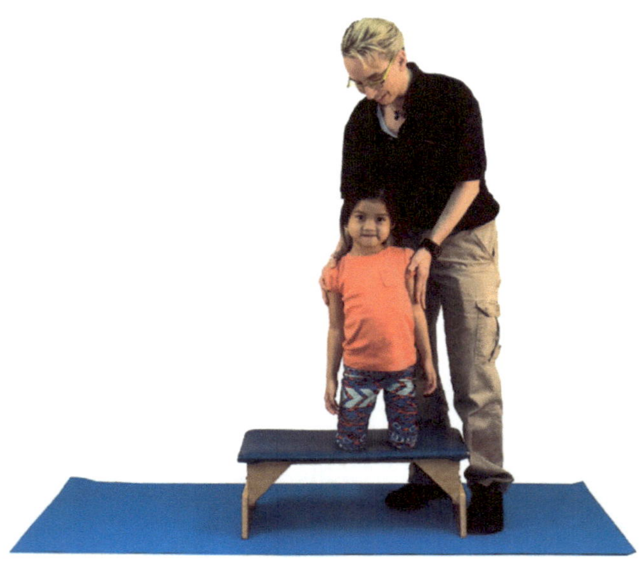

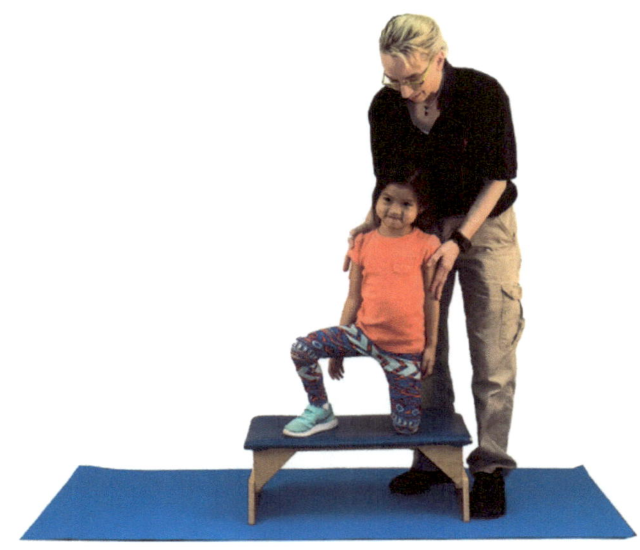

22. HALF KNEEL STAMP PROGRESSIVELY WIDER

I like using squeak toys to have a child stamp on, but anything will do. This exercise elicits abduction on the leg with the knee down as well as on the stamping leg. Stamping the leg wider makes this activity trickier.

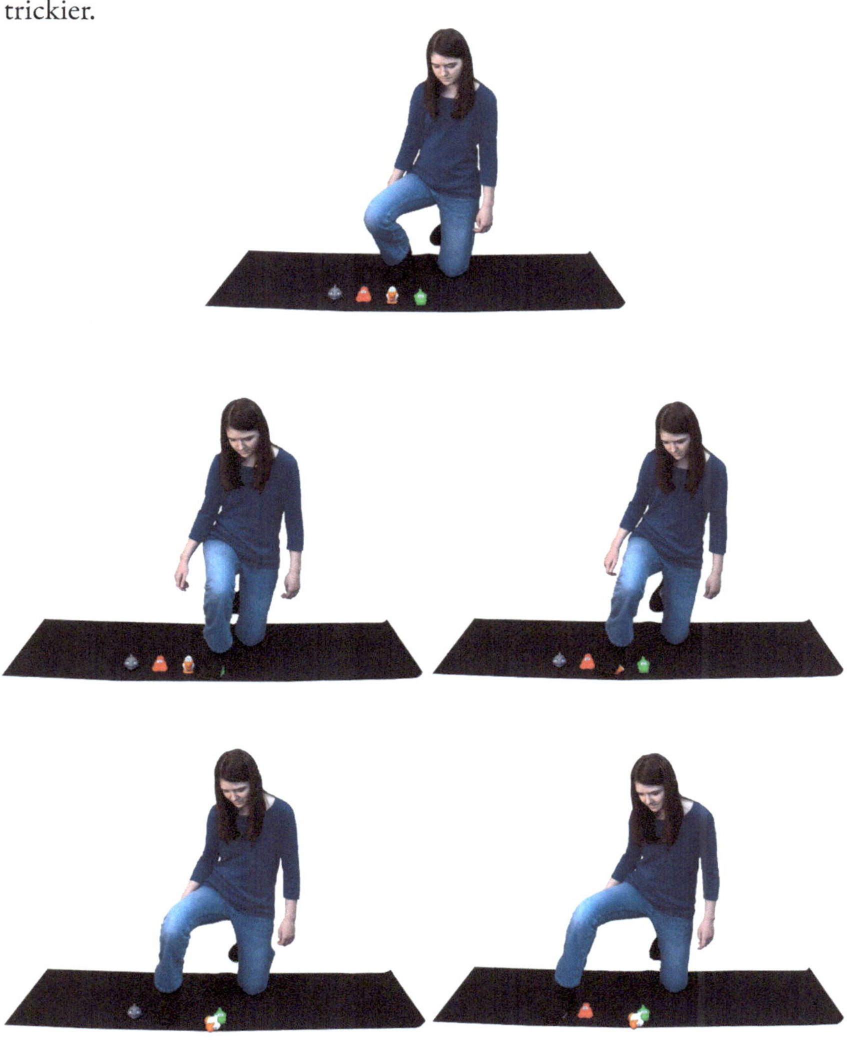

23. HALF KNEEL KICK PROGRESSIVELY WIDER

This exercise is a trickier version of the previous one. If the client has to sustain balance on her left knee while kicking, then this activity becomes very hard.

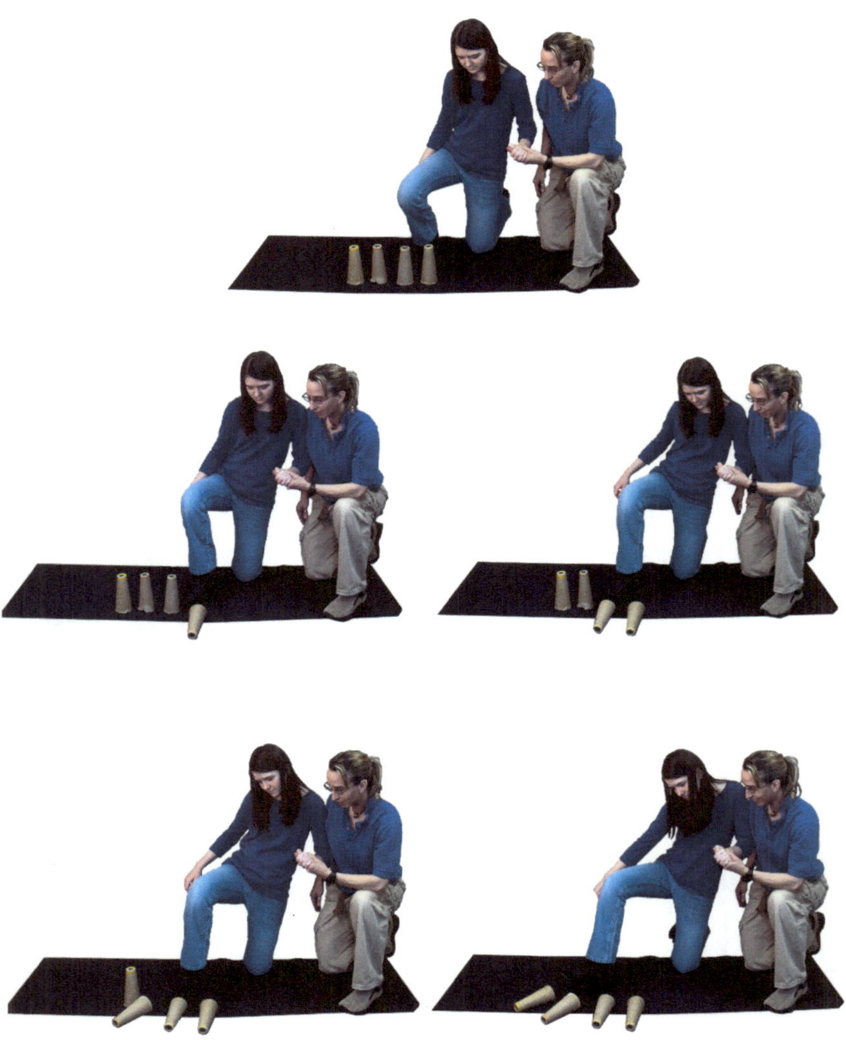

24. QUADRUPED ON THE ROCKERBOARD

This exercise gets abduction/adduction of the upper and lower extremities and lots of core work too! Speed matters! I like to start this exercise with small ranges and slow tilts. Then I ramp up the tilt angle and the speed.

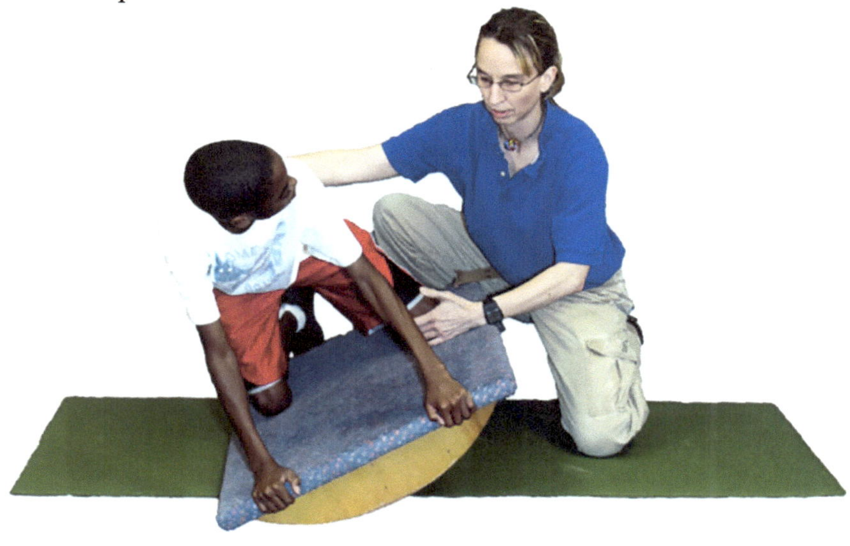

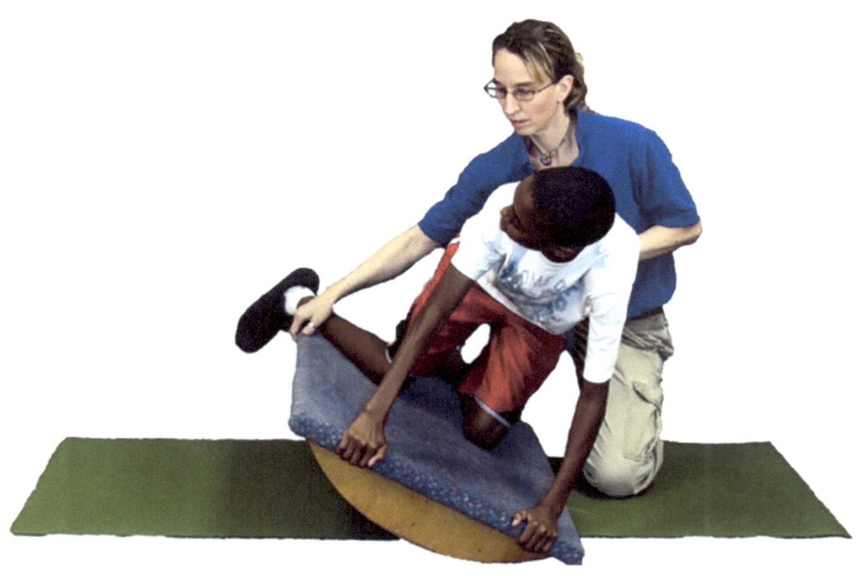

25. TALL KNEEL ON THE ROCKERBOARD

This one is dramatically harder than the previous exercise. Rocking side to side strongly engages adductors and abductors.

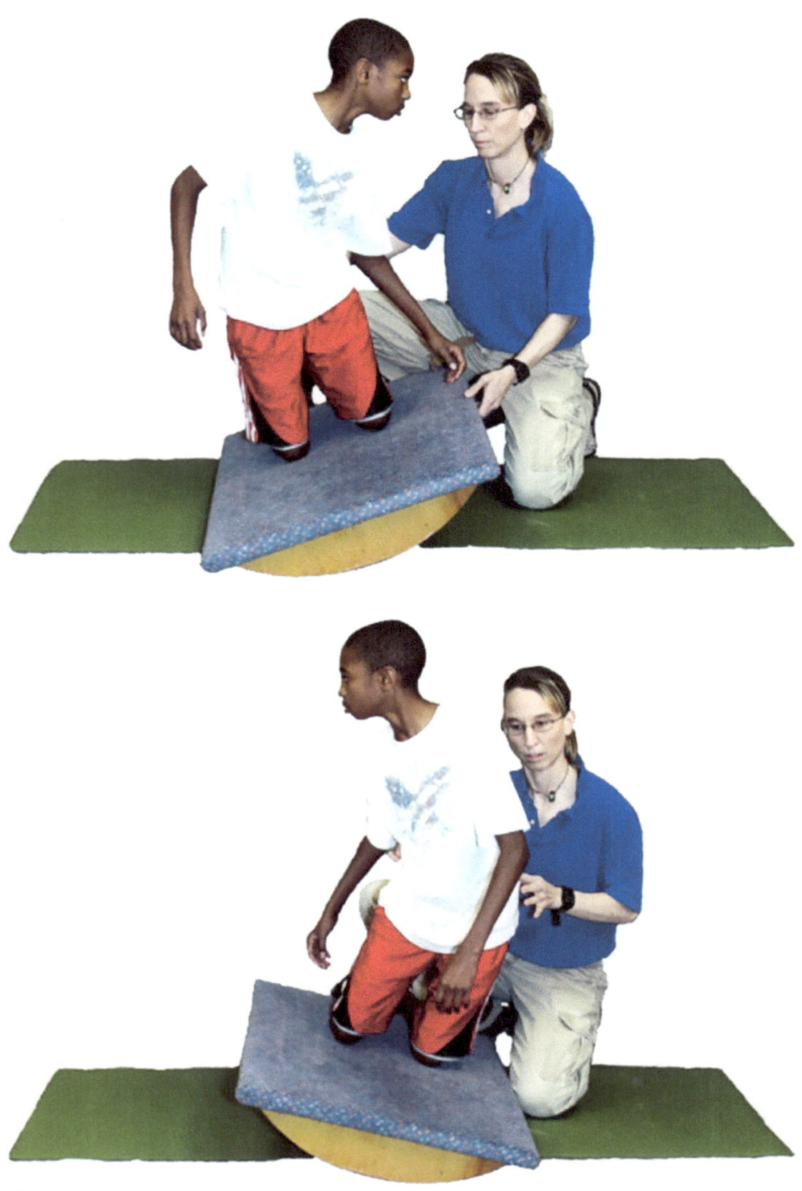

26.HALF KNEEL ON A ROCKERBOARD

As if the previous exercise wasn't enough, this one is even harder. If the child has an easier side, I always let her do the easy side first to get the feel of the movement.

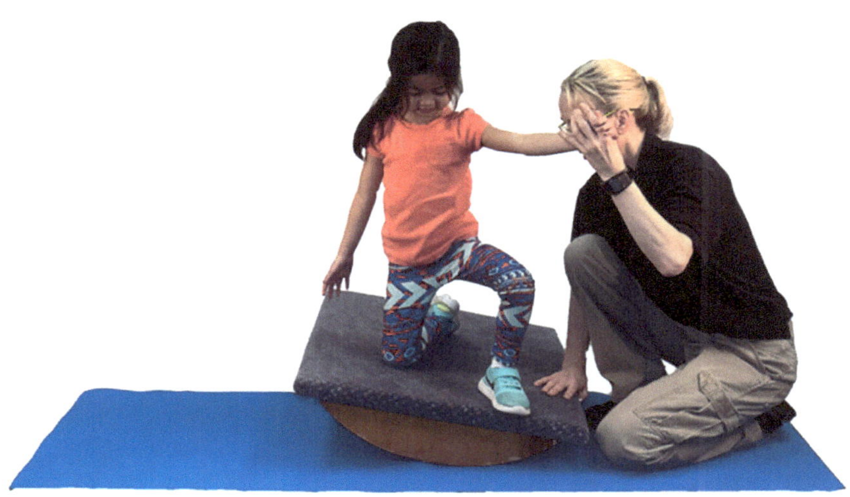

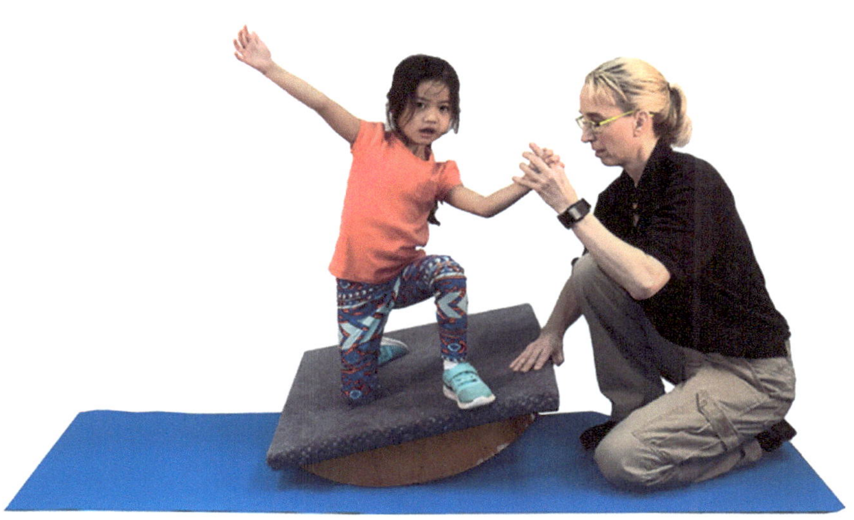

27. STANDING ON ROCKERBOARD

This is much more challenging. I have 2 short benches that I tuck under each side of the rockerboard to stabilize it for a client who has trouble stepping on or off a wobbly rockerboard. Once he is safely on, I remove the benches to allow the rockerboard to rock freely. If the client is very challenged, I have him hold onto wall grips for stability while I rock the rockerboard. As the client gets more confident, then I have the client rock the rockerboard on his own. To encourage end range rocking, I put a piano keyboard or a squeak toy under one side or each side of the rockerboard. I encourage my client to rock far enough to play the piano. Keep a close spot on your client. Rockerboards get wild fast.

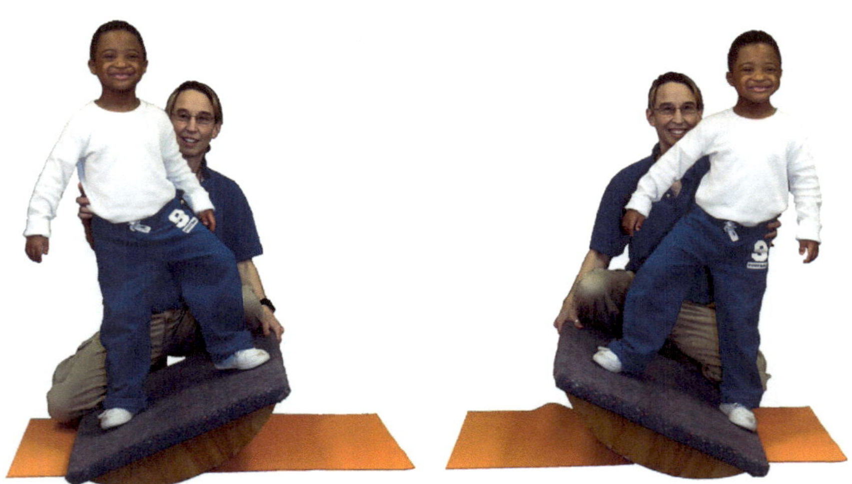

28. STANDING WITH KNEES APART

I feel that an adducted alignment in stance and gait is a often the result of a weakness in both abductors and external rotators. I have some kids work simply on standing with knees apart. I put my hand between her knees and say, “Keep your knees off my hands.” I may put a small electronic keyboard between my client’s knees to give auditory cues for when the knees fall back together. I also love to play the game on the trampoline. My client can hold wall grips for balance as needed. As I bounce them or they bounce themselves, they keep their knees apart to a ten count or however long I feel like counting. Sometimes we go for records of minutes at a time with knees apart.

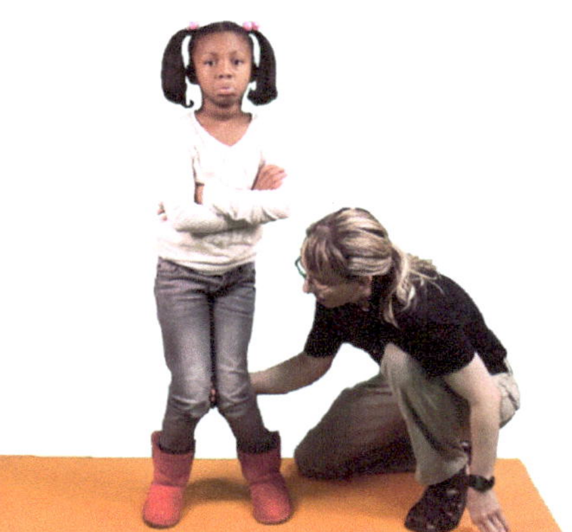

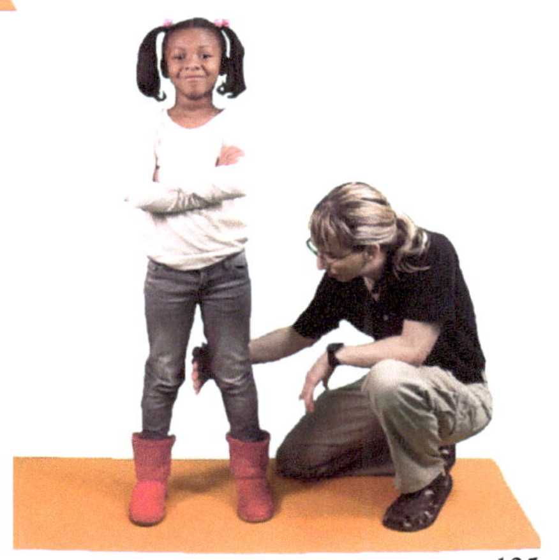

29. ABDUCTION STANDING OPEN CHAIN

This girl makes it look easy, but the clients I have who need to work on this have a harder time. I perform this activity a variety of ways. Sometimes I have the client hold the stabilized vertical poles or wall grips, or just place her hands on the wall. Then I have her lift her leg in abduction, sometimes to hit a target such as my hand, a wall, a ball, or a block. A block is advantageous since it doesn't roll away. Often I see substitution of hip flexion. If that is the case then I may have her stand with her back to the wall and encourage her to keep her leg along the wall as she abducts. I usually have to remind them to "Lead with your heel not your toes." I often have to physically assist to keep the toes pointing straight out from the wall.

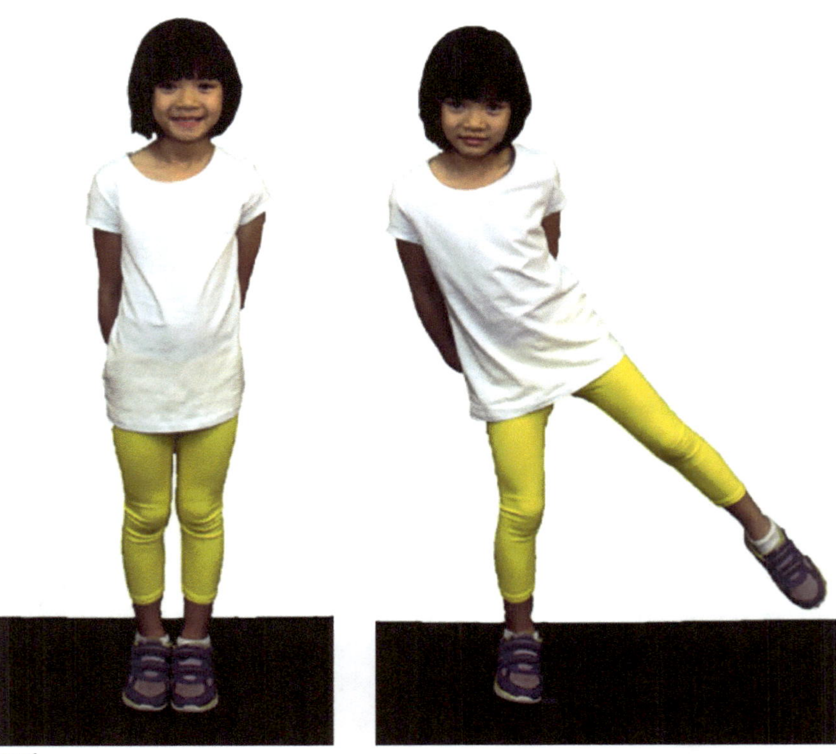

30. SIDE SLIDE OUT AND IN UNILATERALLY

I find something that slides easily for my client put his foot on. Here I have simply used a piece of paper. You can use baby powder to make it slide easier. He simply slides his foot out and back. A target such as a line on the floor is always helpful. You can provide upper extremity support as needed.

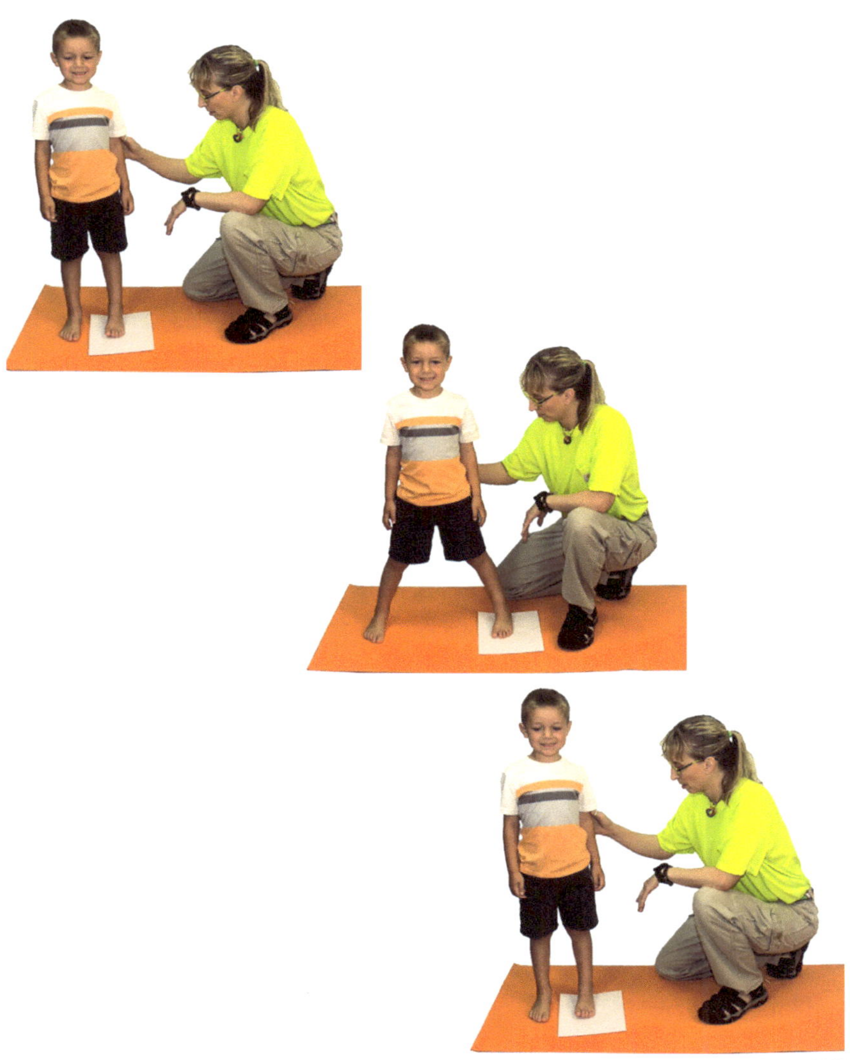

31. PENDULUM ABDUCTION STANDING

This can be done with or without weights. The leg can move in front of or behind the stance leg or even alternating between the two, but I prefer in front. Ankle weights increase the difficulty of this exercise. Many clients need upper extremity support for success with this activity.

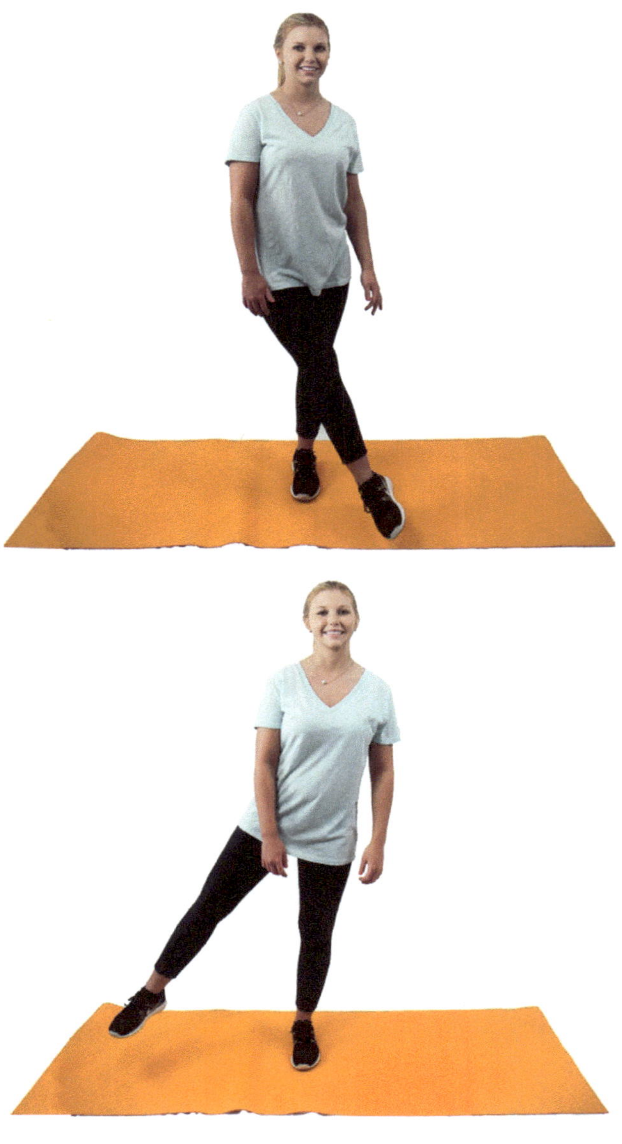

32. TETHER BALL ABDUCTION STANDING

This is similar to the previous exercise. I can hold the tether ball rope or my client can. I can also hook it up to the ceiling to add less reproducibility in the abduction kicks. Weights on the ankles make this activity harder. External support is often needed.

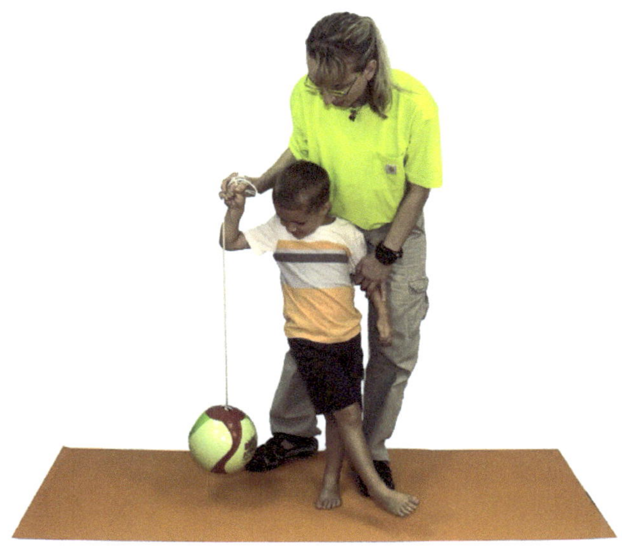

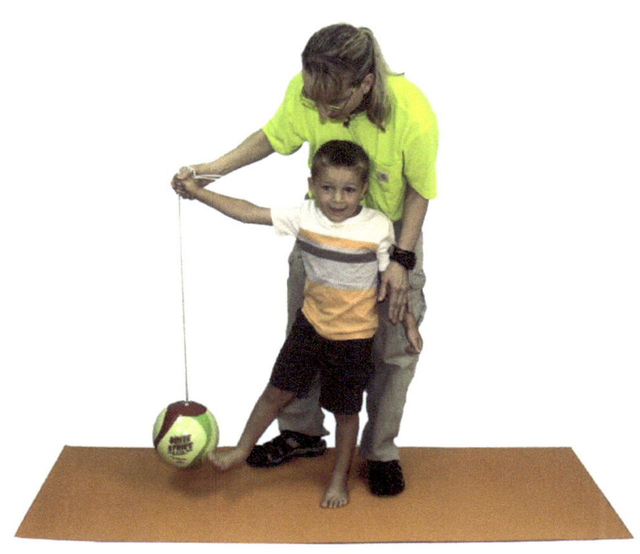

33. RESISTED STANDING WITH A LATERAL PUSH

This actually works abduction and adduction depending on the leg. I usually give ten discreet pushes or I push for a duration of ten seconds. Kids love this. If he successfully withstands my push, then I always let the kid push me-much to their glee. Where I push with restraint, they never do.

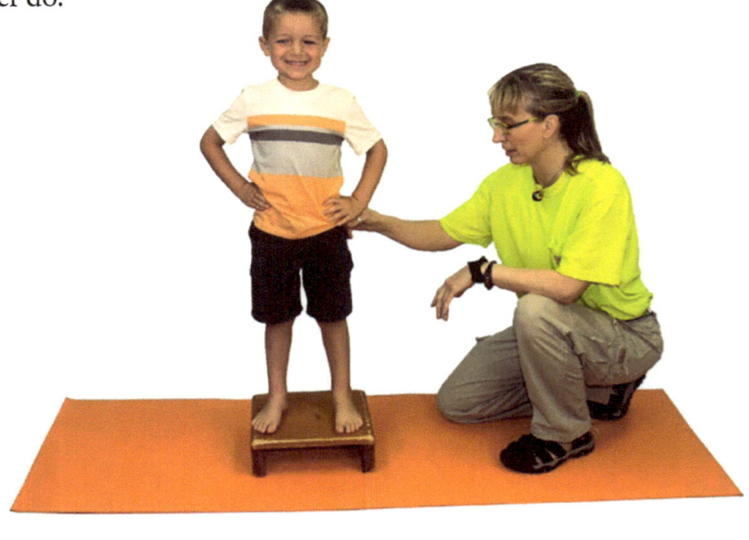

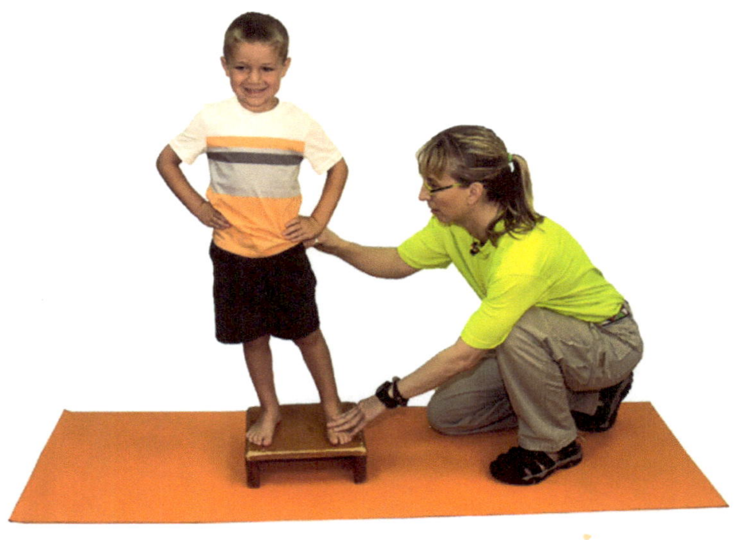

34. SIT TO STAND WITH ABDUCTED LEGS

For children with diplegic or quadriplegic cerebral palsy, this can be a very difficult exercise. I put my hand or an electronic keyboard between the client's knees and have him move from sitting to standing and back down again keeping knees apart. If the client is having a hard time, make the bench higher or give hand support.

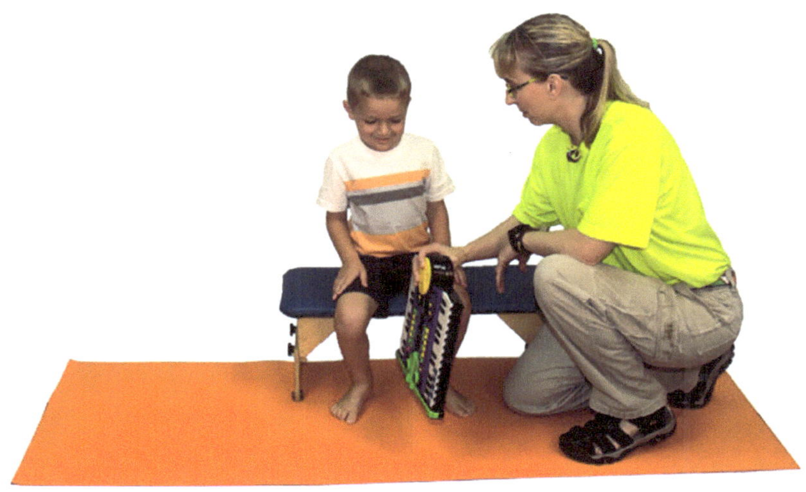

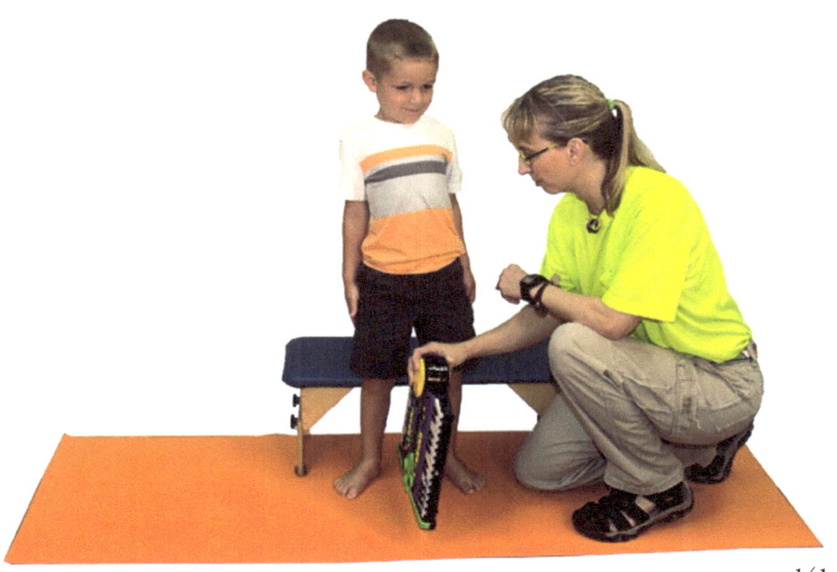

35. BOUNCE WITH KNEES APART

This is also a tricky exercise for clients with cerebral palsy. I usually have to let the client hold onto a wall grip or someone's hands. He simply bends and straightens his knees keeping his knees apart. I like this activity particularly on the trampoline. I count to see how many bounces he can get with his knees apart.

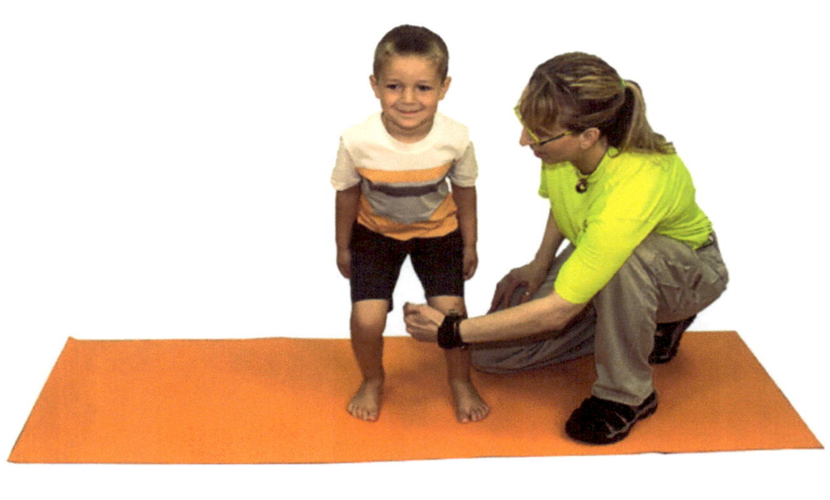

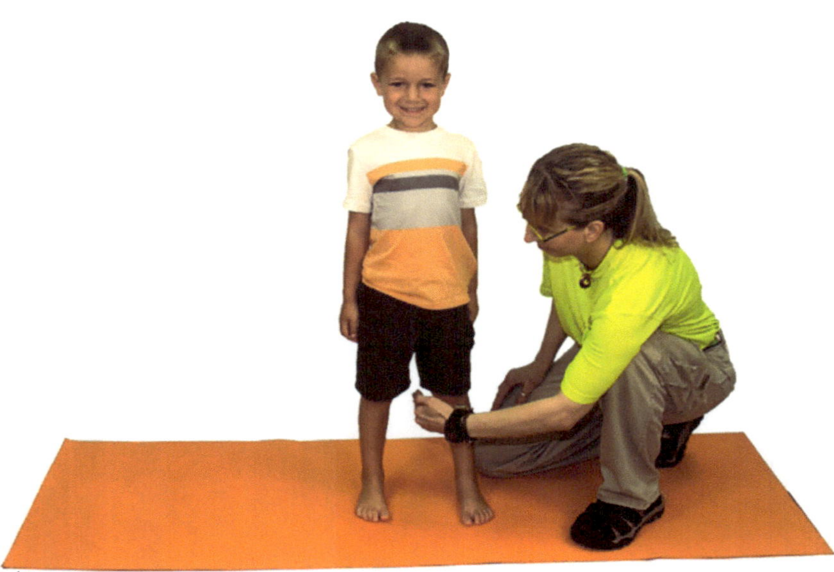

36. JUMP WITH KNEES APART

This is basically the same exercise as the previous one, except this time the client bounces hard enough to clear the floor or the trampoline, depending on the standing surface.

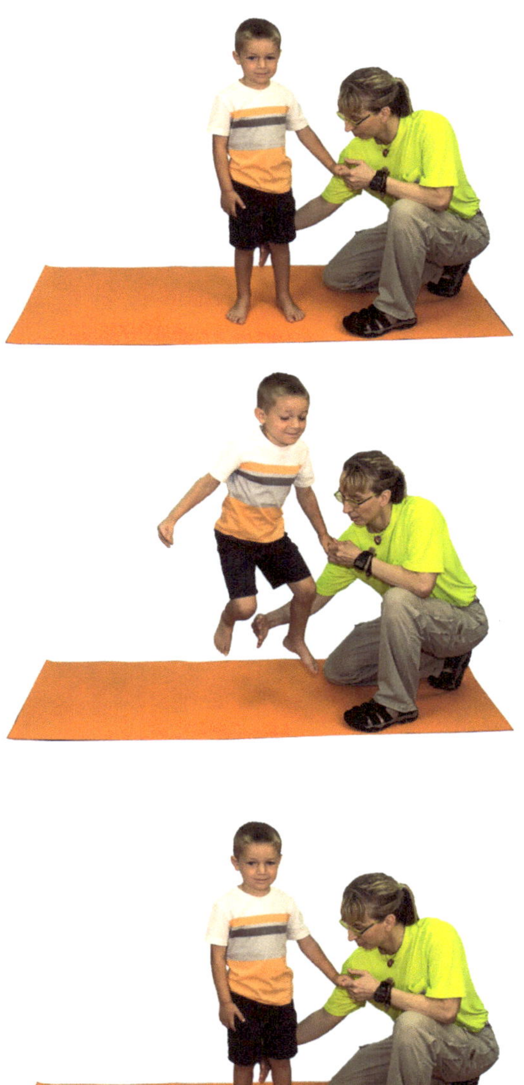

37. STANDING SIDE PICK UP TO BENCHES

Picking up to the side engages the trunk but also adductors and abductors, depending on the leg. The lower the child reaches the more challenging this activity is. Here the legs are placed symmetrically.

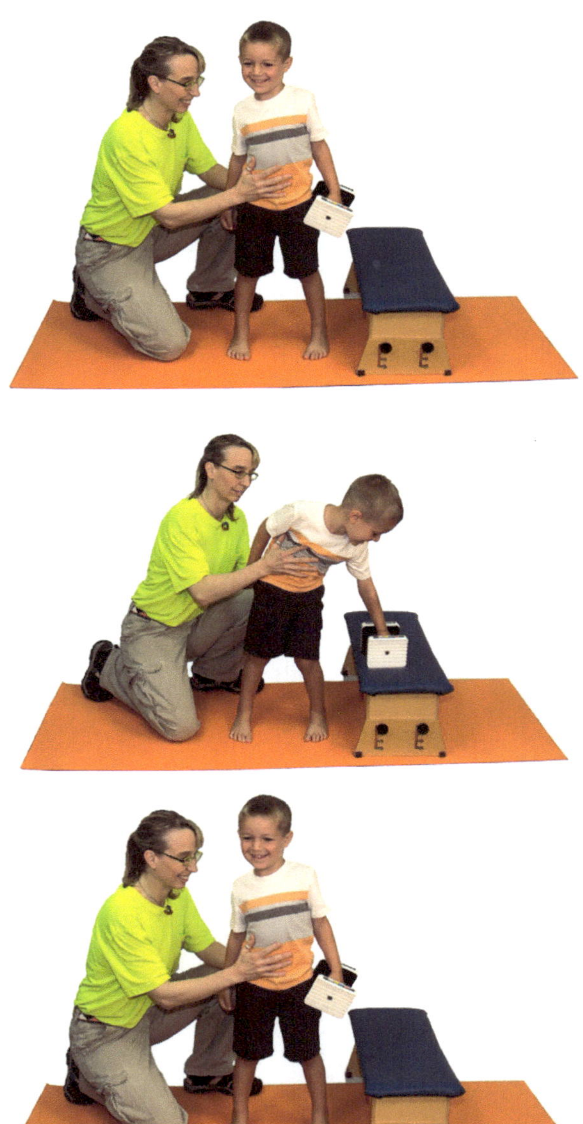

38. ONE FOOT ON A BENCH, SIDE PICK UP

To get abduction with this exercise, you have to make sure you set up the exercise so the child is moving laterally to pick up the toy on the ground. This is great with clients with hemiplegia. With one foot up on a bench, the client is immediately more likely to put more weight on the leg on the floor. I have watched more than a few kids try to figure this exercise out without putting more weight on the leg on the floor. For these kids I often support the knee on the down leg to guide the weight shift over to pick up the object. The weight is shifted to the down more on the lower leg as the upper leg is place on a progressively higher bench. Some clients need trunk support, a hand held, or a bench in front of them to stabilize on to complete this activity. I may initially not put the toy all the way on the ground. I measure progress by how close to the floor I can hold the toy and the child still be able to pick it up and return to upright.

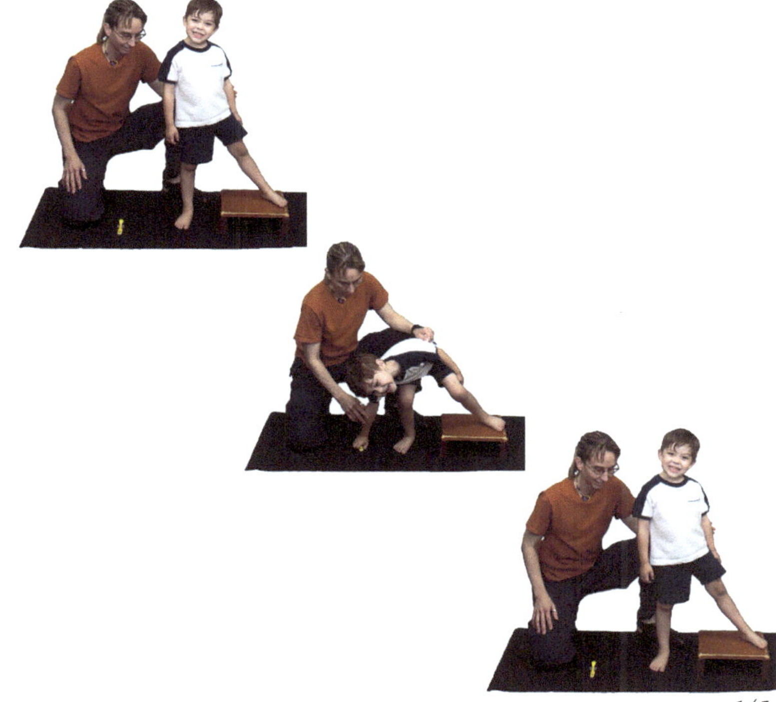

39. IN LINE STRIDE STANDING

Simply standing in the position of in line stride requires co-contraction of the adductors and abductors. To make this easier allow the foot placement to be progressively wider laterally. Often I measure progress by the duration the position can be held.

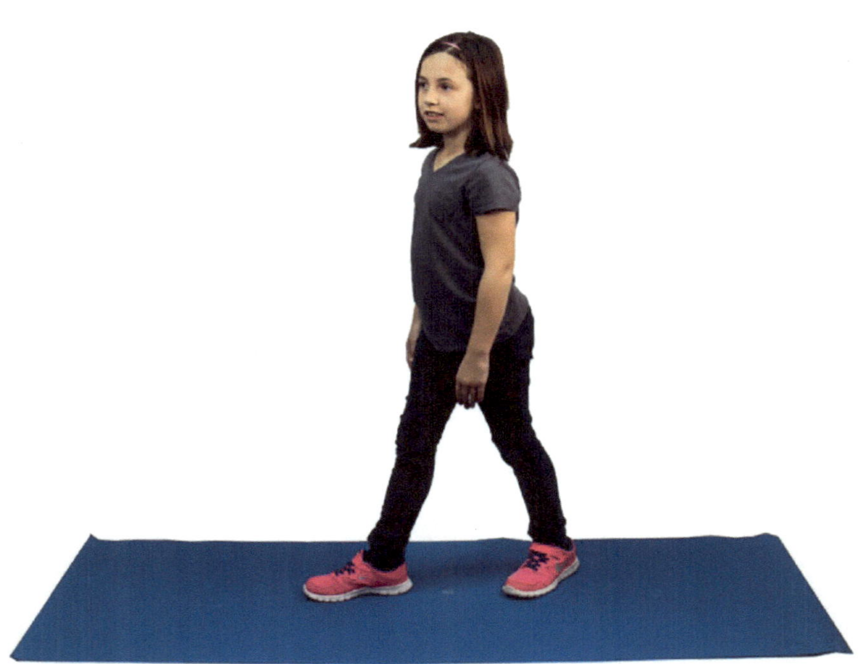

40. IN LINE STRIDE SIDE PICK UP TO FLOOR

Make sure you put the object/weight slightly behind the child's lateral midline. Encourage only a side movement. Many of my children cheat by leaning forward and then reaching back with their arm. Lifting heavier objects causes more muscle activation. To make this easier, simply have the child step forward with one leg into stride. In line stride makes this activity much more challenging. To make this easier, put the object on a bench. This activity is easier with a higher bench.

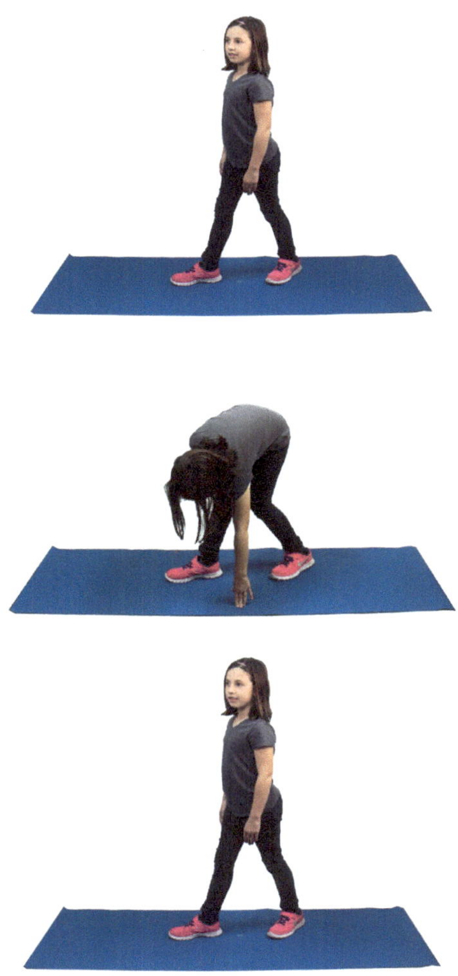

41. SIDE STEPPING

I usually have the client side step along a line. At the clinic we use Velcro lines on the carpet. For clients who have trouble and substitute with hip flexion, the line keeps the child from creeping forward as she moves sideways. The same clients often externally rotate their leg to lead toes first. I often find I have to remind them to lead with their heel to encourage the child to more correctly side step with abduction. To make this easier, I may allow the child to lean back against a wall. The parent, the child,and I all line up with our backs to the wall usually holding hands. To make this activity harder, use elastic bands or tubing around the lower thigh. I love sideways walking on the treadmill. Side stepping is important for side protective stepping reactions for fall prevention in emerging ambulating clients. In a smaller client this activity could be as simple as cruising sideways from one end of the couch, dining room table or counter top to the other. A well placed toy always helps.

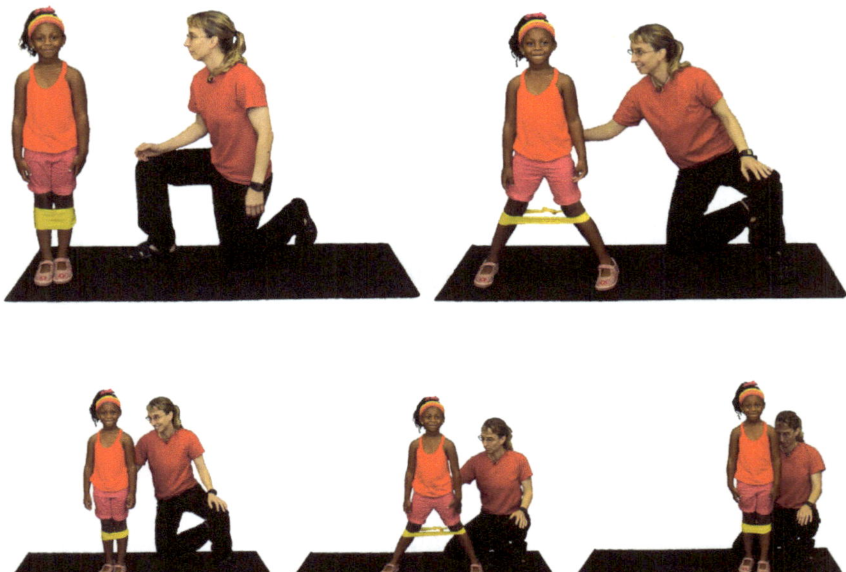

42. CROUCHING SIDE STEP WITH ARM SUPPORT

This is a variation of the prior exercise. The crouch adds more quad activation to this abduction exercise. This child needed upper extremity support to be able to perform it accurately.

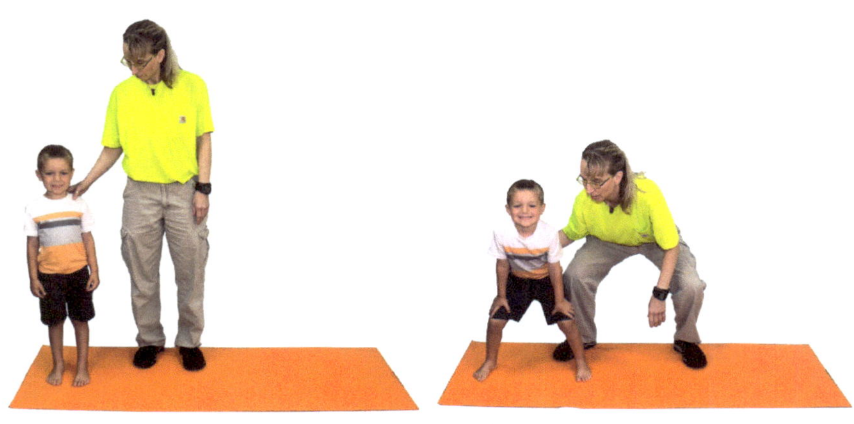

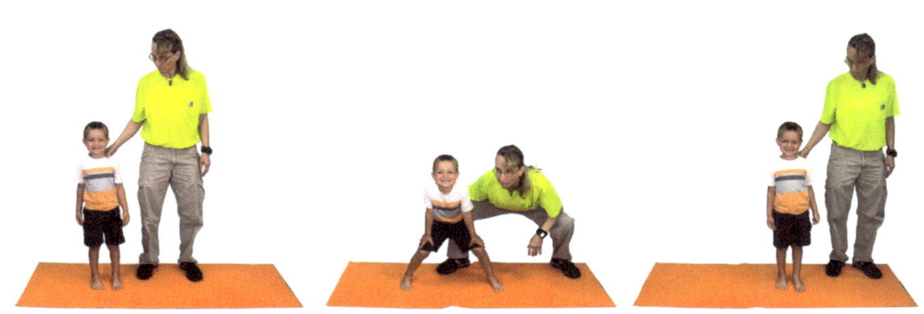

43. CROUCHING SIDE STEP, HANDS FREE

This is the variation with hands free. This provides a strong quad and abductor work out. I used elastic bands to increase the difficulty.

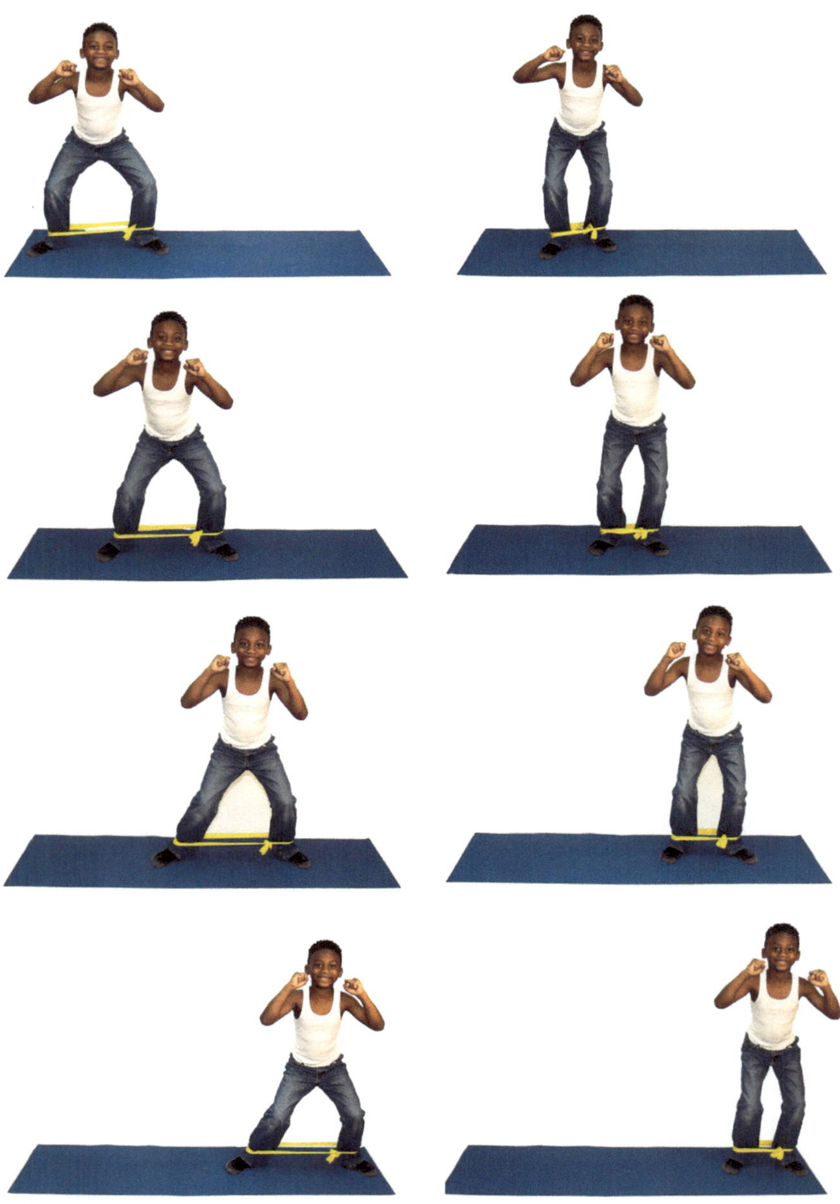

44. SIDE SLIDE

This can be easy or hard according to how easily the object the child is sliding moves along the floor. Slick surfaces like vinyl, tile and wood floors make this easier while carpet makes it harder.

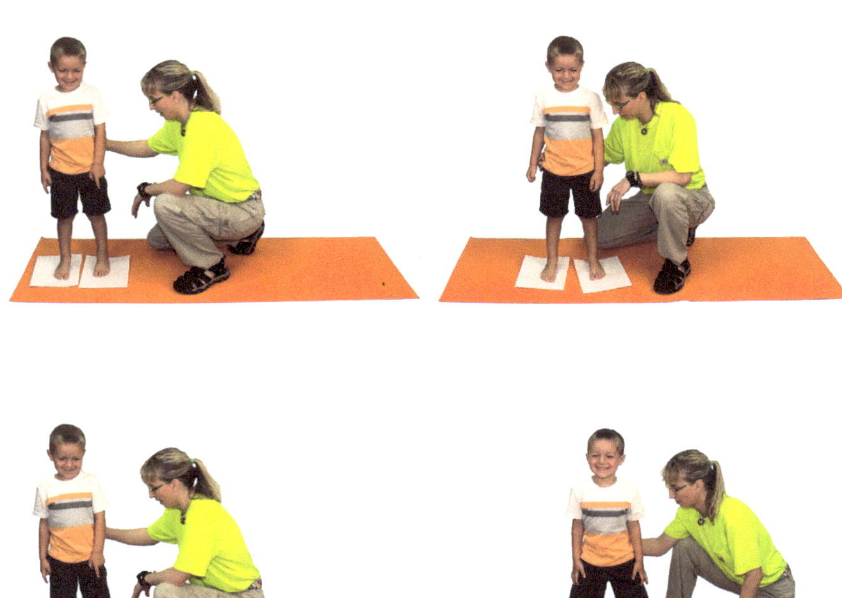

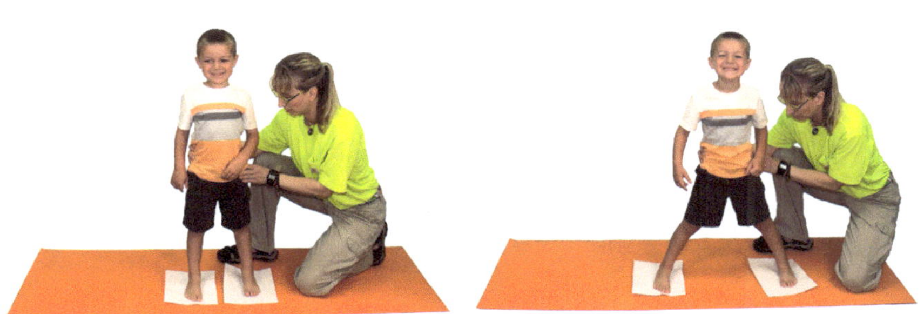

45. DIAGONAL SIDE STEP FORWARD

These are otherwise known as monster walks. The client steps forward and then out wide into abduction. If my client is having a hard time, I draw chalk diagonal lines down on the ground as guides for how wide she needs to step. The wider apart the lines are the harder this activity becomes. Elastic bands or tubing around the lower thigh increases the difficulty.

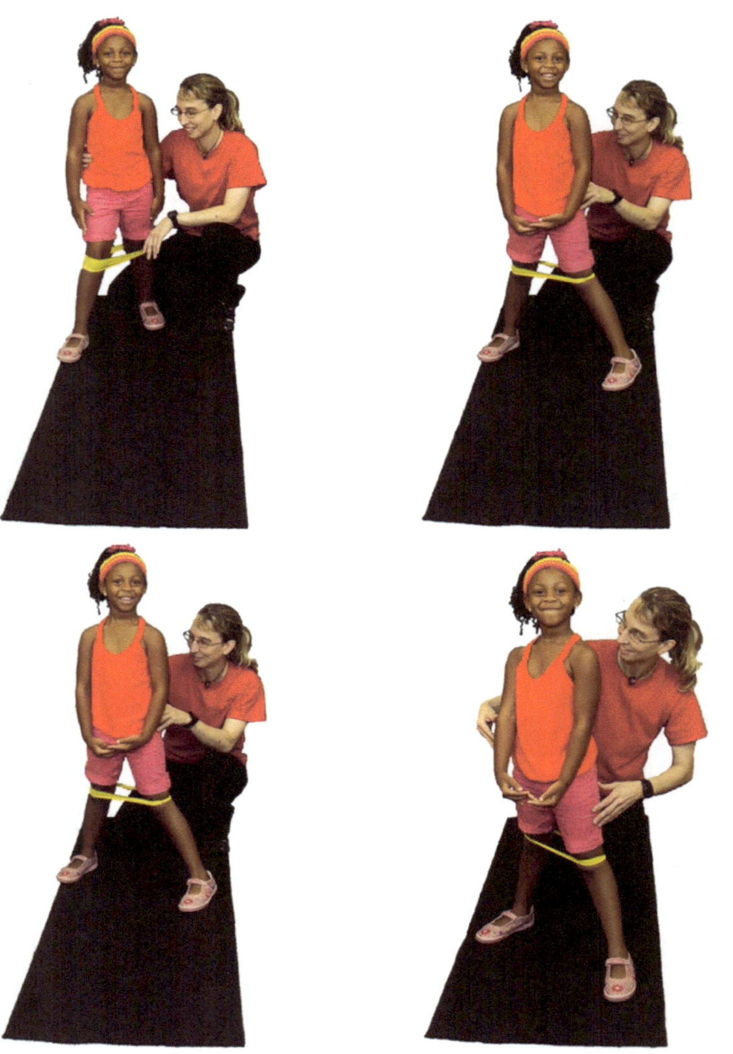

46. WALK WITH A HOOP OUTSIDE OF LEGS

This activity increases in difficulty using a progressively wider hoop. Kids always seem to like this. I have my client walk across the room or down the hall trying not to drop the hoop.

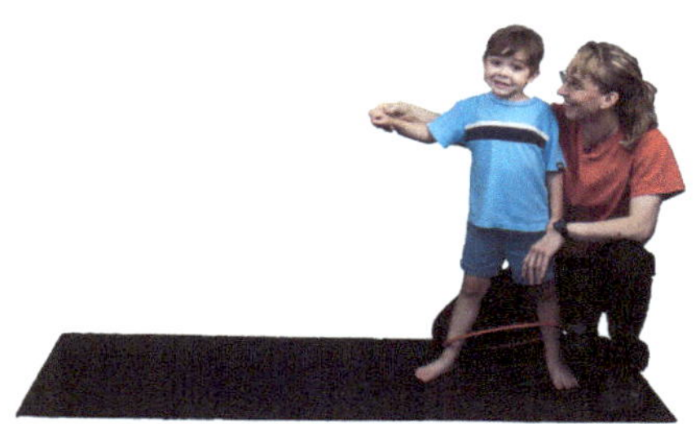
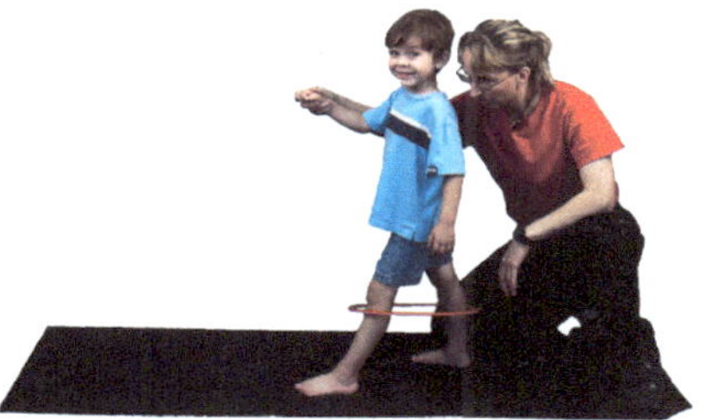

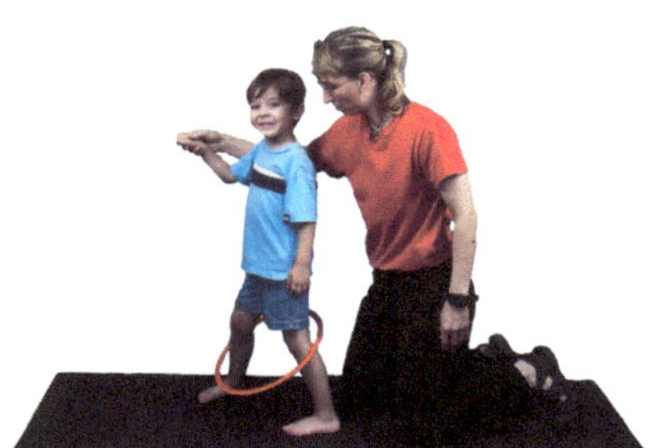
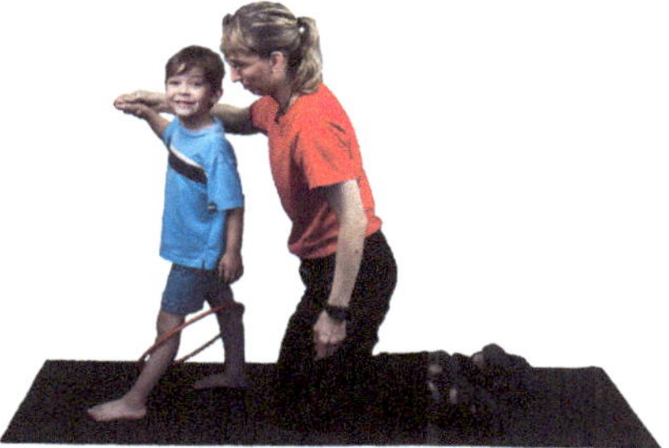

47. SIDEWAYS BALANCE BEAM WALK WITH ANKLE WEIGHTS

I have balance beams that are two inches (5 cm) wide, four inches (10 cm) wide, six inches (15 cm) wide and ten inches (25 cm) wide. Walking on a balance beam generally discourages the child from substituting with hip flexion. A smaller balance beam encourages a balance component. Using elastic bands at the thigh or ankle weights makes this activity harder. I often get the mother to hold her son's hands, and I hold hand over ankles keeping his legs in neutral rotation. I may also assist the movement. My clients often substitute hip flexion and external rotation for straight abduction.

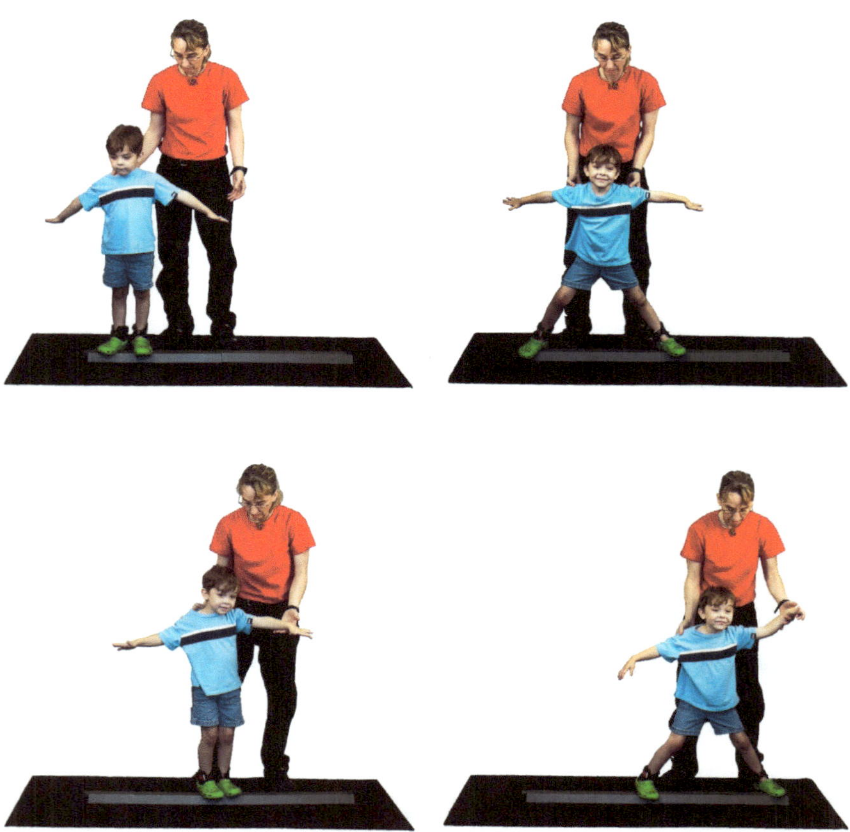

48. SIDE SLIDE OUT AND IN BILATERAL

It is challenging to move both pieces of paper/slippery spots simultaneously. I have to bounce up as I pull the pieces of paper together when I try it. This is a phenomenal exercise to strengthen adductors and abductors. Perform this on slick floor!

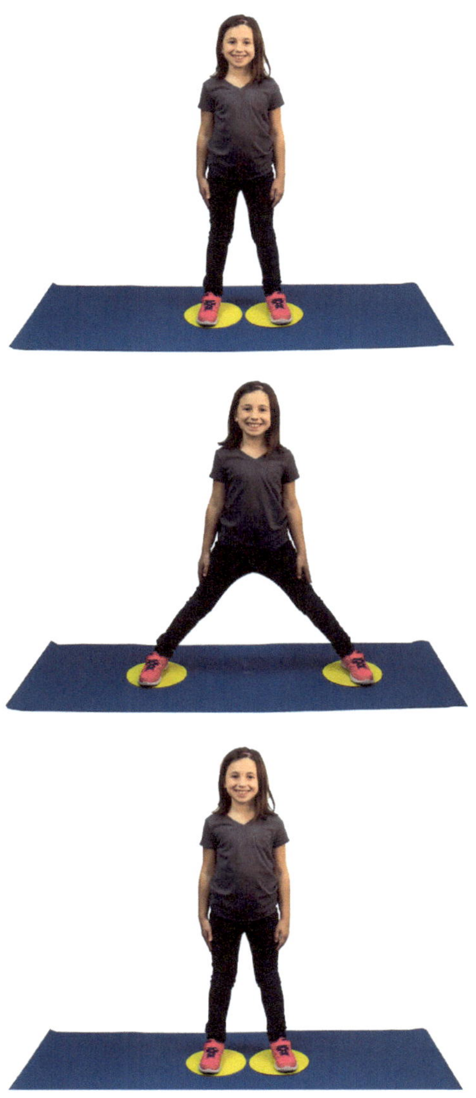

49. SCOOTERBOARD STAND UNILATERAL ABDUCTION

This is dramatically easier with upper extremity support. The flooring surface also affects how easy or difficult this activity is. Standing on scooterboards is potentially dangerous, so make sure you spot closely.

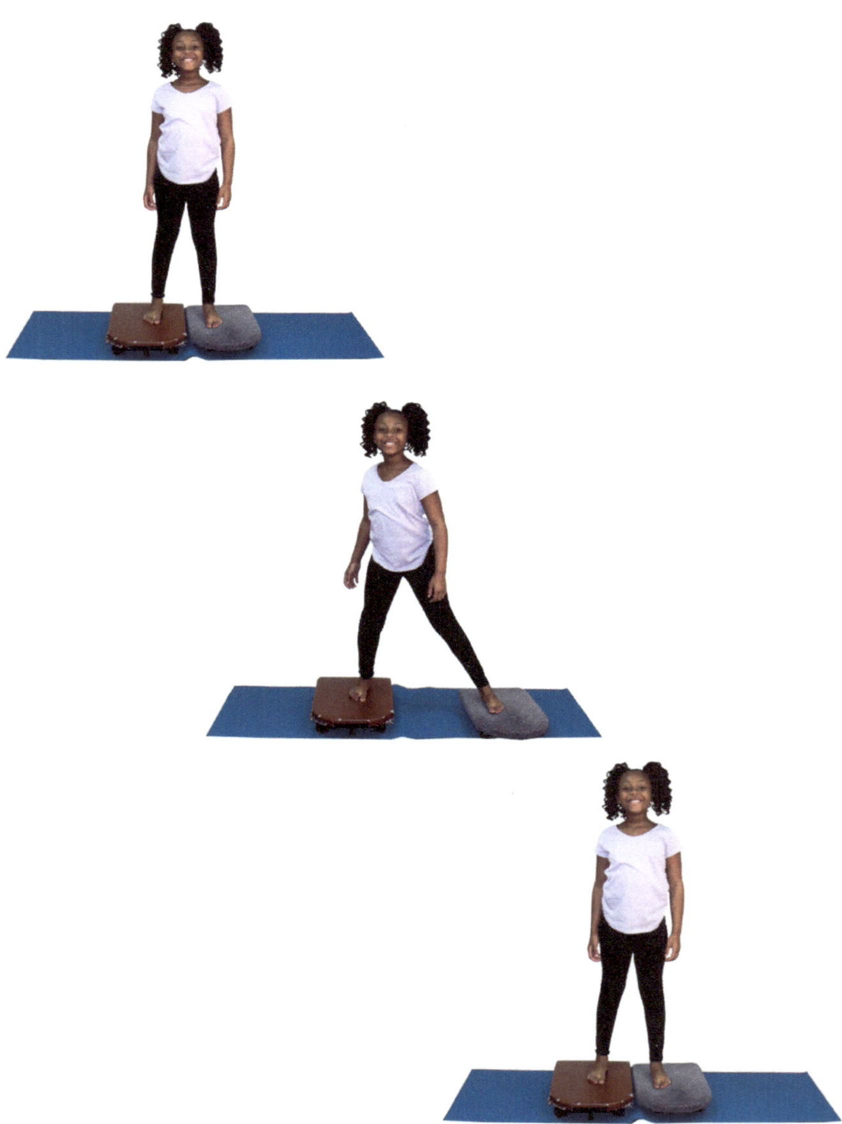

50. SCOOTERBOARD STAND BILATERAL ABDUCTION

Moving one leg was risky, but abducting both legs while standing on the scooterboards is much trickier. Contact guard spotting (or more) is recommended.

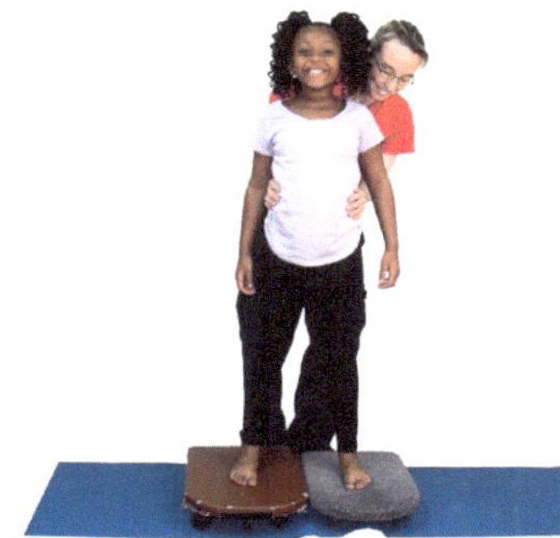

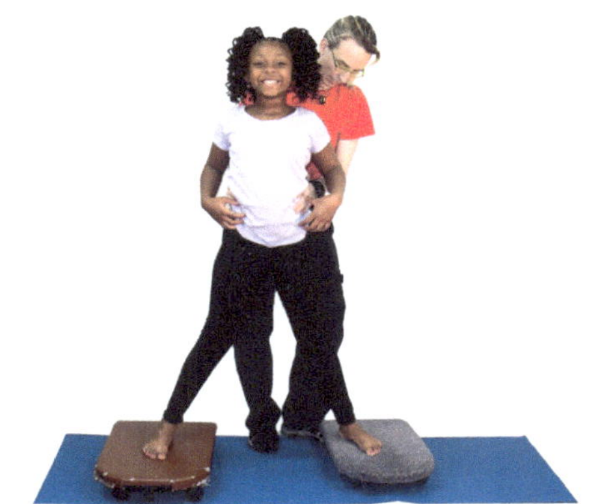

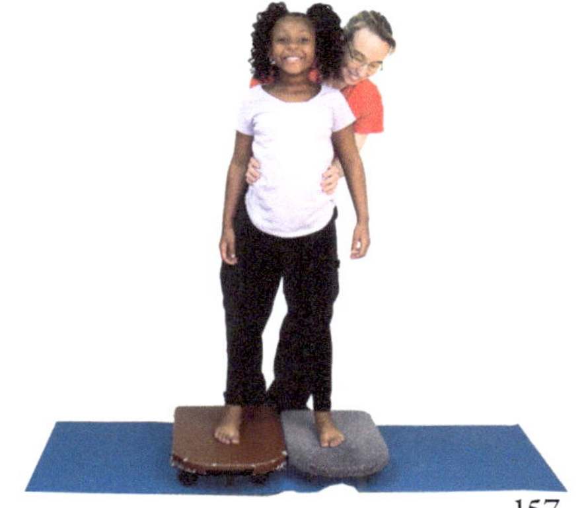

51. BENCH KICKS

This exercise targets the weakness that causes a Trendelenburg gait pattern. Here my client holds single leg stance, kicks a cone off a bench and then puts the foot back down on the floor. This is harder if you make the bench higher or you put the cone/object to be kicked further back on the bench. You can also make it harder by placing multiple cones on the bench that she has to kick down before she can set her foot back down on the floor. Make sure you spot your client closely. Loss of balance is common.

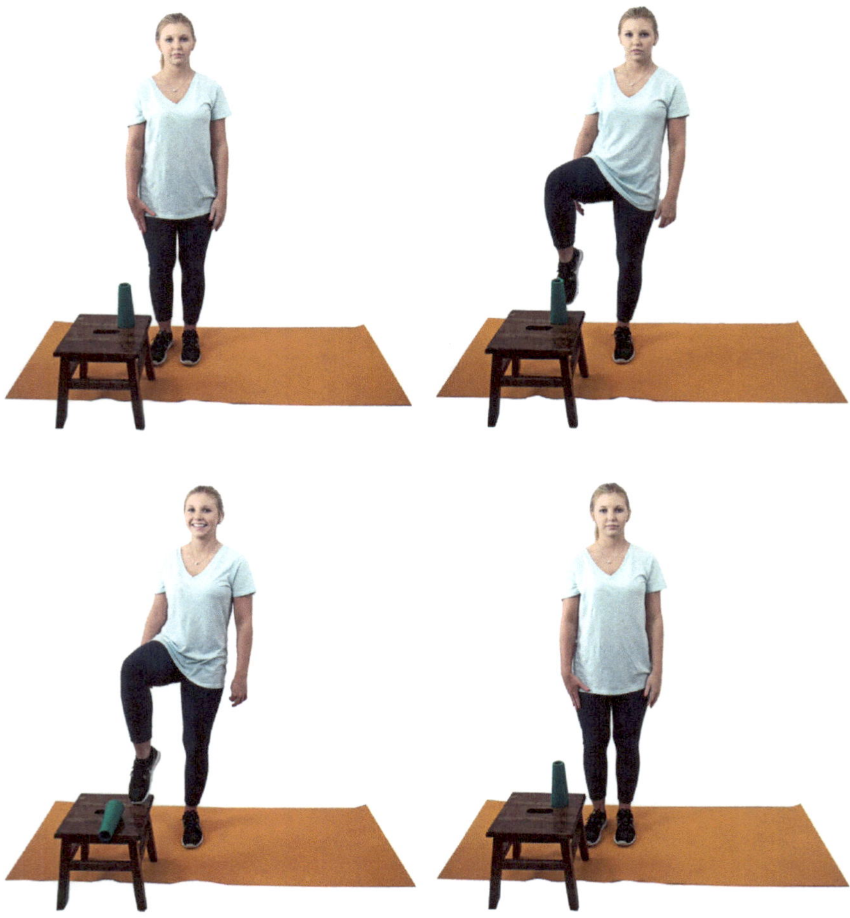

52. DIP KICKS

This is another exercise that targets the abductor weakness that causes the Trendelenburg gait pattern. The client is having to support single leg stance and perform an activity with the other foot. The client stands on a bench and dips down to kick over an object. A greater height differential between the bench and the object makes this activity harder. Sometimes I require multiple kicks to an object before I allow her to return to standing with both feet on the bench. Sustaining the dip for longer makes this activity more difficult. In this picture, the model required support from an upright pole and a hand held. If the client is strong enough, I perform this activity with only one hand support or no support.

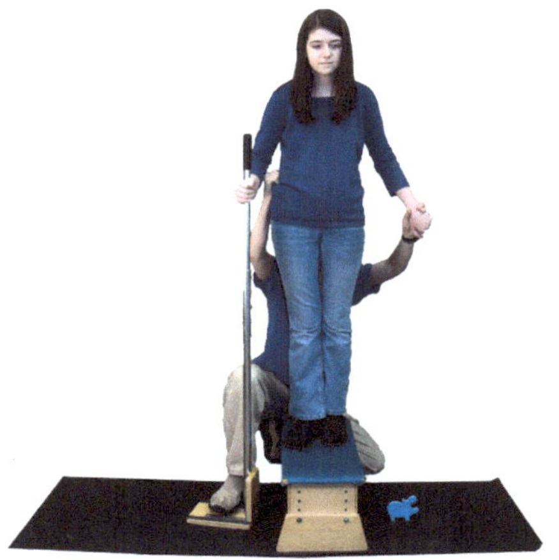

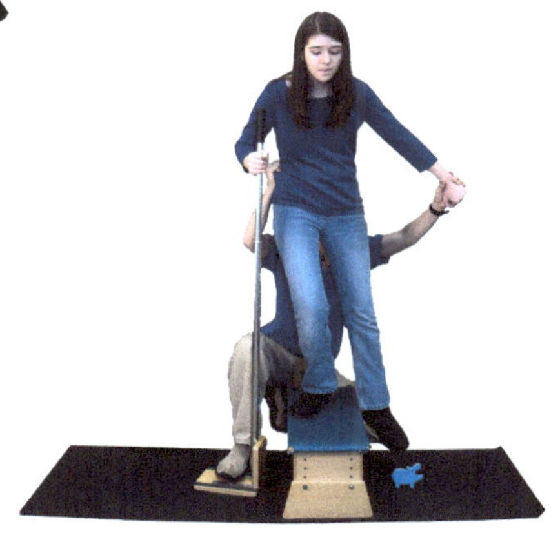

53. SIDE STEP UP AND DOWN

This exercise addresses abduction with hip and knee flexion. The higher the step, the harder this is. I may perform this activity repetitively up and down with a bench, or I may just head to a flight of stairs and have them walk up and down the stairs sideways. According to the client, I allow him to hold the railing with one hand, two hands or no hands. If I need more of a challenge, I add ankle weights. Unless I have a unilateral weakness, I have the client perform both sides.

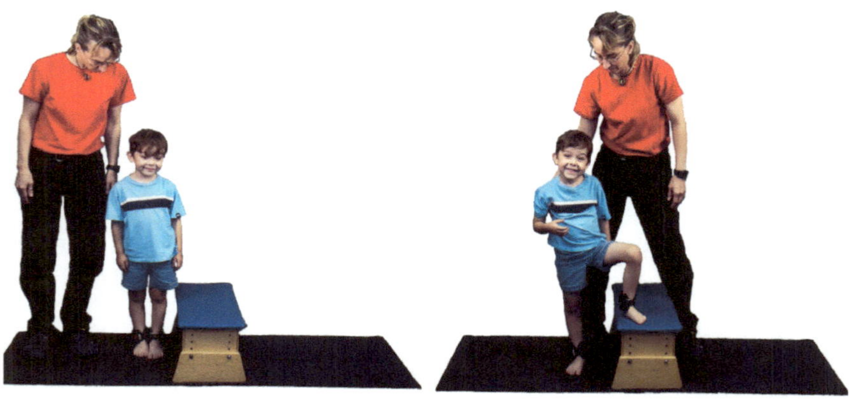

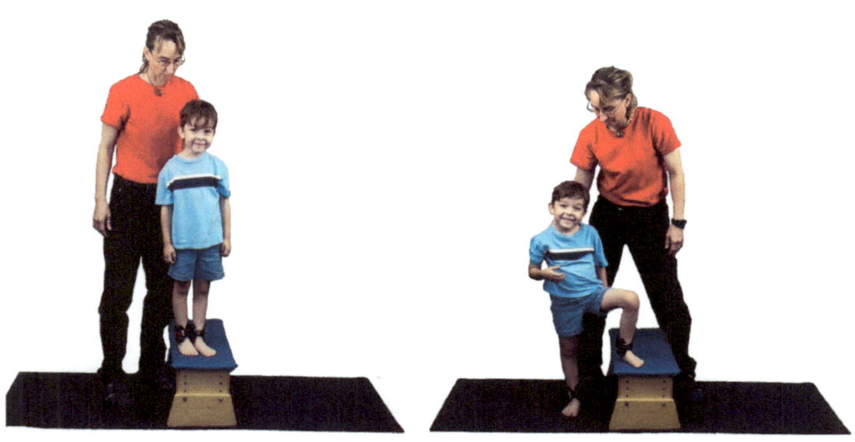

54. SIDE LUNGE AND RETURN

Oh, the dreaded side lunges! You can allow your client to touch hands to the ground or keep arms up. Lunging lower is harder. Having a target to step out to is helpful for most children.

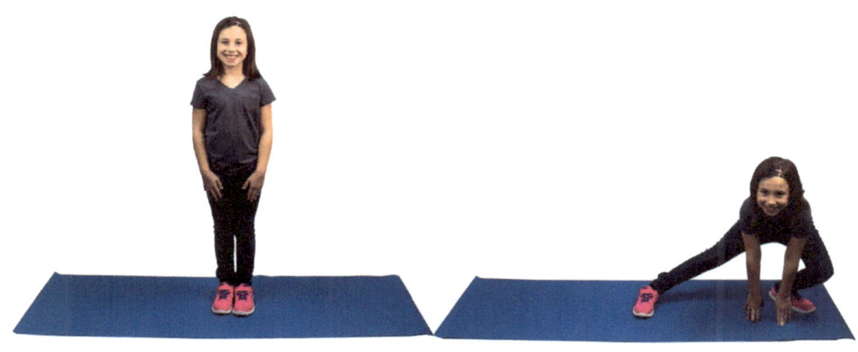

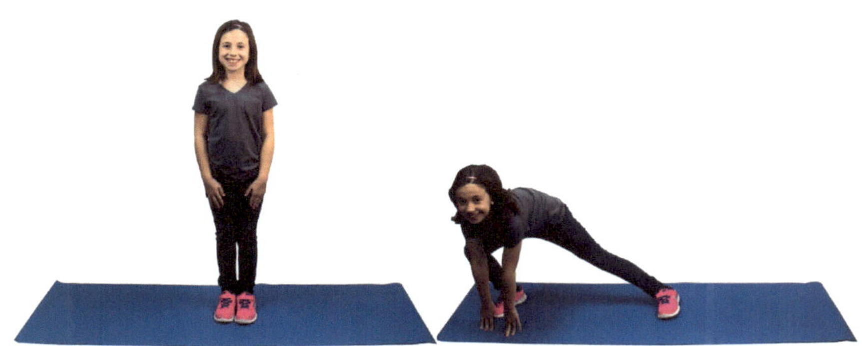

55. CRAB WALK SIDEWAYS

Oh my, this is a tricky activity! With this exercise, I want abduction with hip extension, but I do usually have to prompt the child to lift her hips higher off the floor. I have my client go both directions unless I am only targeting one leg.

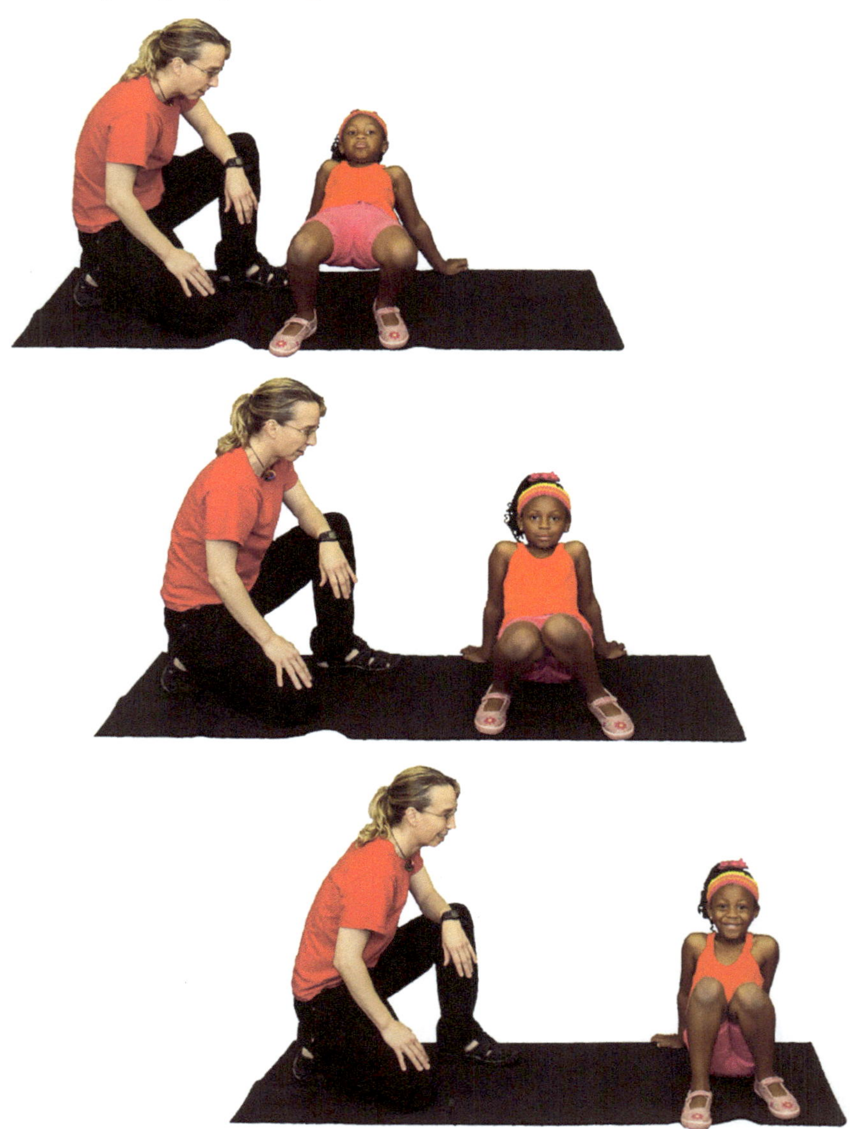

56. SCOOTERBOARD SITTING WITH HEELS PLANTED MOVING SIDE TO SIDE

Have your client sit on a scooterboard. Mark a spot for the child's feet. Now have her move the scooterboard side to side. A line down on the floor helps. This is a challenging exercise. Slick floors makes this easier. Textured or soft floors makes this next to impossible.

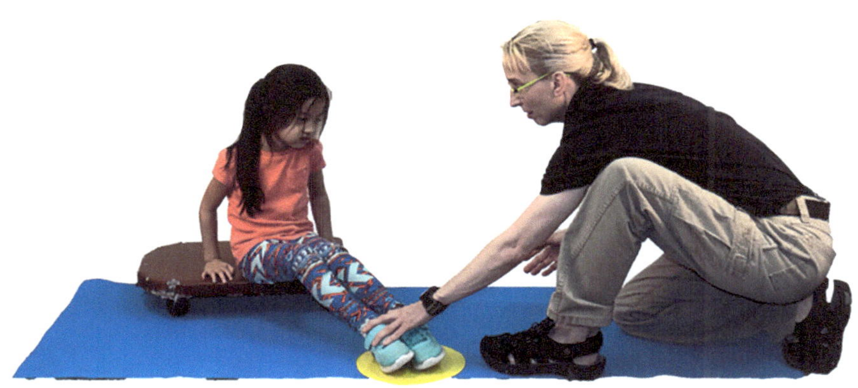

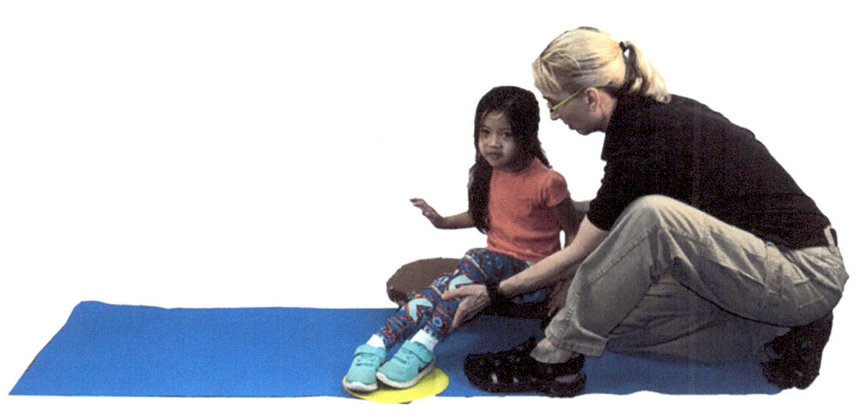

IV. HIP ADDUCTION

* * *

THE HIP ADDUCTORS MOVE THE femur medially toward neutral or midline or conversely the pelvis toward the femur if the femur is stabilized. These movements are in the frontal plane. The hip adductorrs are powerful lower body stabilizers. Weakness or tightness in the hip adductors will affect gait and particularly skill at standing on one foot. This chapter includes a wide variety of exercises to improve hip adduction strength.

* * *

1. SUPINE ADDUCTION WITH LEG IN SLING

The sling minimizes drag and resistance. I may abduct the leg for the child or have her abduct the leg and adduct it.

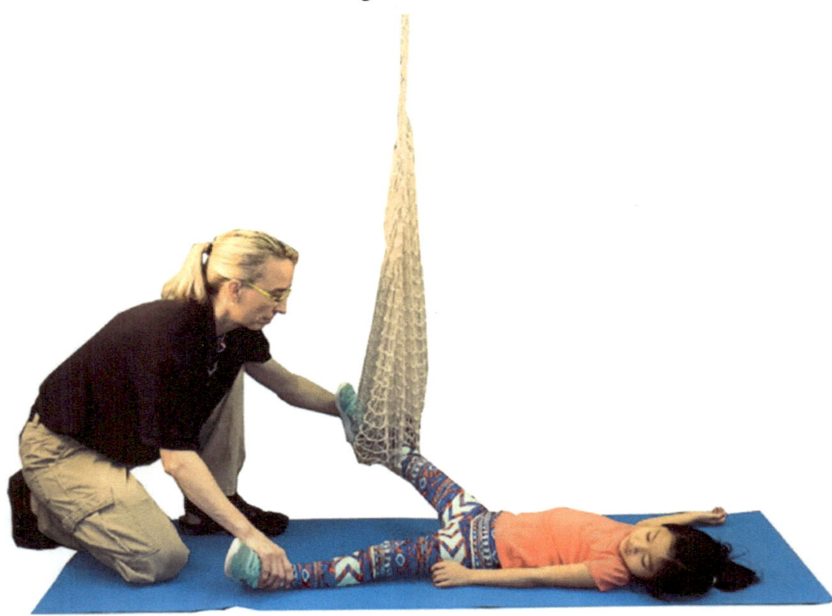

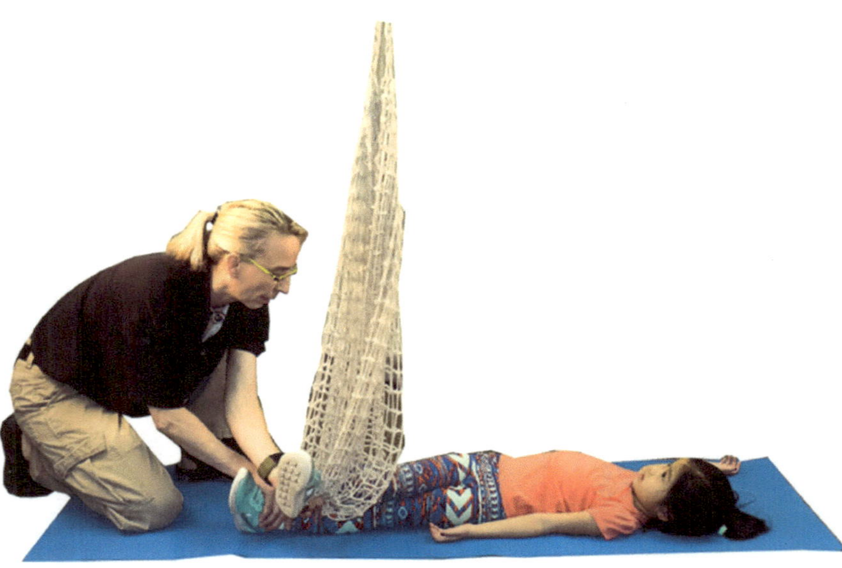

2. SUPINE ADDUCTION UNILATERALLY

Despite the fact that I am working on adduction, I still use the blocks to hit on the way out. If necessary I prop the child's head up on a pillow to allow him to see better. I can resist or assist the movement of adduction as needed. I often find that in part of the range I am resisting and part I am assisting. Ninety-nine percent of the time I am assisting at the end part of the range of adduction as the moving leg approaches the leg staying still. I usually resist manually but I can also add ankle weights. The wider I place the blocks, the harder this activity is. If I want to minimize but not eliminate the resistance, then I may put the leg on a scooterboard. I often take off a shoe so the foot slides easier on the supporting surface.

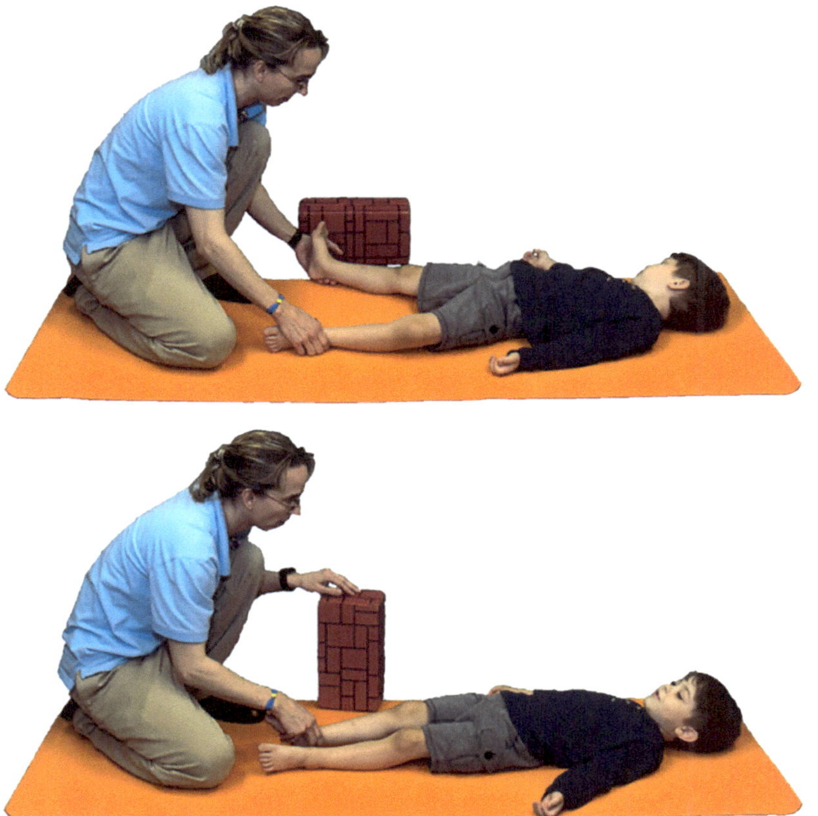

3. SUPINE BILATERAL ADDUCTION

This is the same activity as the unilateral one, but now I am requesting adduction of both legs, either simultaneously or sequentially. My directions are similar to the unilateral version of this exercise. Some clients are actually better at bilateral than they are a unilateral abduction.

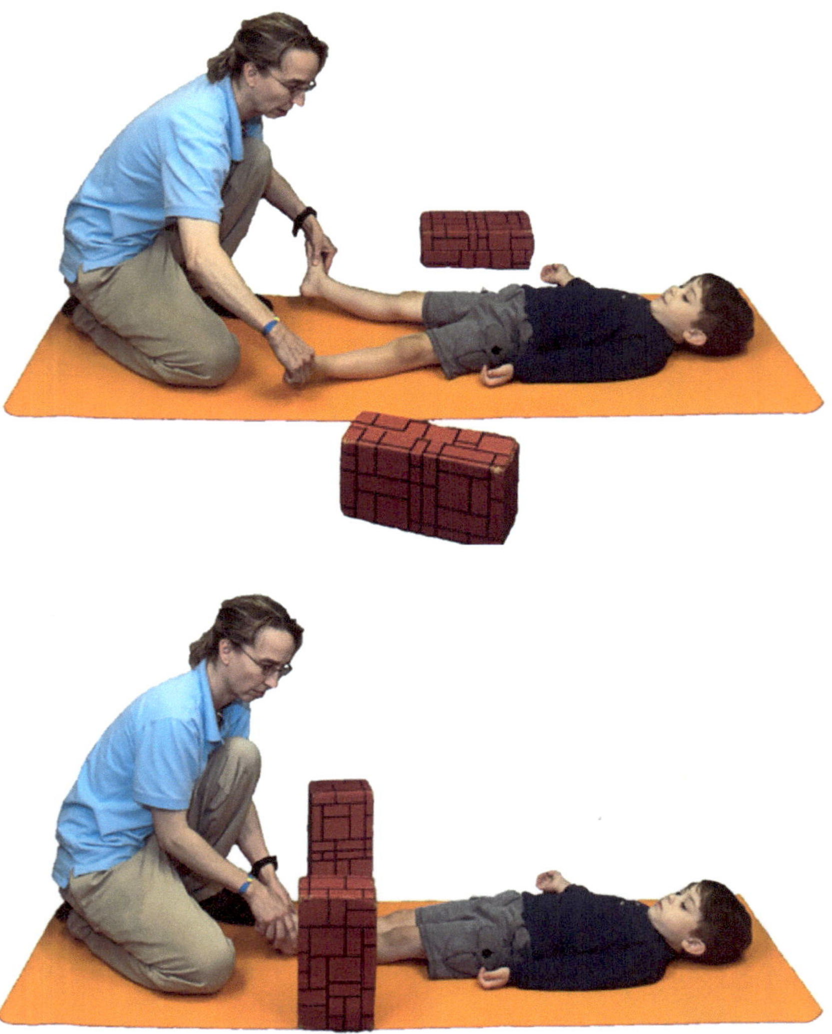

4. SQUEEZE BALLHOOKLYING

Since it is the end range of adduction that I usually see the difficulty with, I like this activity squeezing a ball. This gerdy-style ball is perfect because it deforms and squeezes well. It also glows in the dark which makes it more fun. "Ten Squeezes and we'll turn off the light!" Who wouldn't want to do it?

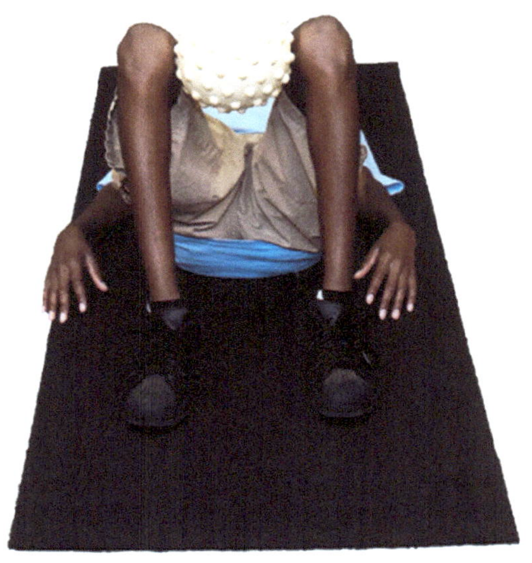

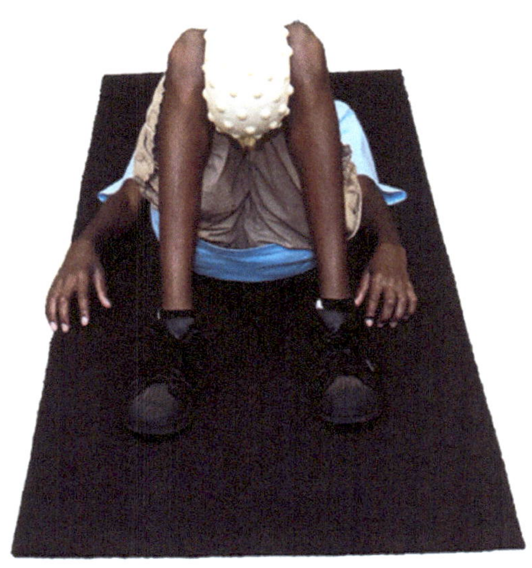

5. SQUEEZE SQUEAK TOY HOOKLYING

I have several squeak toys of different sizes. Different ones require harder or softer squeezes to squeak well. I use the auditory feedback as confirmation that the knees have been squeezed together. I have also used a small keyboard when I thought that a squeeze toy was inappropriate or would not be appreciated. Sound effects make any child work harder. I have performed basically this same activity sitting on a chair or in the wheelchair. End range adduction is often very hard to attain.

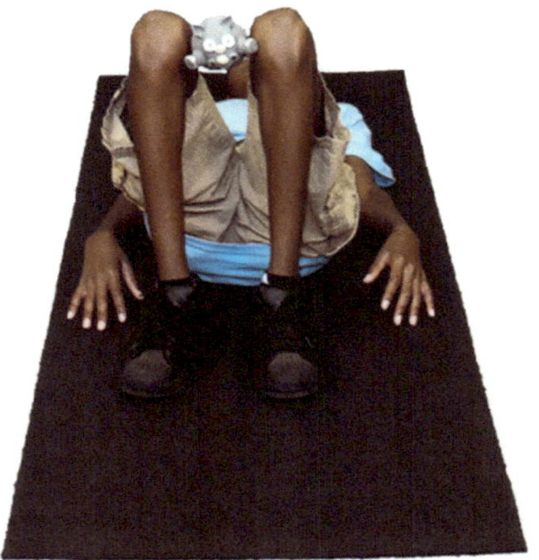

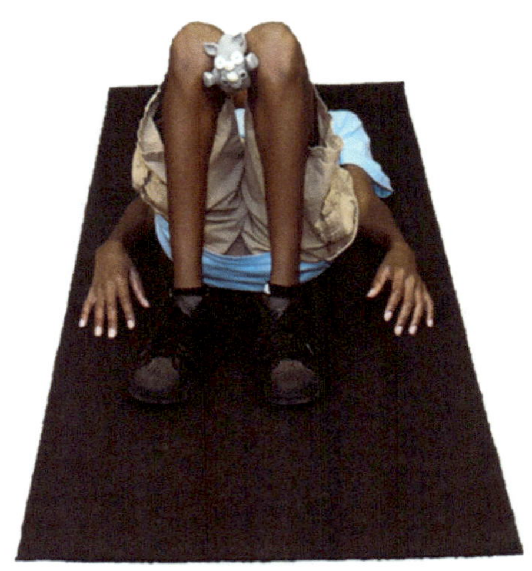

6. SUPINE ADDUCTION WITH AN ELASTIC BAND

The child holds the ends of the elastic band and hooks the bottom of one foot. She can assist or resist herself in performing the adduction movement according to the line of pull. I also feel the elastic band gives proprioceptive feedback to help her feel the movement.

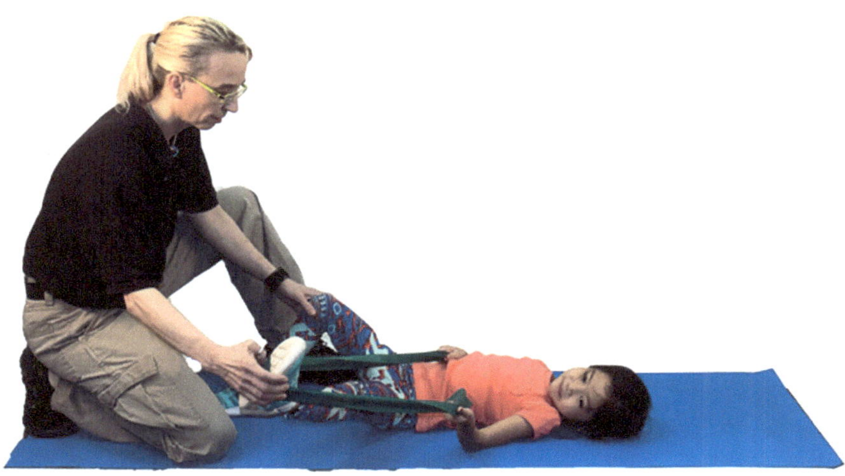

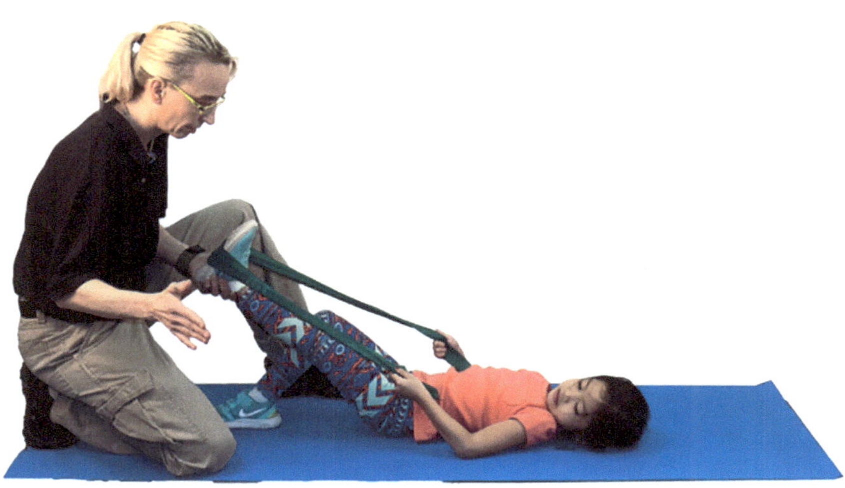

7. SUPINE LEGS UP ADD/ABDUCTION

Adduction just got harder. This exercise is for a child who is ready for more of a challenge. The wider the legs are abducted before the legs are adducted, the harder this activity is. I find children have trouble keeping 90 degrees hip flexion. Having my hands out as a target for the abduction seems to help. You can add weights to your client's ankles or manual resistance to increase the difficulty as well. Document repetitions, range, and resistance/assistance provided.

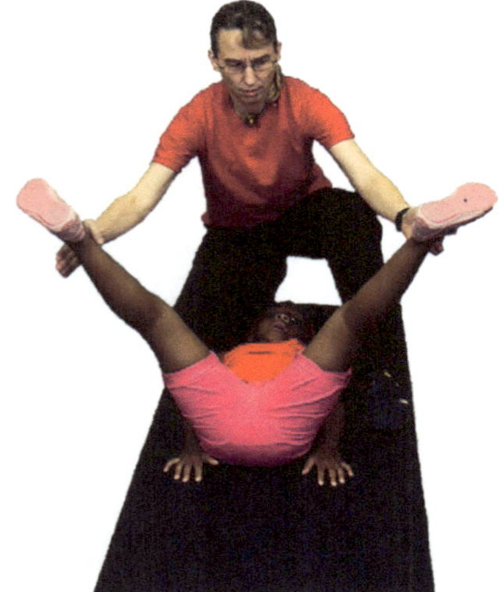

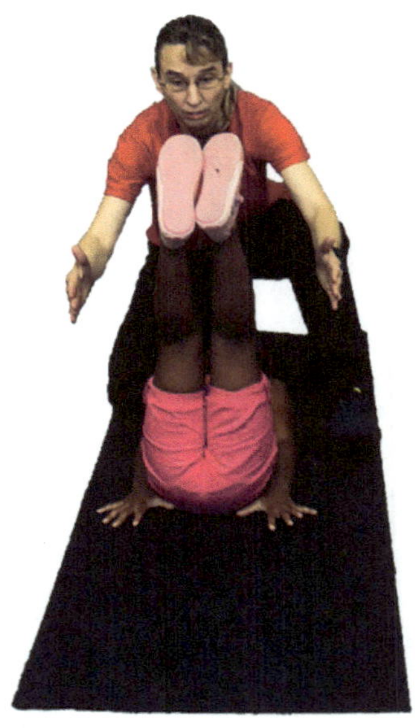

8. SUPINE LEGS UP, FEET BALL SQUEEZE

Another difficult adduction exercise. I like this gerdy type ball because it deforms and squeezes well. It also glows in the dark. "Ten Squeezes and we'll turn off the light!" Who wouldn't want to do it?

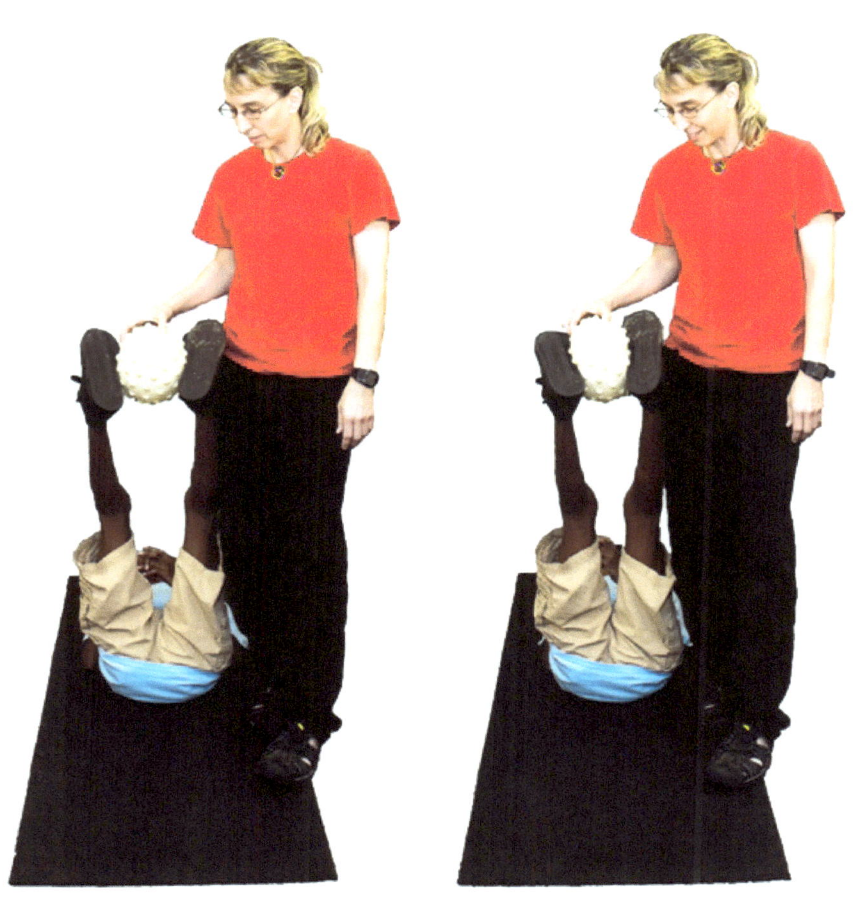

9. DINNER PLATES IN UNILATERAL BRIDGE

This exercise can be performed from raised bridge or lower bridge. From low bridge, the child raises and extends one leg. She moves the raised leg in a circle about the size of a dinner plate. If the child can handle a challenge, I encourage her to try to keep the other leg from moving significantly as the raised leg circles.

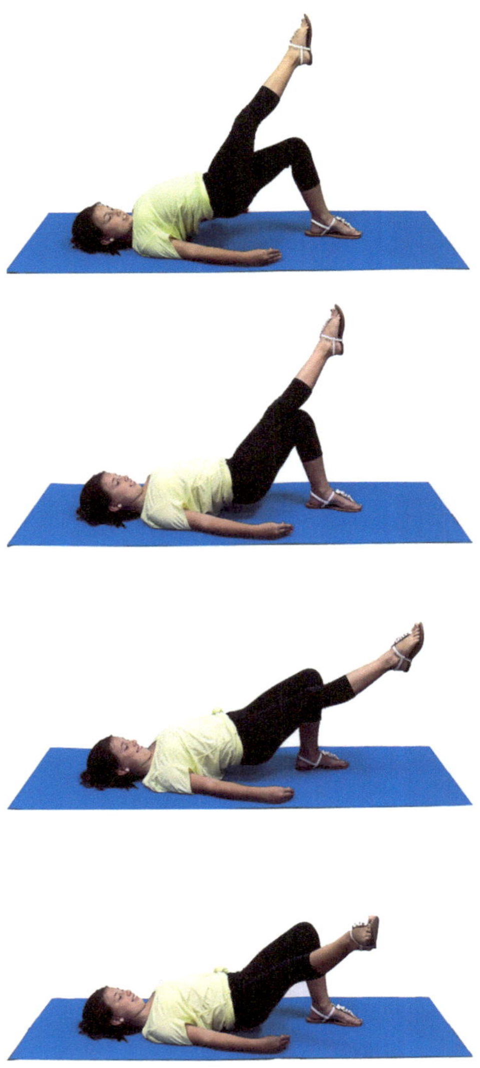

10. SUPINE BALL LIFT, PT AT HEAD

Sometimes adduction with a side order of abdominals is just what the doctor ordered. I usually have the child bring me the ball from laying flat supine with the ball between her legs. Then after the child gives me the ball, I pause for a second after she releases it, and then give it back. I try to get the child to set the ball back down on the floor slowly so as not to lose the ball. All to be able to do it again! There had better be a great reward after this, because this game is hard!

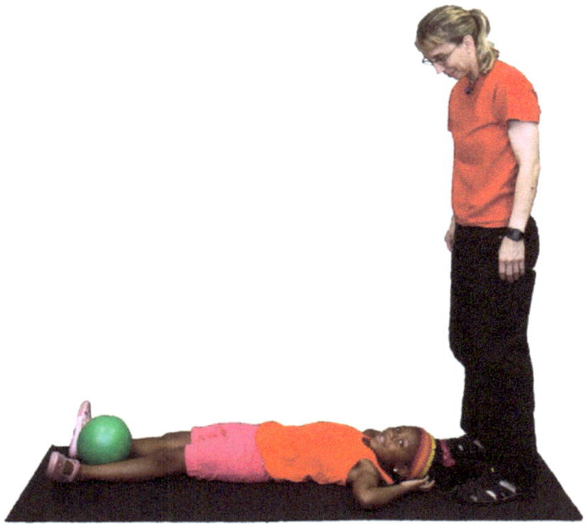

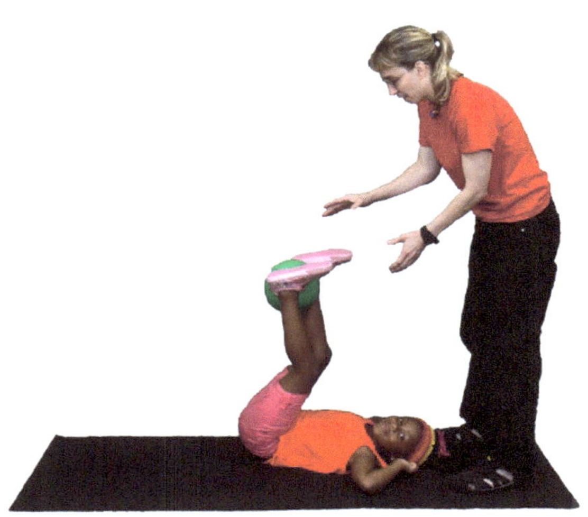

11. HOOKLYING HEEL TOUCH

The client laterally flexes far enough to touch his hand to his heel when he lies hooklying. Abductors and adductors are assisting according to the leg and the direction my client is going. This is a fantastic exercise for my clients with hip diplegia and hemiplegia, and is also good for my common clients with proximal weakness. This exercise is easiest on slick floors, harder on mats, and quite difficult on carpeting.

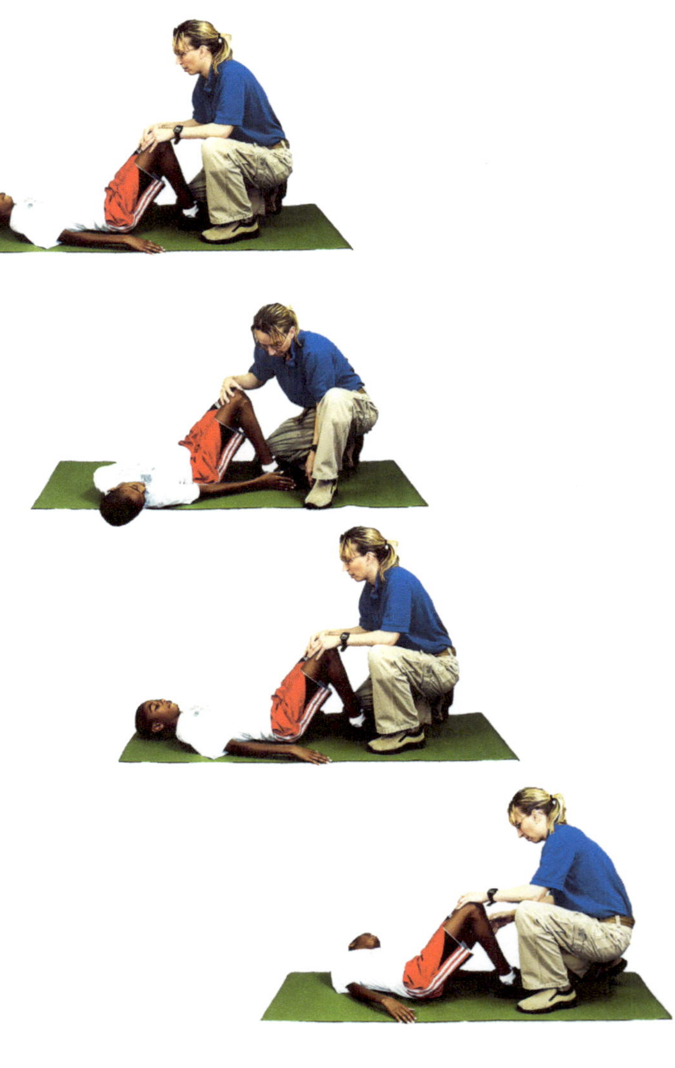

12. BENCH BRIDGE, BALL BETWEEN KNEES

This exercise takes a traditional hip extension exercise and adds adduction and core work by adding the gerdy ball between the knees. Any soft, medium size ball will do.

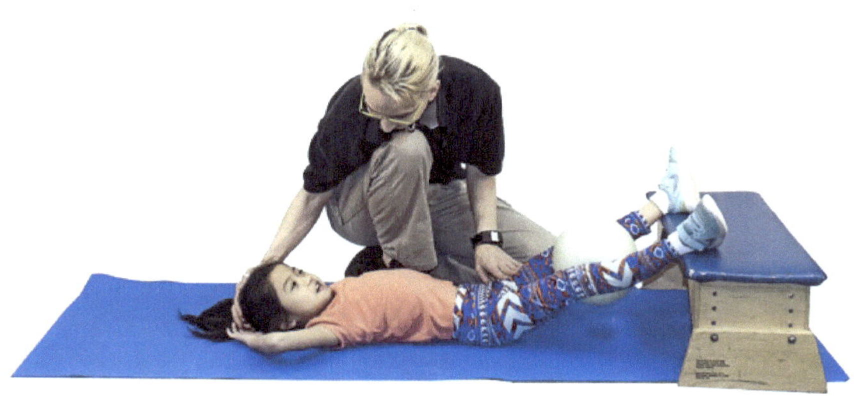

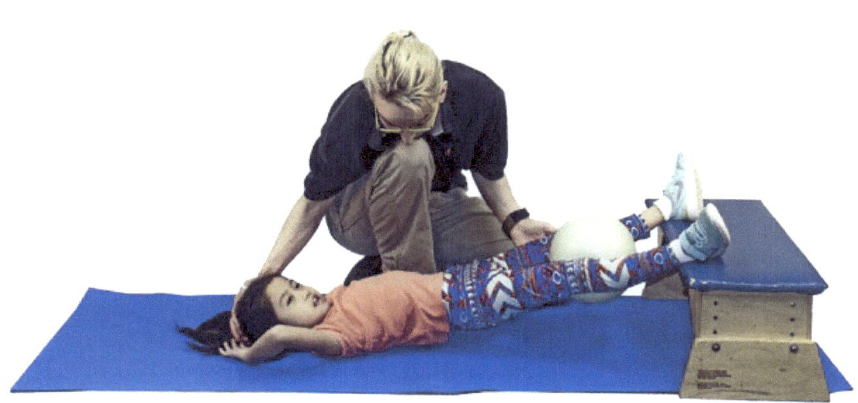

13. BRIDGE ON A GERDY BALL

This exercise is deceptively hard. You have to extend your hips in end range, but also squeeze your feet on top of the gerdy ball. With your adductors and abductors, you control the ball from rolling side to side.

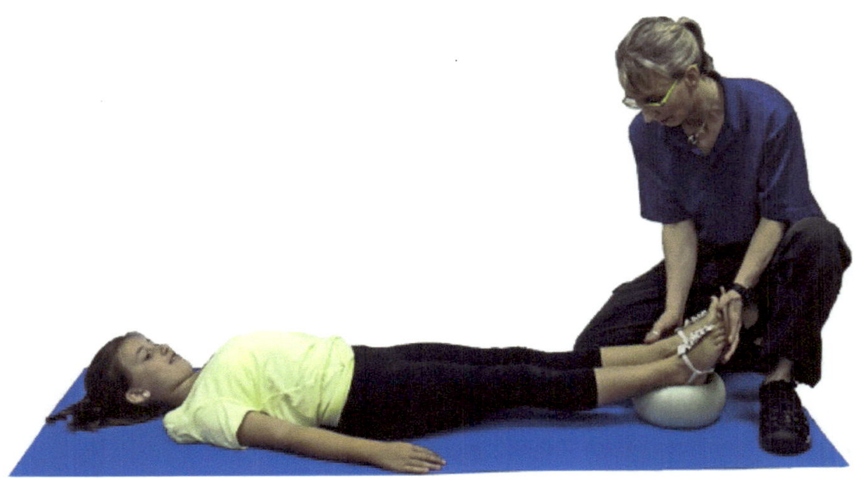

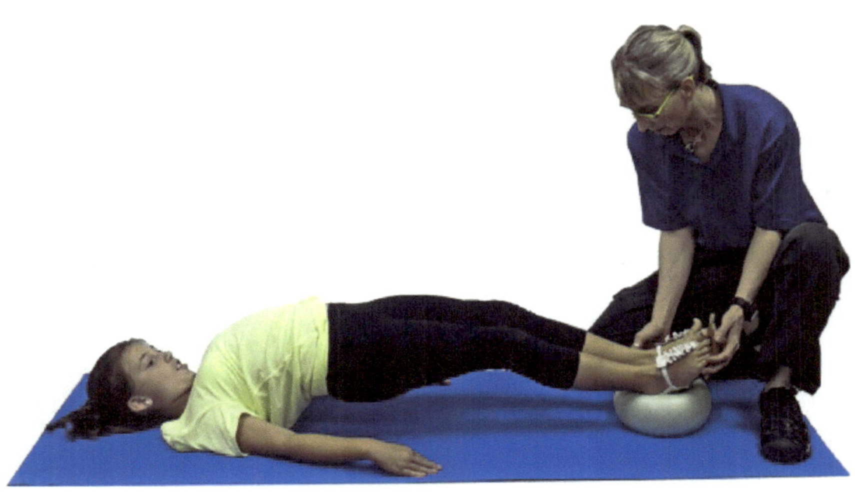

14. PLANK WITH A BALL BETWEEN KNEES

By adding the gerdy ball between the knees, this classic core and upper body activity effectively increases dramatically adduction and core work.

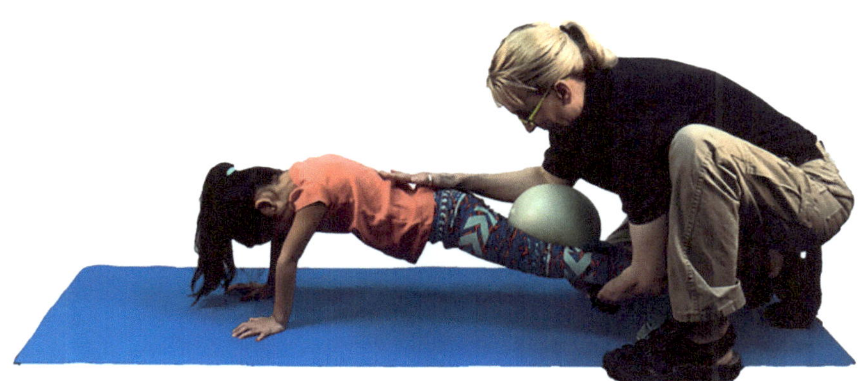

15. STRAIGHT ARM SIDE PLANK ON WALL

For an easy way to start side planks, have the client lean against an upright stable surface. Imagine the mats are a wall in this picture. Keep your client's body moving only in the frontal plane. The elbow should stay straight.

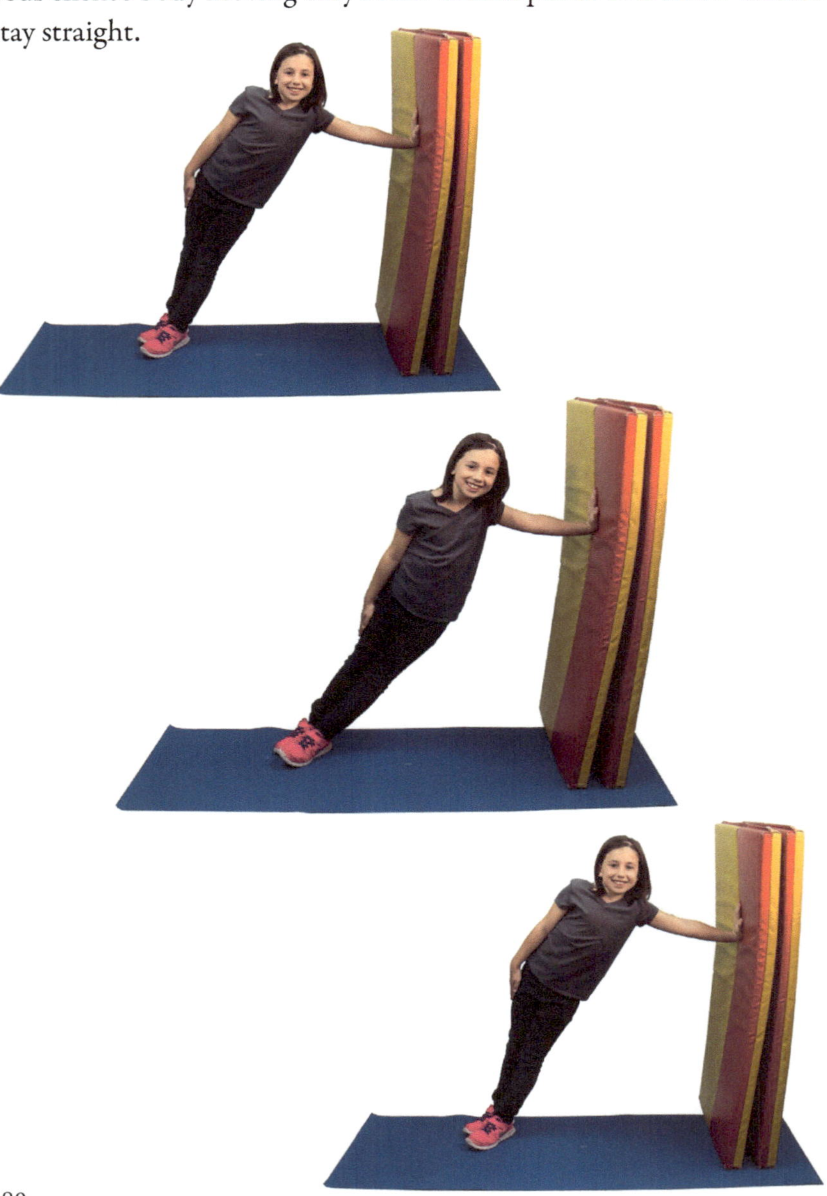

16. STRAIGHT ARM SIDE PLANK ON BENCH

After the client masters the wall side planks, work slowly progressively lower. Instead of going straight to the floor, I use benches, stacked if necessary, to achieve an intermediate level of difficulty.

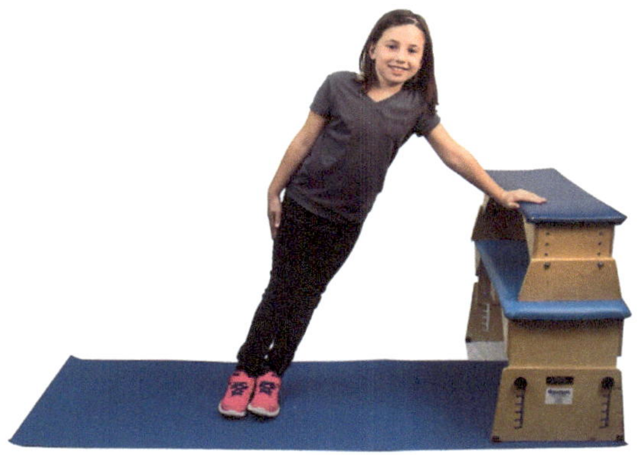

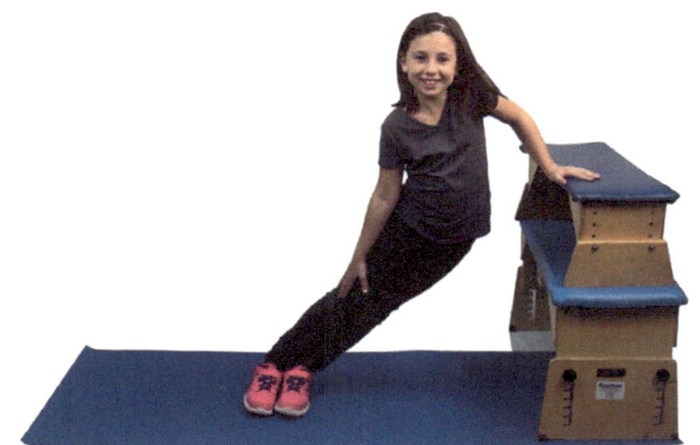

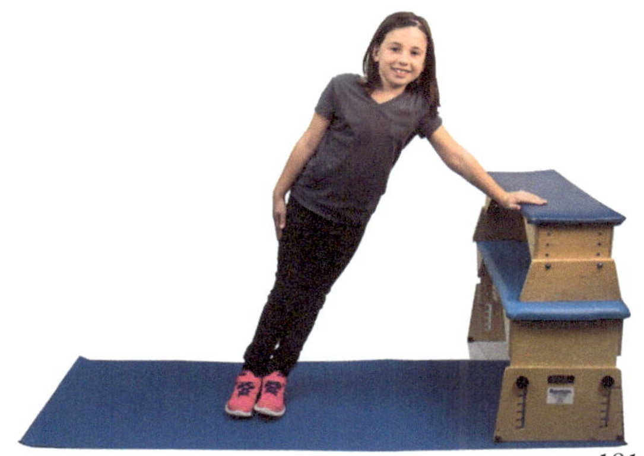

17. FOREARM SIDE KNEE PLANK

This exercise encourages abduction on the lower leg and adduction on the upper leg. With the forearm support, the client is lower to the floor and working hard against gravity but more supported by the forearm than an extended arm.

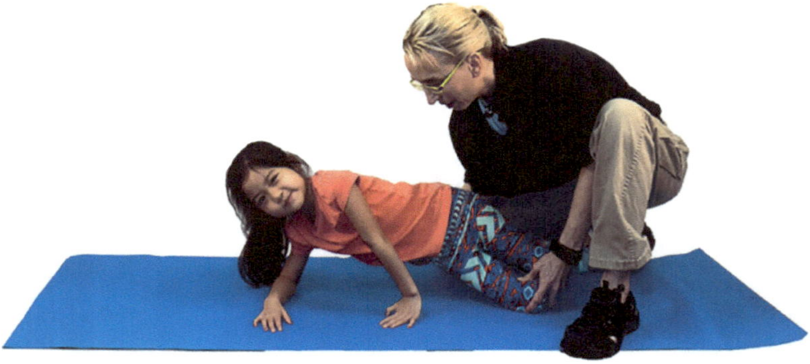

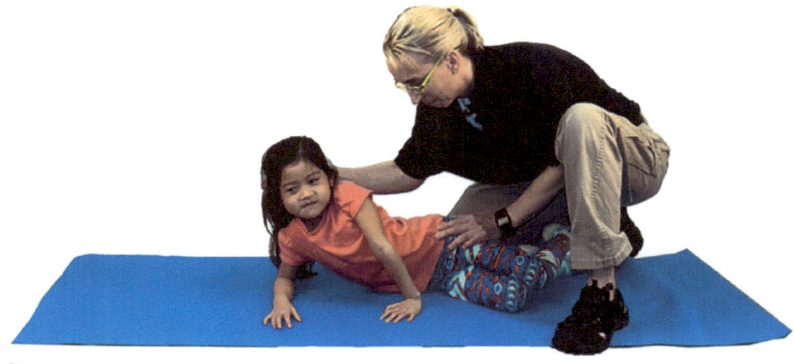

18. STRAIGHT ARM KNEE SIDE PLANK

This side plank is harder for some and easier for others. The extended arm allows a greater range of movement into adduction. The shoulder and tricep work is much harder and the client is potentially more unstable

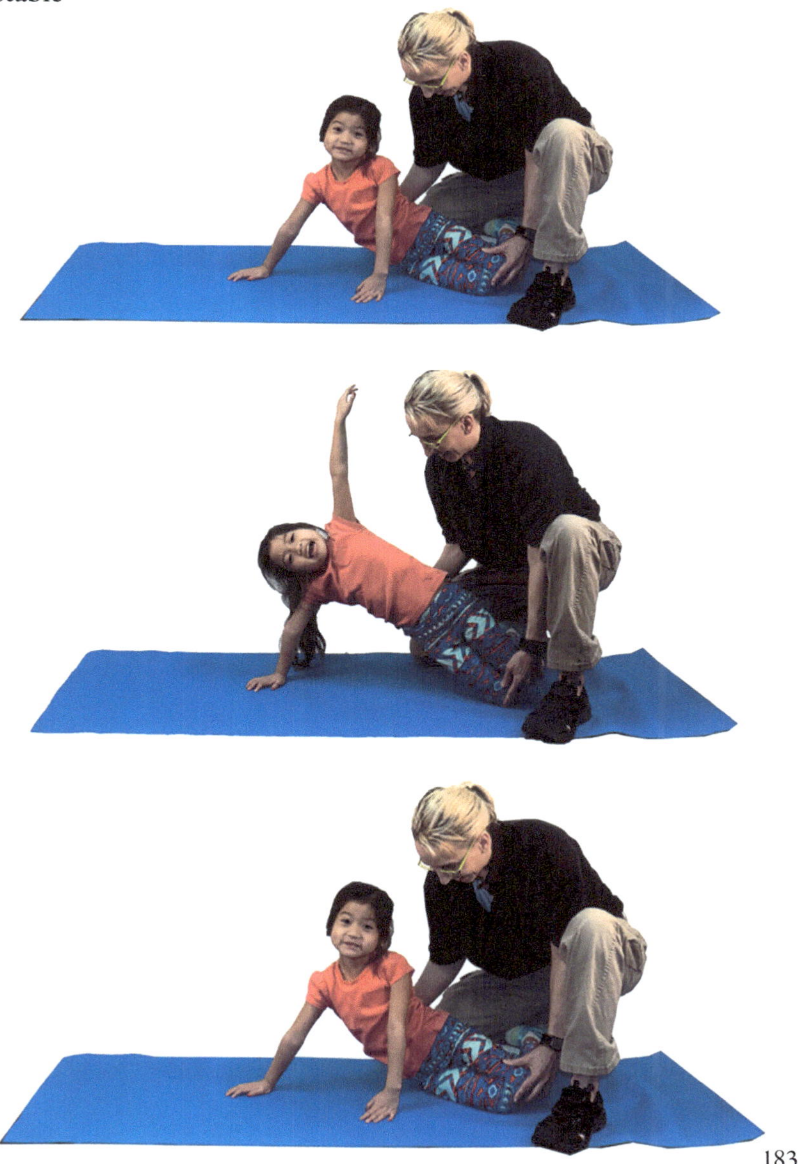

19. FOREARM SIDE PLANK

Oh my goodness, this is a tough exercise! It is a great general body toner. This requires core strength and abduction/adduction activation depending on the leg. This exercise is marginally easier on a forearm than on a straight arm. For my clients who will tolerate it, I love it for those trying to hold off scoliosis surgery or who persistently shorten one side. I often see the client kind of roll forward instead of lifting his hips straight up toward the ceiling. When this is the case, I have him start lying down with his back to the wall. I ask him to lift his hips up straight along the wall. It is then visually obvious to everyone when he rolls forward instead.

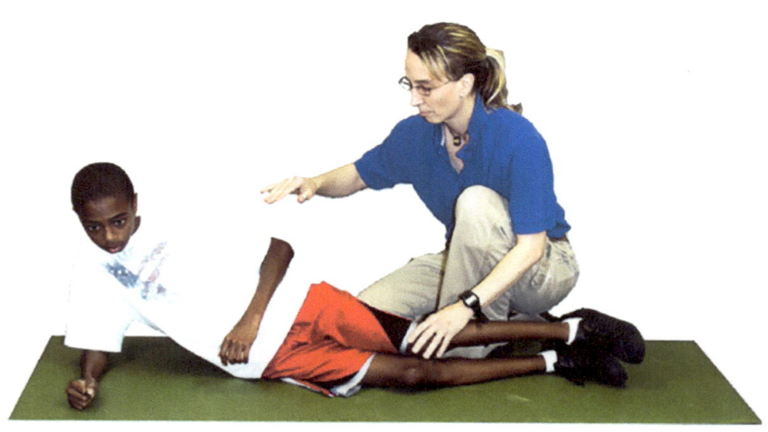

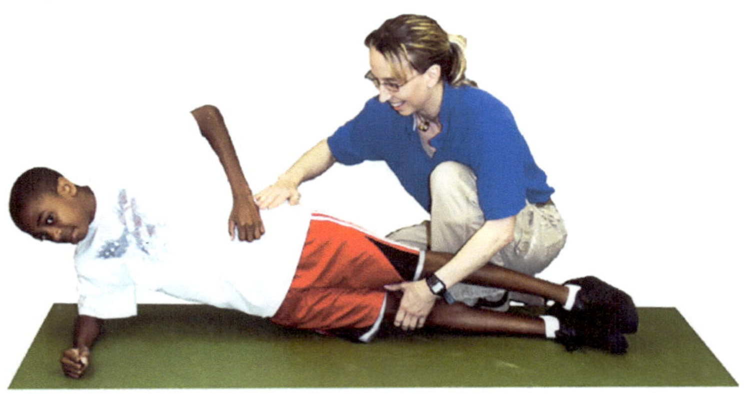

20. STRAIGHT ARM SIDE PLANK

Oh my goodness, this is a tougher exercise! The straight arm adds a greater arc to the movement and more instability requiring co-contraction. I often have my client perform this exercise next to a wall to improve form.

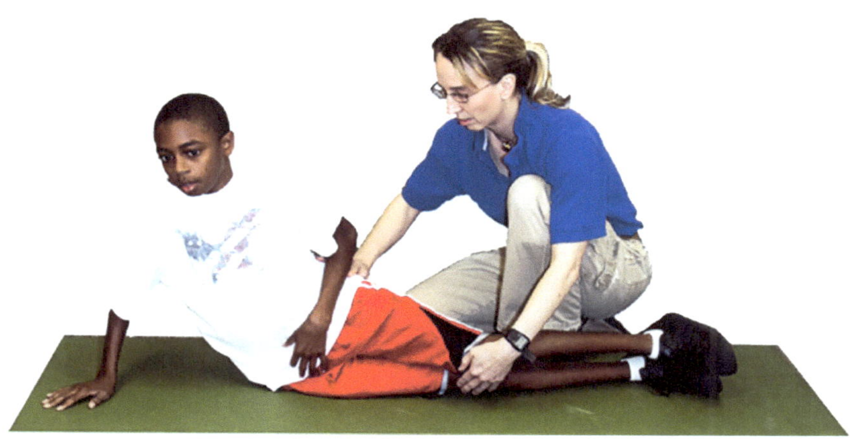

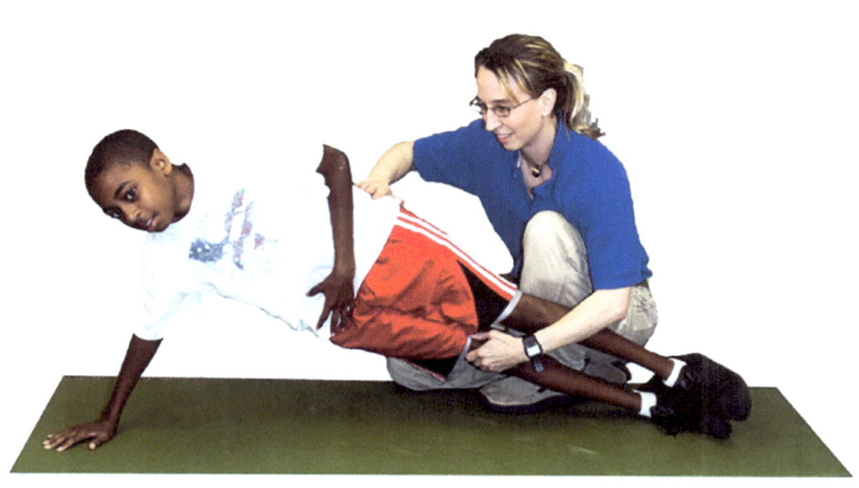

21. LONG SITTING HIP WALK

I call these butt walks. This exercise works adductors with the femur stabilized and the pelvis moves. Kids usually like this exercise. If the child is capable of performing these independently, I butt walk with them. Keep the knees straight to help prevent cheating.

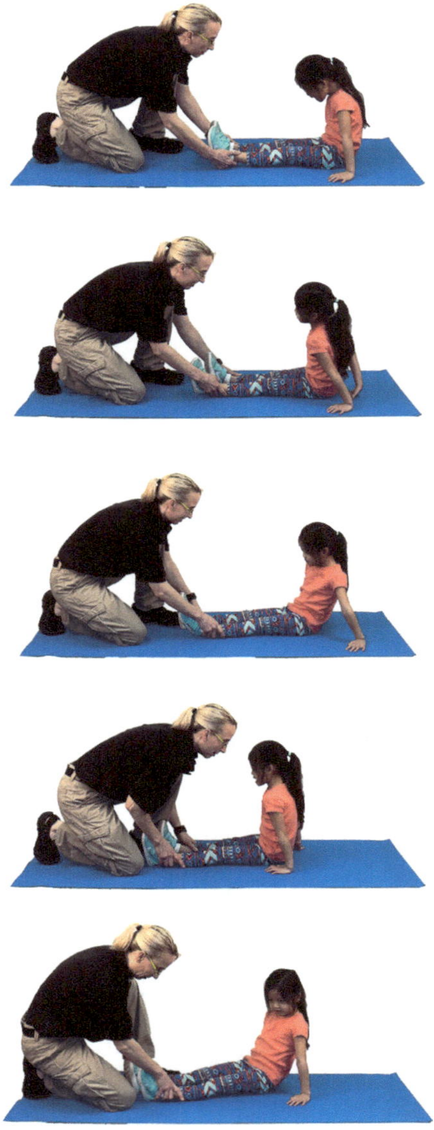

22. SIDE SIT, KNEES PROGRESSIVELY CLOSER

If a child sits side sit with his knee spread as wide as possible, the pelvis is fairly level. As the child put his knees closer together the pelvis becomes more tilted. When the knees are completely on top of each other in side sit the pelvis is very angled. The more angled the pelvis is the more challenging a position the side sit is to hold. This exercise requires lateral flexion, internal/external rotation and hip abduction/adduction strength depending on the leg referenced. I typically start with the child's knees very wide. I may start with two hands held, then one hand held, to two hands propping on the floor, then 1 hand propping on the floor, and finally hands free. Once a child can hold a position for ten seconds or for ten claps, I have the child move his knees a little closer. I perform the exact same activity with the child on a trampoline, rockerboard, a ball or even a platform swing for higher balance challenges with small/medium/large bounces/rocks/swings.

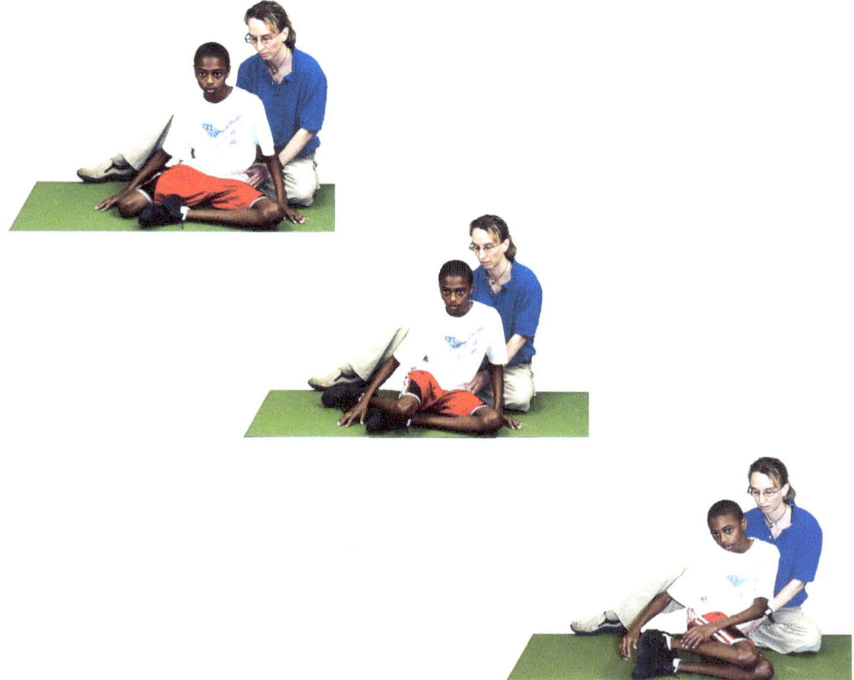

23. SIDESIT TO TALL KNEEL

Often this is a very difficult transition for my clients. It requires lateral flexion, hip internal/external rotation and hip adduction/abduction depending on the leg. I may place a four inch bench for the client to sit down to from tall kneel to make it easier. If he is successful from the bench, I will often double a pillow for him to sit down on. If he can do that, then I put a single thickness pillow down. From there, he goes down to the floor. This exercise is quite hard in general...but if you need to challenge your client more, have him cross his arms on his chest.

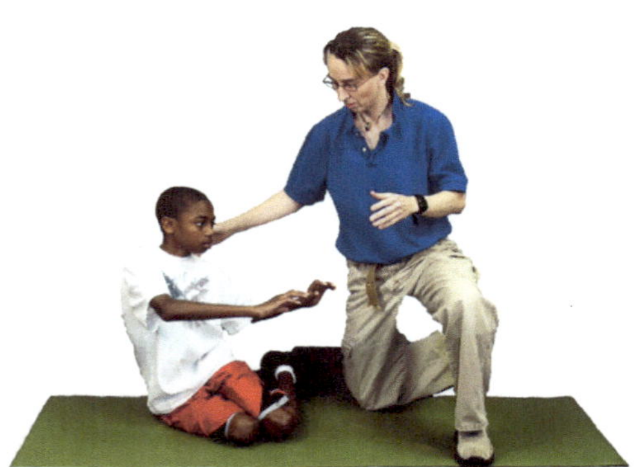

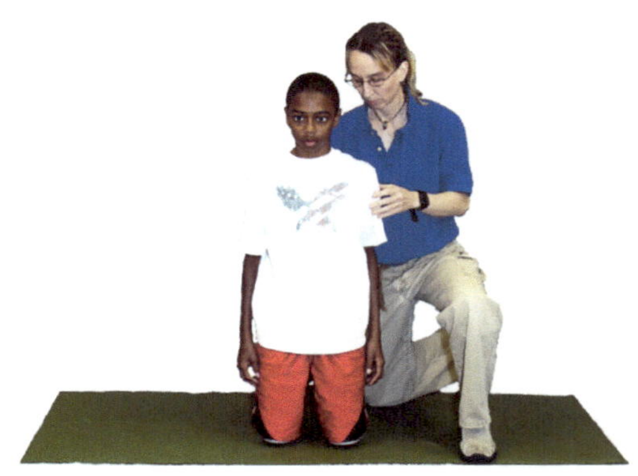

24. SIDE SIT TO TALL KNEEL HANDS ON BENCH KNEES ON BALL

This is quite a tricky exercise. I have physical therapy interns who have difficulty performing this exercise. Always spot closely. I often keep a hand on my client and on the ball. Sometimes I guide the movement through the ball so the client gets the feel of it. Often my clients don't keep 90 degrees hip flexion-either falling into too much flexion or extension. I remind them when upright to keep the knees under the hips.

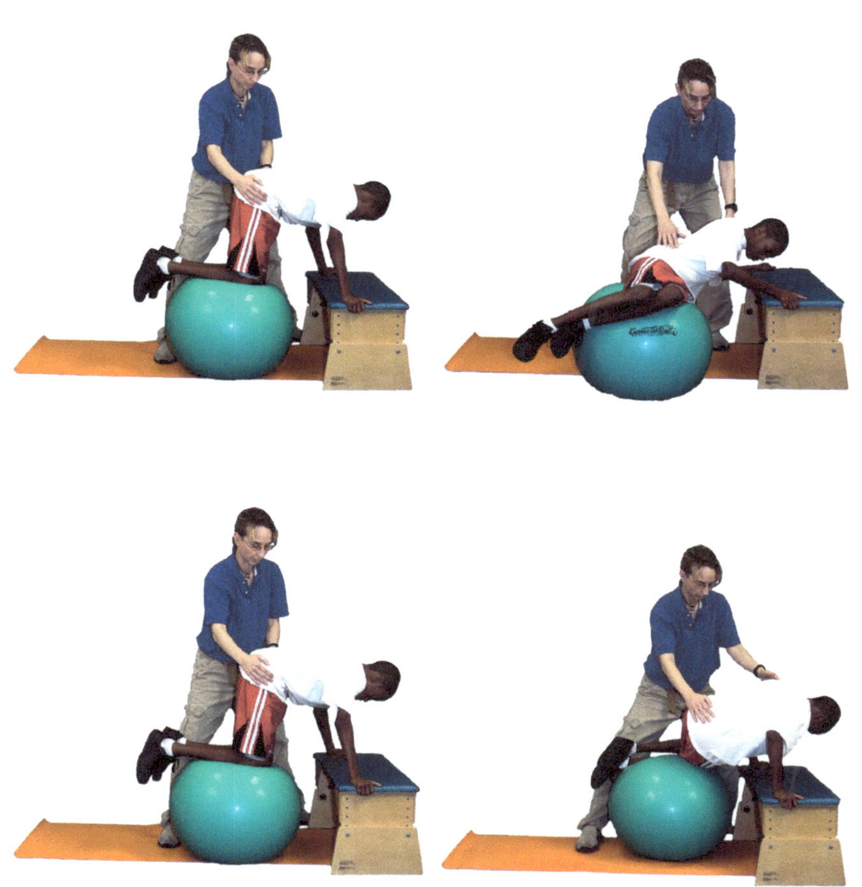

25. SIDEWAYS KNEE WALK

This picture shows the model knee walking sideways holding my hand, but, I rarely do sideways knee walking this way. I usually put the mat down next to a wall and have the child knee walk sideways facing the wall with two hands on the wall/mirror. Sideways walking looking at the mirror seems to work since children love to look at themselves. It is worth cleaning the mirror later. Unless I am targeting only one leg, I have the client go to the right and to the left.

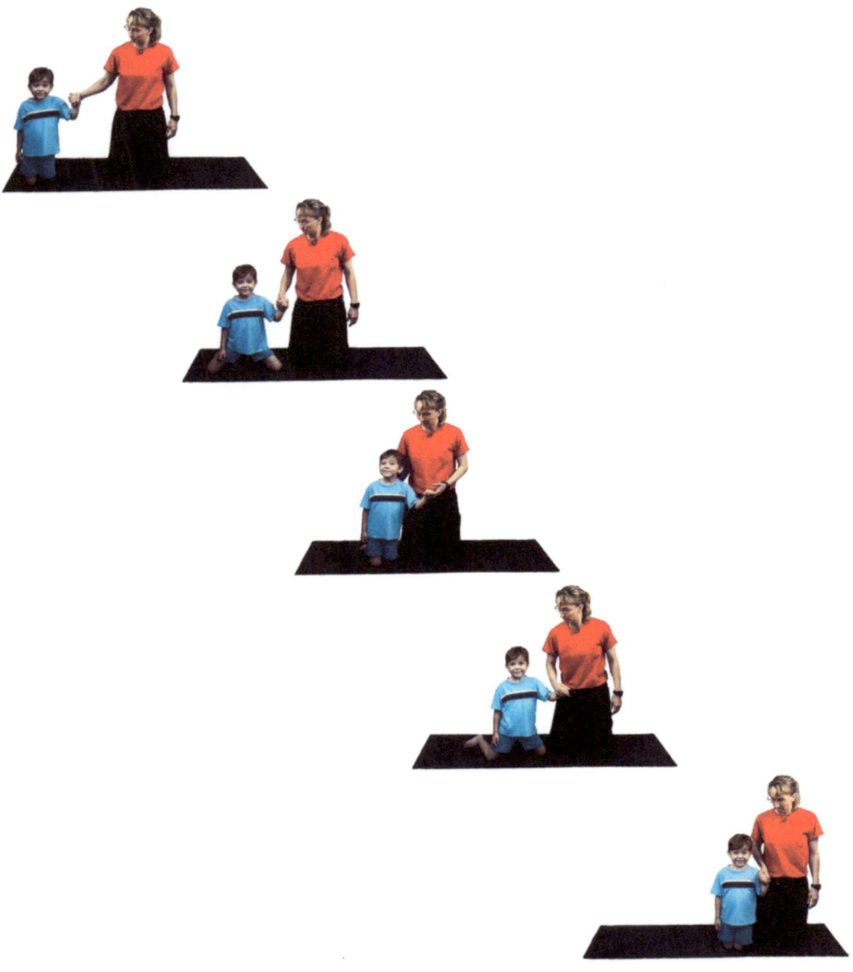

26. SIDESTEPPING

I have the client side step along a line, wall or board. The parent, the child, and I all line up together. The parent and I may hold the child's hand as we walk sideways with the child between us. Put ankle weights on the child to make this harder. I like sideways walking on the treadmill with upper extremity or trunk support if needed. Side stepping is an important skill for side protective stepping reactions for fall prevention in emerging ambulating clients. In a smaller client, this activity could be as simple as cruising sideways to get a toy from one end of the couch, dining room table or counter top to the other.

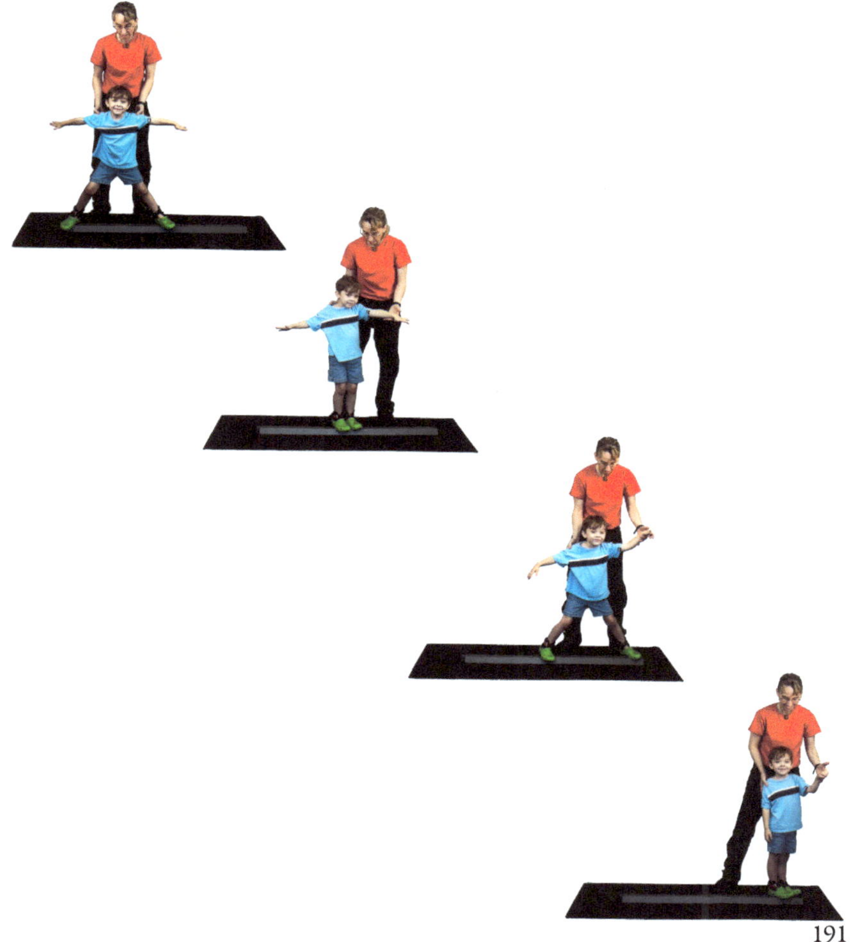

27. STANDING SIDE PICK UP TO BENCH

On the exercise, the closer leg to the side your client is leaning to works adduction concentrically on the movement back up to standing. The further leg works concentrically in abduction.

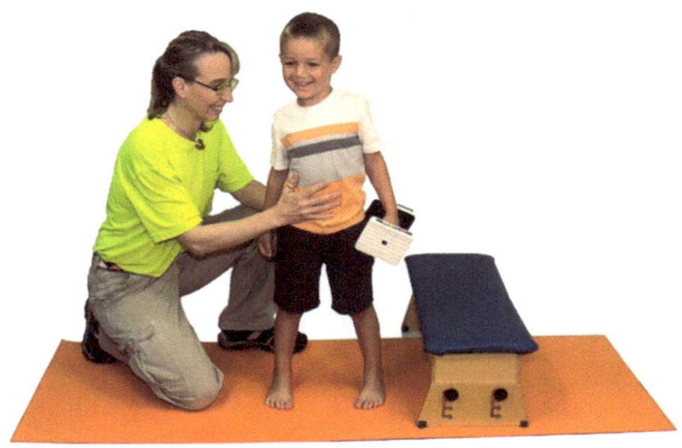

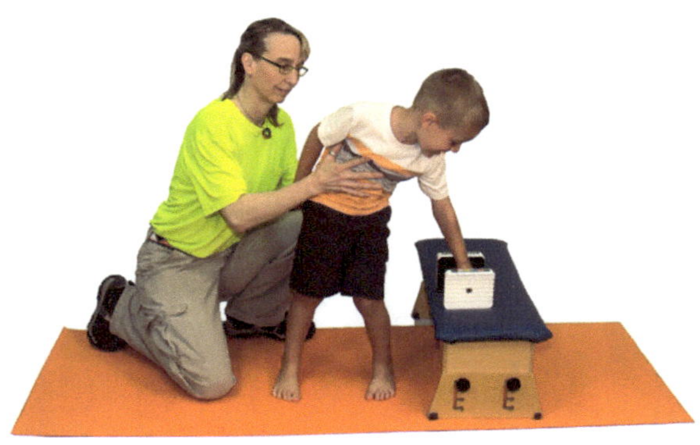

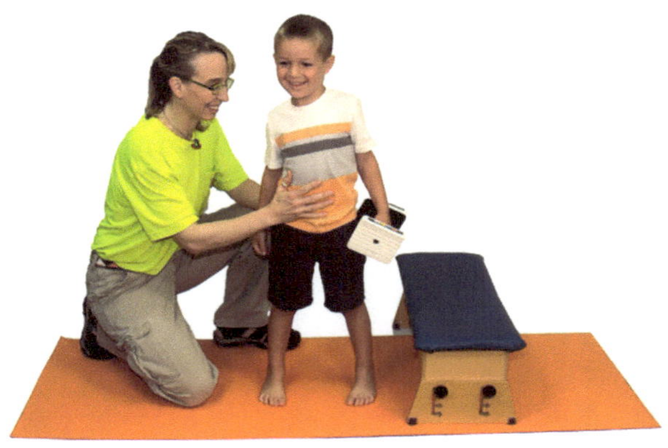

28. TETHER BALL KICK WITH ADDUCTION

This activity requires some coordination so you may need to provide upper body support for success with this activity. By adding a weight to your client's ankle, you can add a strengthening component.

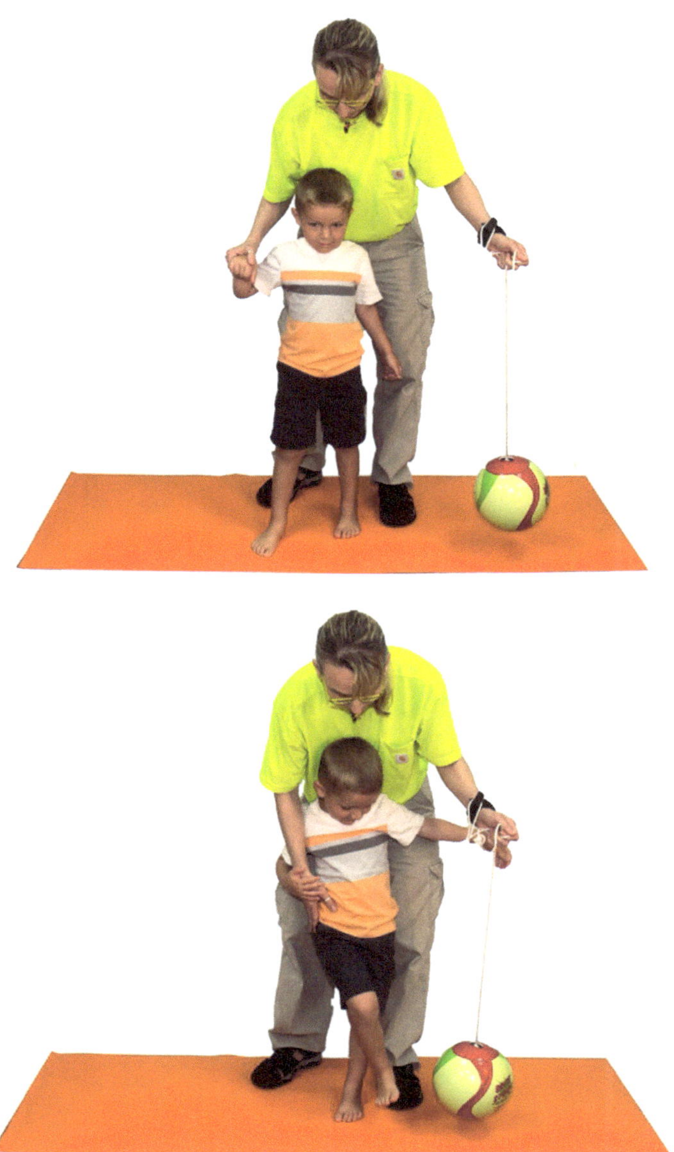

29. PENDULUM SWINGS ADDUCTION/ ADDUCTION

You may need to provide upper extremity support for this exercise. I have more success with my clients swinging their leg in front of their body as opposed to behind but technically either would work. I feel the adduction work more powerfully personally when I swing the leg behind the other leg. The wider the excursion the more strength this activity requires. You may need to set up targets to get the range you need. Ankle weights would greatly increase the difficulty of this exercise.

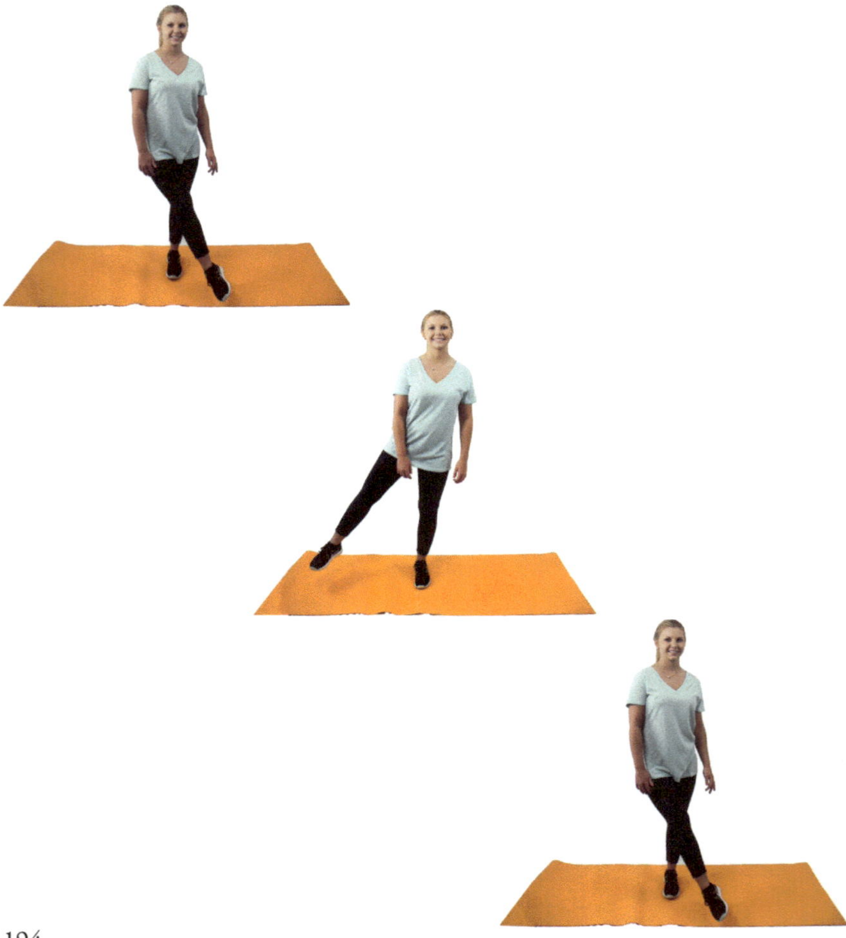

30. IN LINE STRIDE

Simply standing in the position of in line stride requires co-contraction of the adductors and abductors. To make this easier allow the foot placement to be progressively wider laterally.

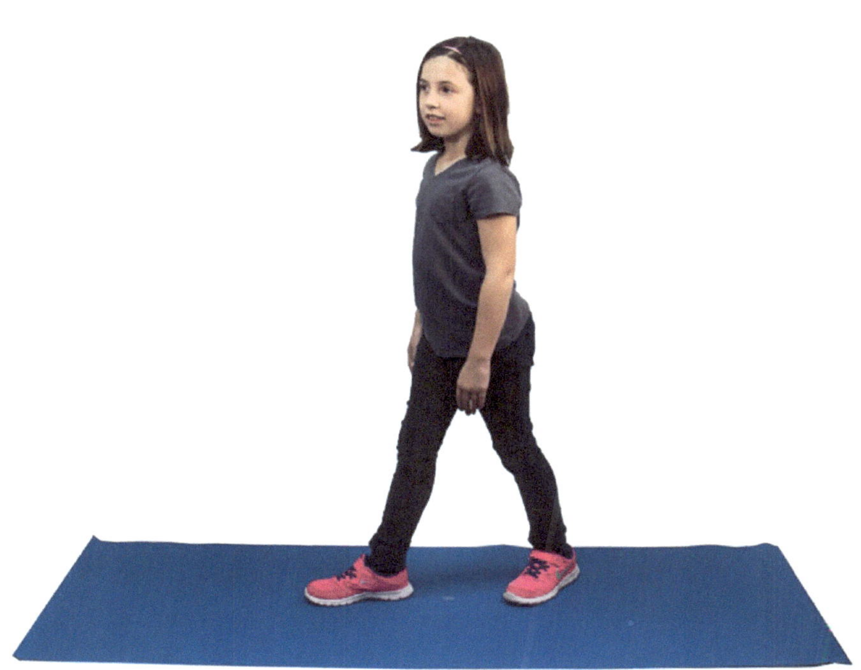

31. IN LINE STRIDE SIDE PICK UP TO FLOOR

For the best results, put the object/weight slightly behind the child's lateral midline. Encourage only a side movement. Many of my children cheat by leaning forward and then reaching back with their arm. The heavier the object lifted, the greater the muscle activation. To make this easier, simply have the child step forward with one leg into stride. In line stride makes this activity much more challenging. To make this easier, put the object on a bench. The higher the bench, the easier this activity is.

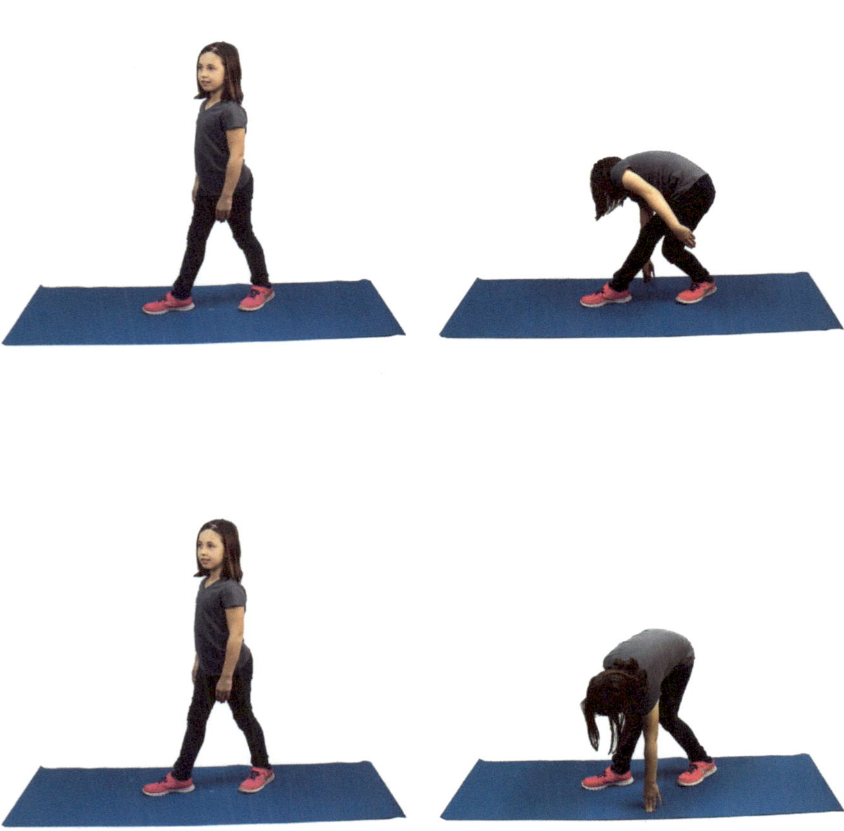

32. ONE FOOT ON BENCH, SIDE PICK UP

For adduction, make sure you set up the exercise so the child is moving laterally to pick up the toy on the ground. One leg is getting abduction and one leg is getting adduction. The lower leg is getting adduction, eccentrically on the way down and concentric ally on the way up. This is particularly good with clients with hemiplegia. With one foot on a bench, the client is more likely to put more weight on the foot on the floor. I have watched more than a few kids figure this exercise out without putting more weight on the foot on the floor. For these clients, I often support the knee on the down leg to guide the weight shift over to pick up the object. The higher the bench the other foot is on, the more the weight is shifted to the down leg. Any child who can cruise is ready to start working on this game with a support in front of him. I may initially not put the toy all the way on the ground. I measure progress by how close to the floor I can hold the toy and the child still be able to pick it up and return to upright.

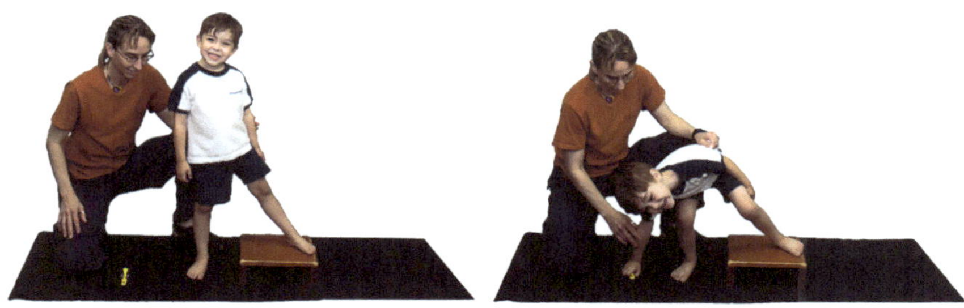

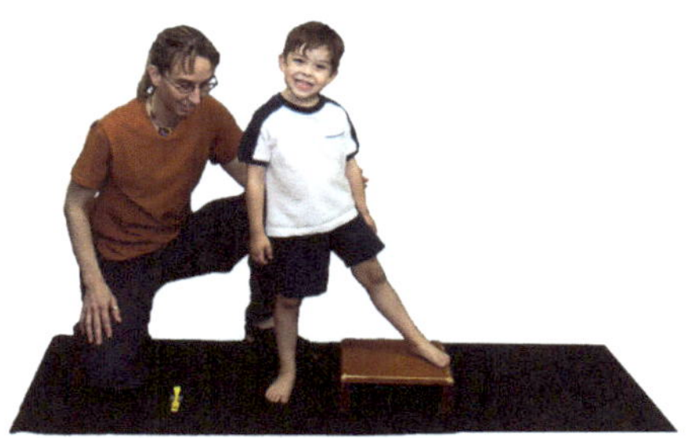

33. SIDE SLIDE OUT AND IN, UNILATERAL

I find something that slides easily to have my client put his foot on. Here I have simply used a piece of paper. You can put baby powder down to make it slide easier. He simply slides his foot out and back. A target, like a line on the floor, is always helpful.

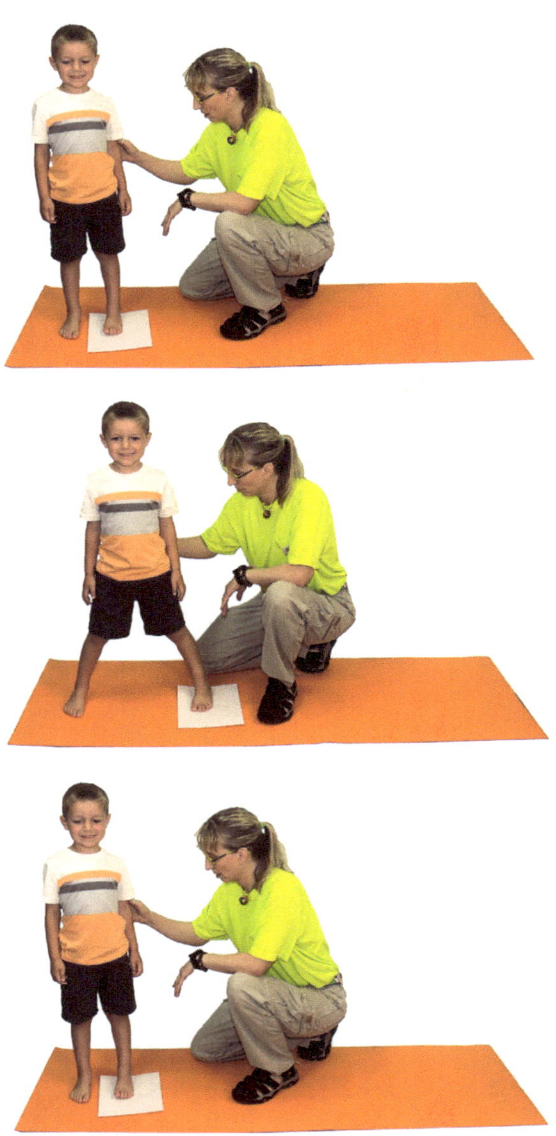

34. SIDE STEP WITH CROUCH AND PROPPING

This is a variation of the prior exercise. The crouch adds more quad activation to this abduction exercise. This child needed upper extremity support to be able to perform it accurately.

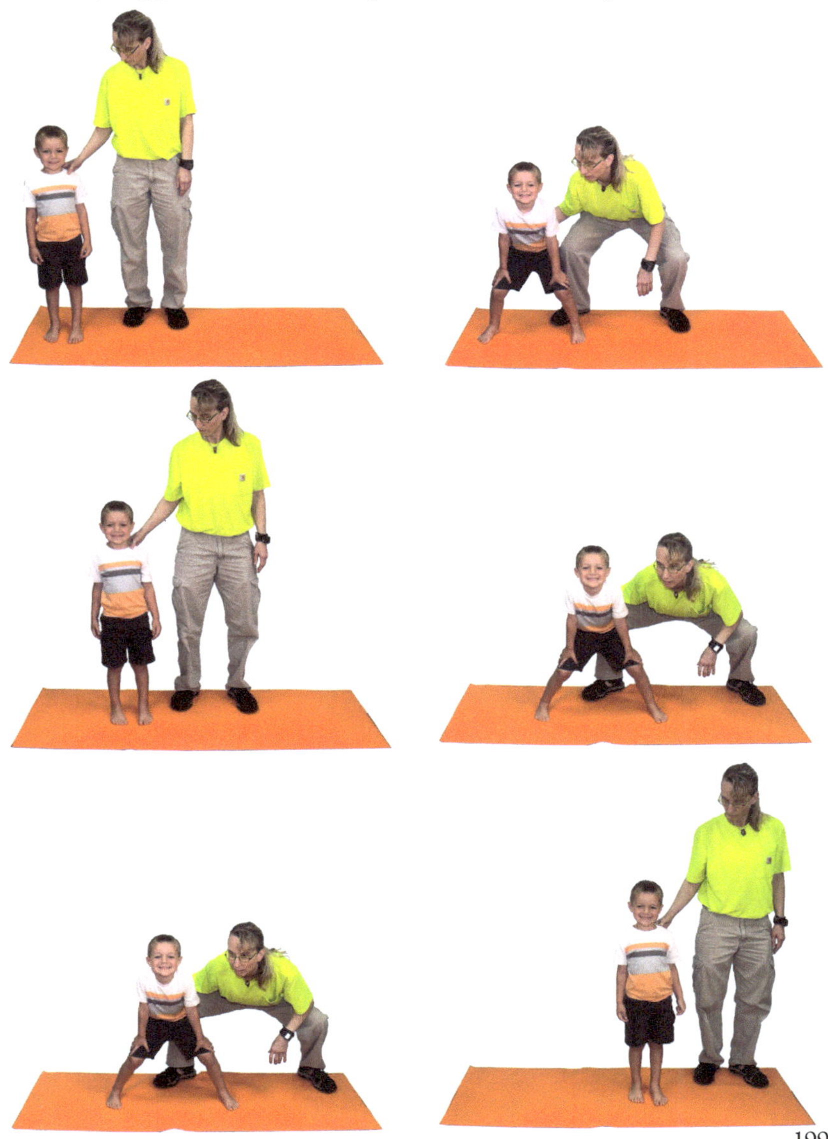

35. SIDESTEP WITH CROUCH HANDS FREE

Here is the variation with hands free. This provides a strong quad and abductor/adductor work out.

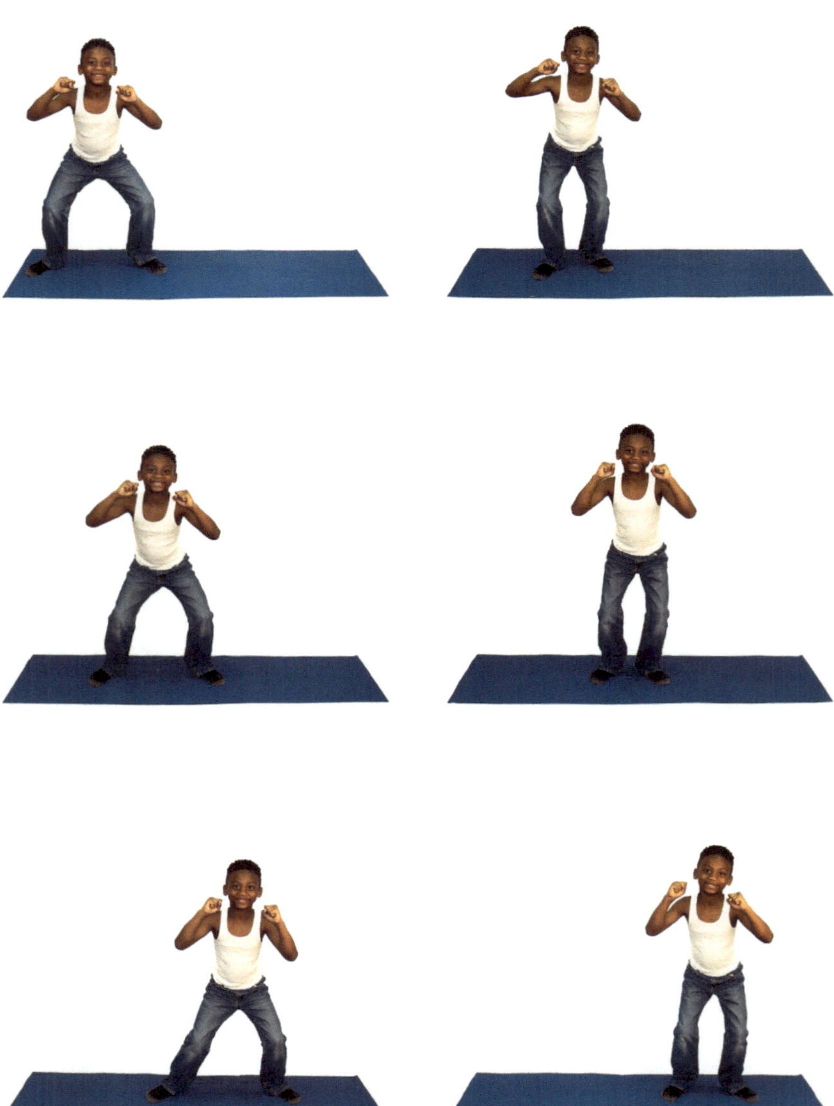

36. SIDE SLIDE

This can be easy or hard according to how easily the object the child is sliding moves along the floor. Slick surfaces like vinyl tile and wood floors make this easier while carpet makes it harder.

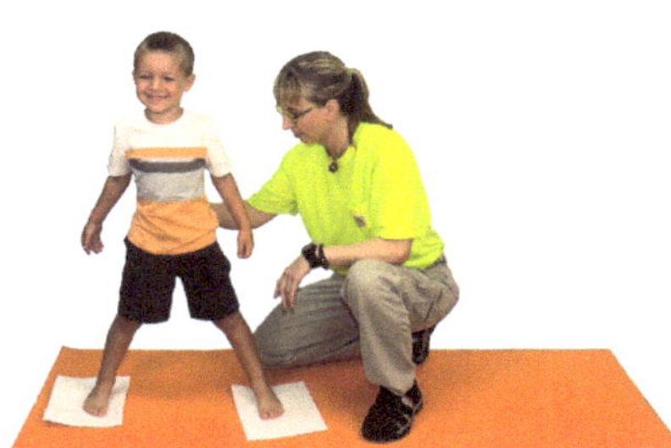

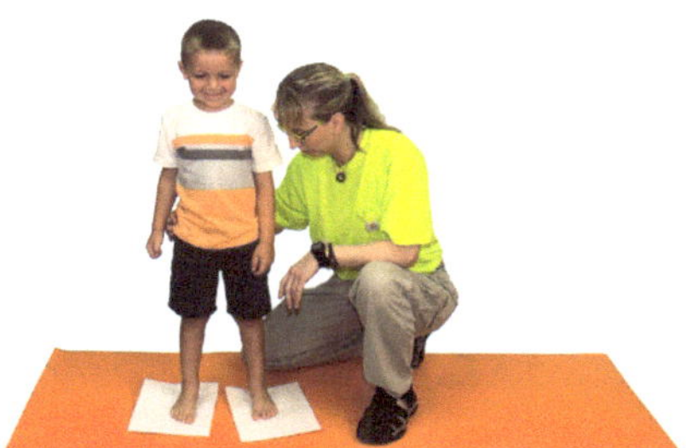

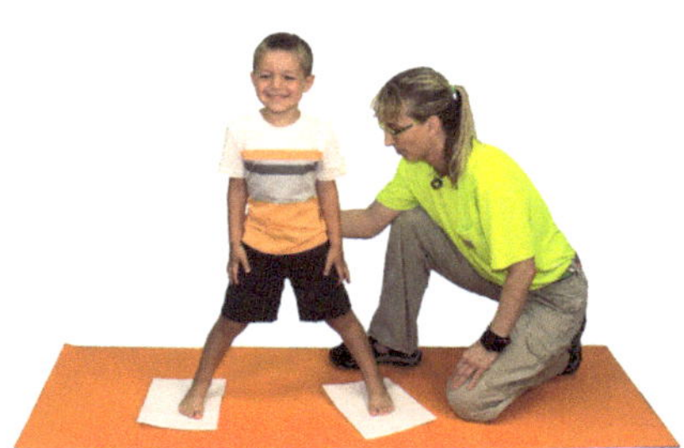

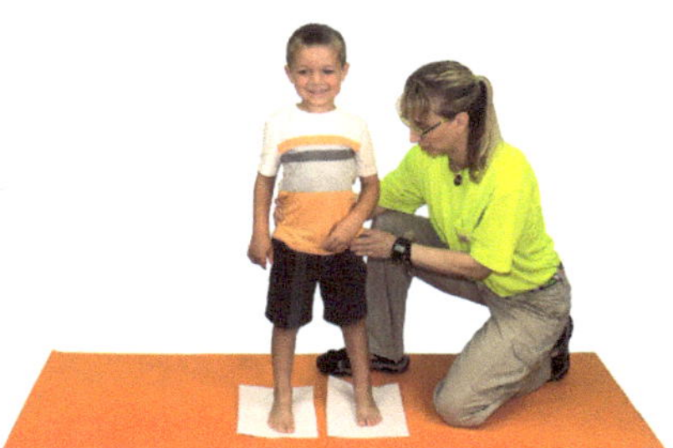

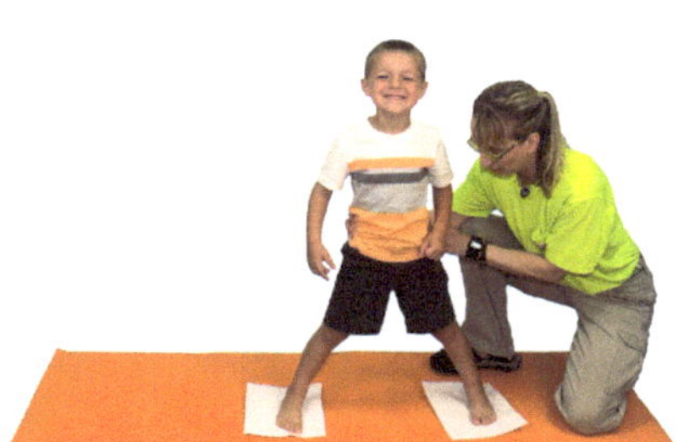

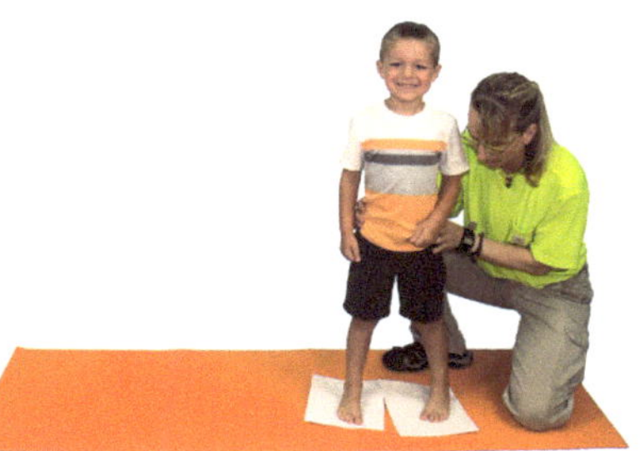

37. SCOOTERBOARD STAND UNILATERAL ADDUCTION

I usually provide physical support to perform this activity for safety. Since both feet are on unstable surfaces, this is a challenging activity. You can always have the child stand with the stationary foot on a similar height surface such as a bench to increase the safety/stability.

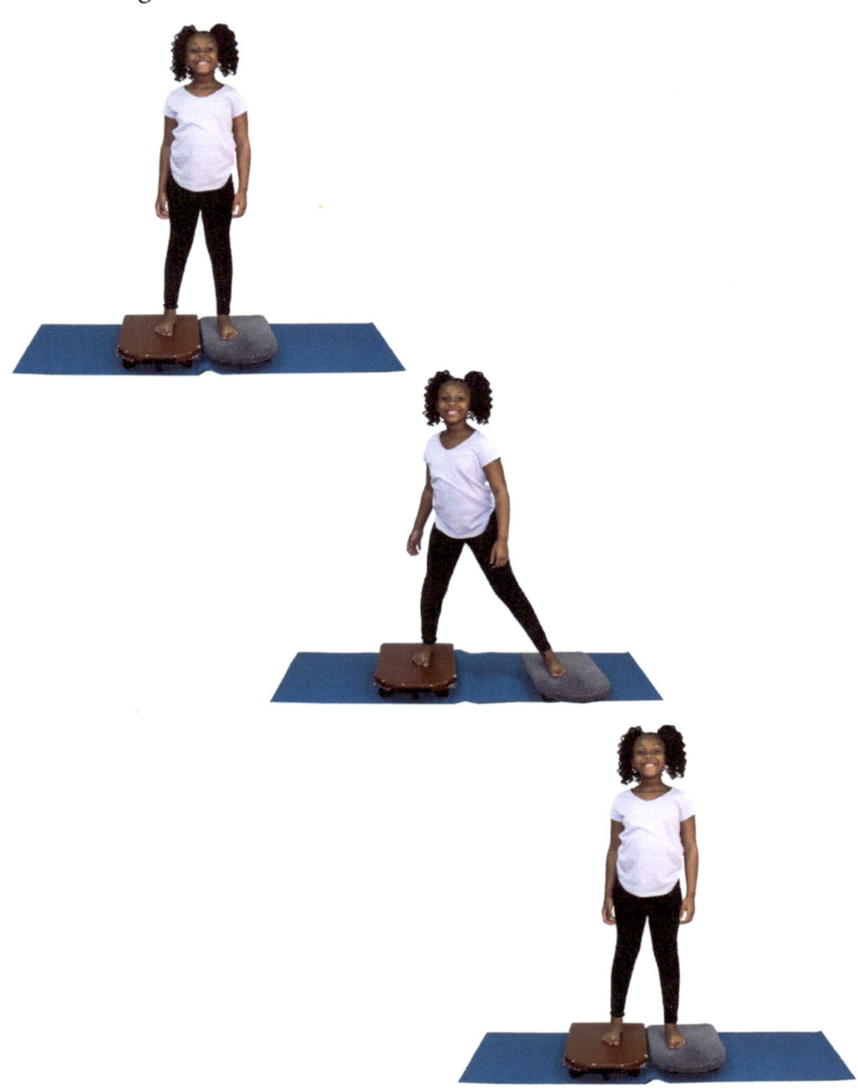

38. SCOOTERBOARD STAND BILATERAL ADDUCTION

This is a challenging exercise with both legs moving. I strongly recommend giving hand support or at minimum a spot for safety with my very capable model. It is actually a little easier on carpeting due to the traction.

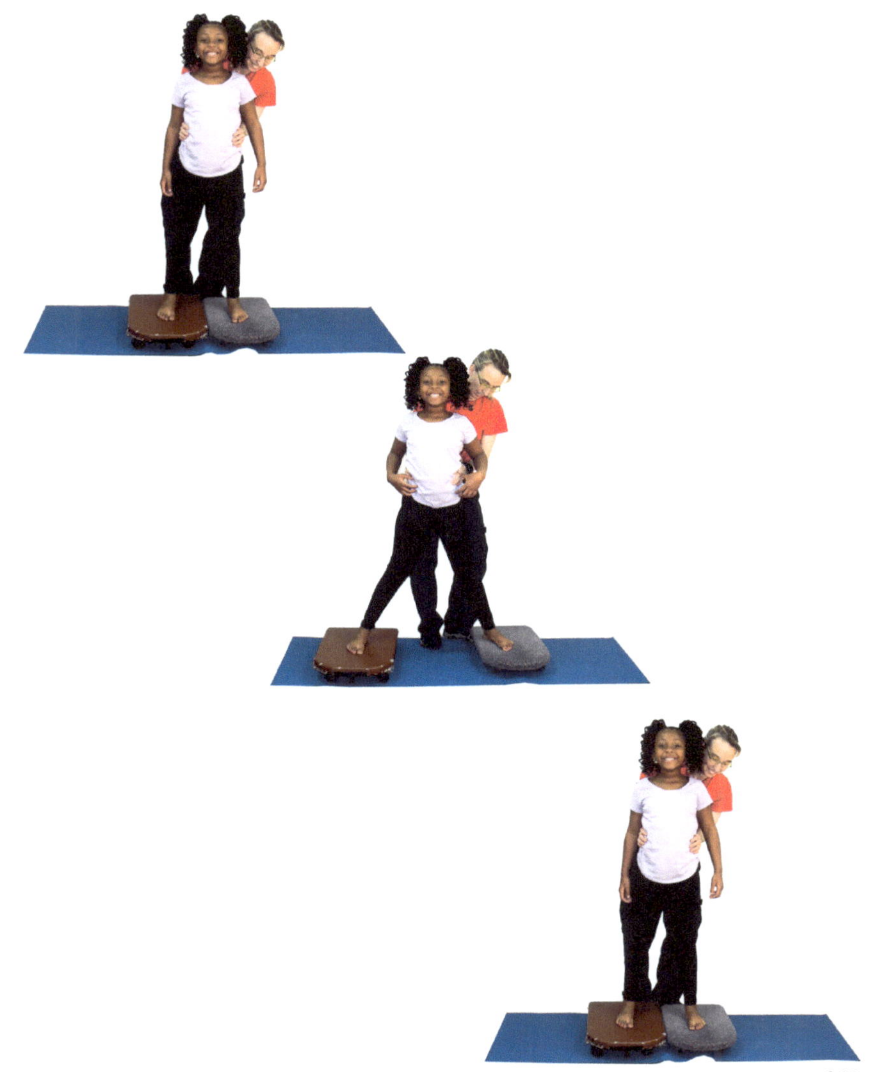

39. WALK WITH BALL BETWEEN KNEES

I have several clients who have a wide base of support with walking. This is one of the exercises I use to practice walking with a more narrow base of support or with a more adducted gait. I love gerdy style balls for this but in this picture I have a ball that has sound effects. It squeaks a little as he walks. Holding the ball at the thighs is easier while at the ankles is much harder.

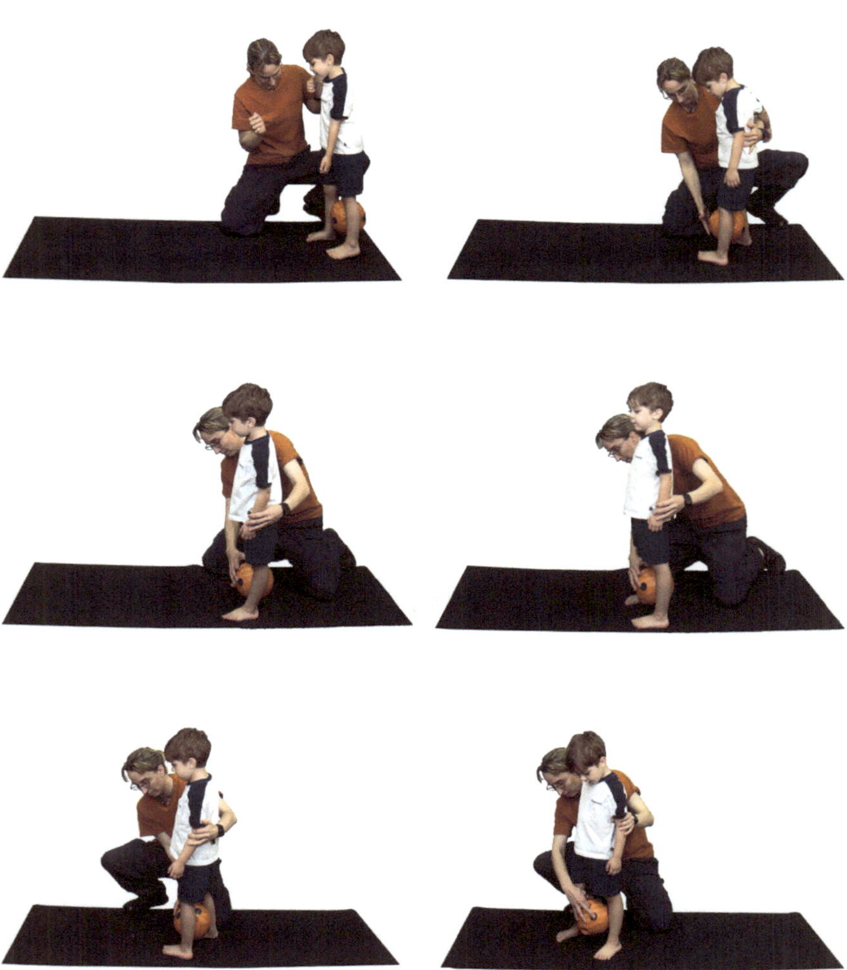

40. SIDE STEP UP AND DOWN

The higher the step, the harder this is. I may perform this activity repetitively up and down with a bench, or I may just head to a flight of stairs and have them walk up and down the stairs sideways. According to the client, I allow him to hold the railing with one or two hands or none. If I need more of a challenge, I add ankle weights. Unless I have a unilateral weakness, I have the client lead with both sides.

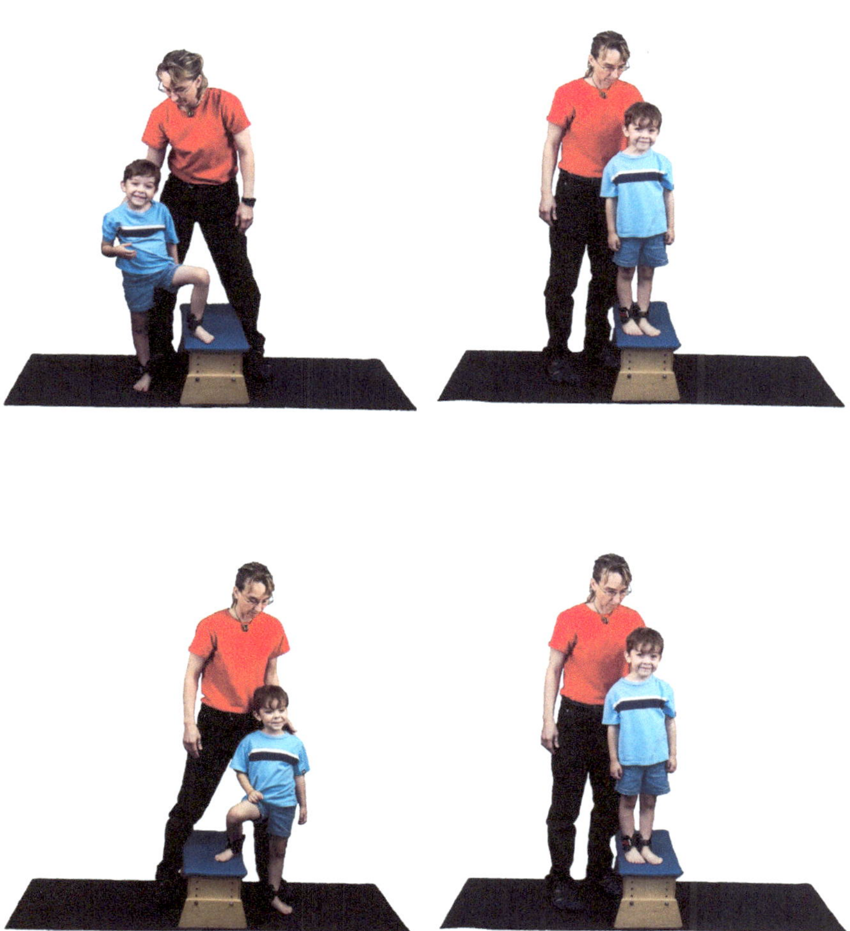

41. SIDE LUNGES

The wider the lunge, the harder this activity is. I often have the child step onto a target to prevent cheating. Here I am having the child touch the floor to increase the difficulty.

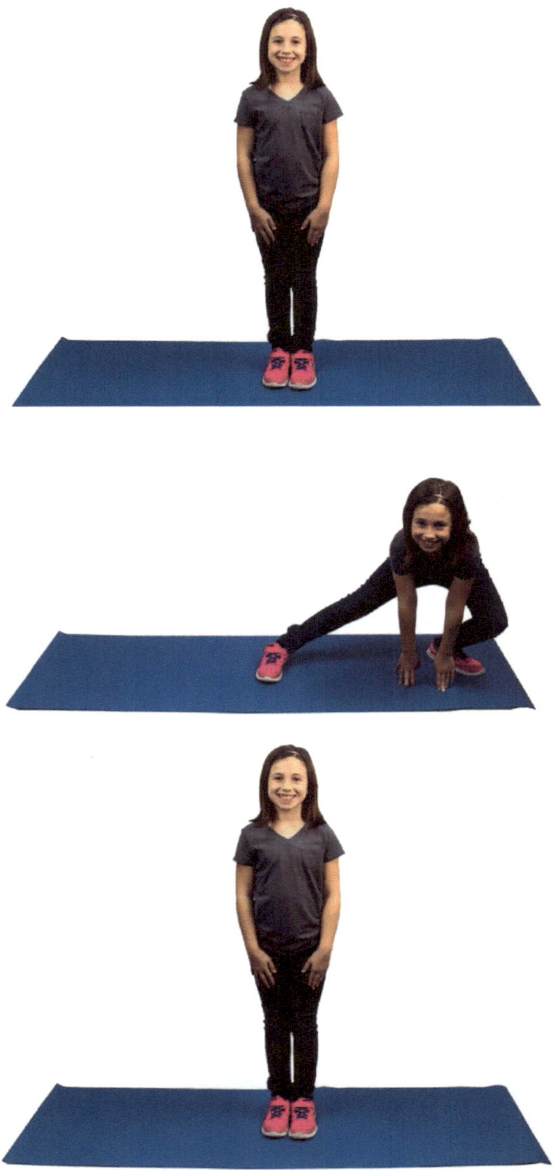

42. JUMP WITH BALL BETWEEN KNEES

This is always fun, even if it is hard. I have many children who have one stronger leg. They have trouble jumping with a two foot take off and landing. They kind of leap one foot at a time instead. This is a go to exercise to teach a child how to keep her legs together when she jumps. Jumping in place is easier than jumping forward.

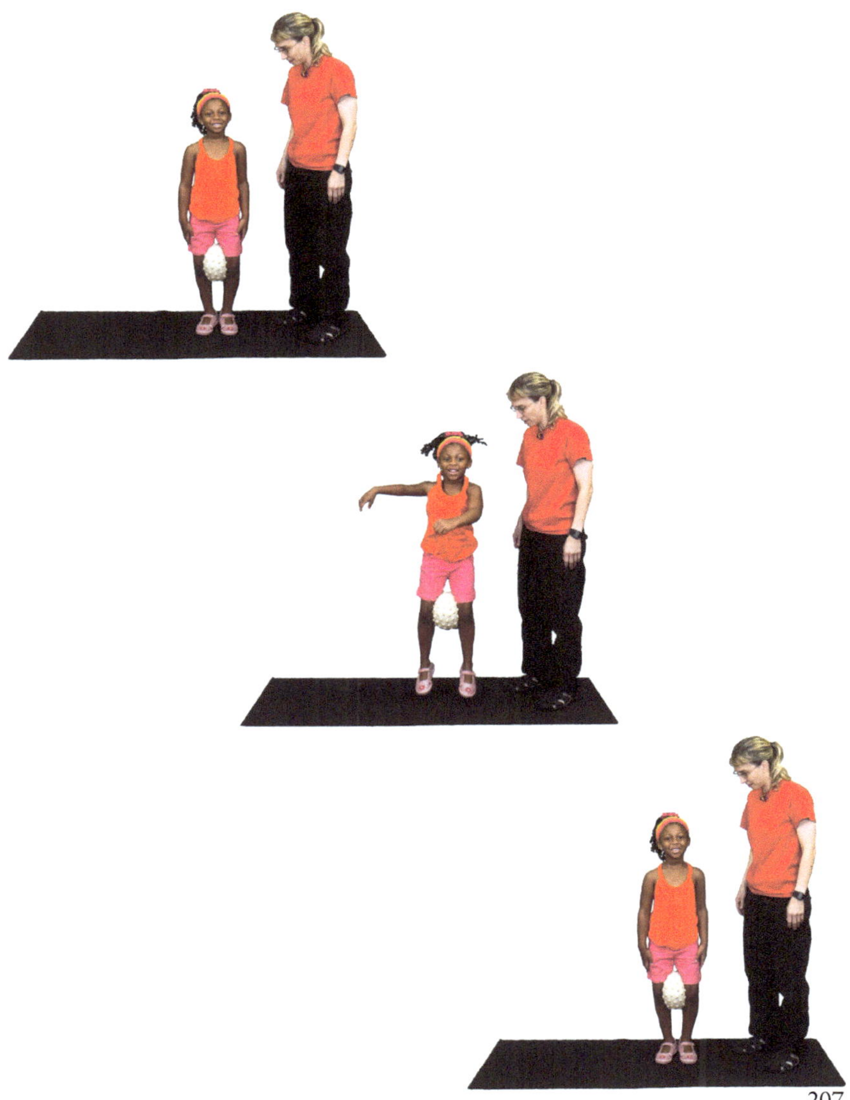

43. JUMPING FORWARD BALL BETWEEN KNEES

This is slightly more difficult, because she jumps forward, but she does not have to jump a distance that will completely clear her own foot length.

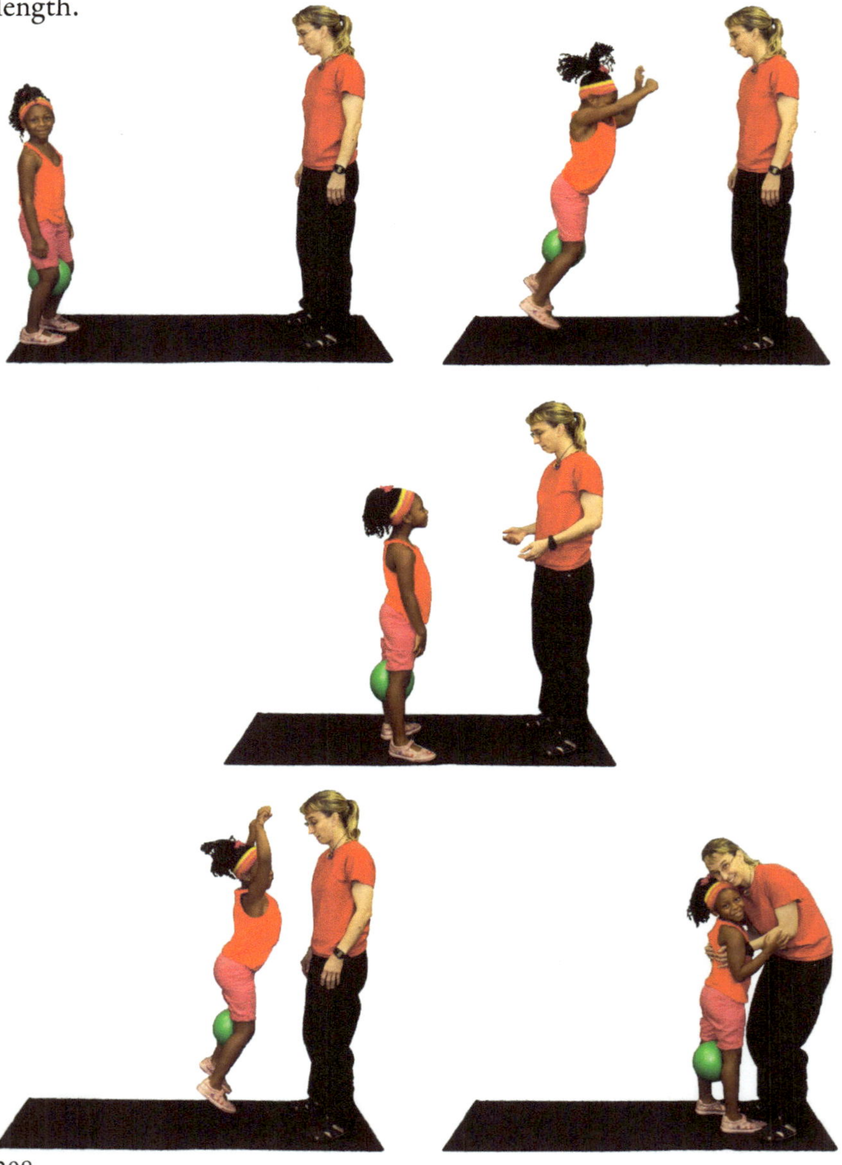

44. JUMPING DOWN WITH BALL BETWEEN KNEES

This is much more difficult, because she has to jump forward a distance that will completely clear her own foot length. Then on the deceleration of landing, she must also maintain control of the ball.

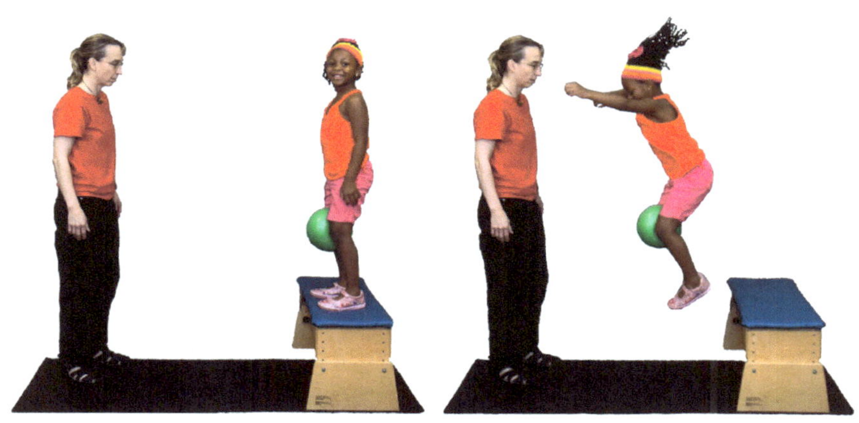

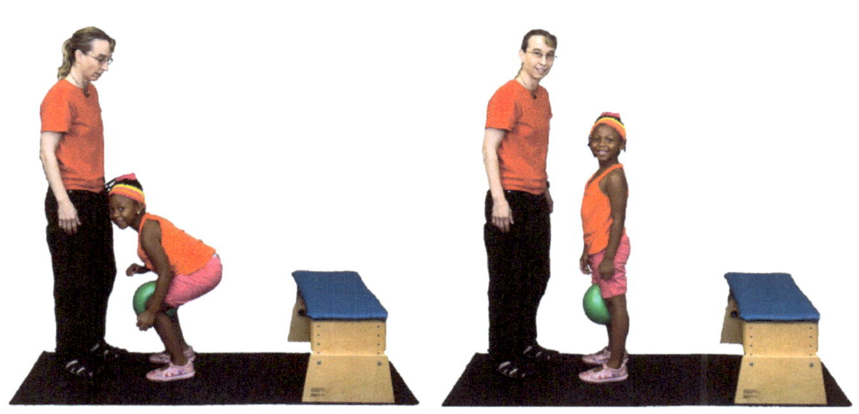

45. BOLSTER SWING SITTING

I love this exercise for adduction. It is fun and kids never know they are working hard. The more you wiggle and shake the swing the harder they have to hold on. I start by sitting on the swing behind the child. If the child is having a hard time, I let him put his hands down on the swing in front of him. I swing the bolster swing forward/back in a challenge ten times to see if he can keep his balance. If he is successful with the forward/back excursions, then I try side to side excursions, then circles and then what I call zig zags. If the child needs a greater challenge, I get off of the swing and try the same series of swings without my weight stabilizing it for him. Make sure a mat is down on the floor because it is not uncommon for a child to fall off. The wilder the excursions, the harder the child must hold on with his adductors. Adding an upper extremity challenge like putting in cups or throwing a ball while swinging would encourage more weight shift and a stronger adduction contraction in the legs to stabilize to keep his balance.

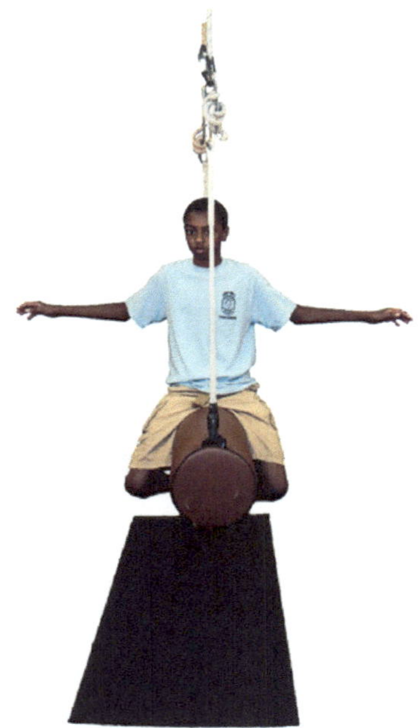

46. POGO BALL JUMP

This only works adductors with pogo balls, not pogo sticks. I usually start out letting my client sit down on a chair to get set up and his feet placed correctly. He holds my hands to stand up. I often first let the child experiment with rocking the ball forward and back and side to side, then bounce and finally jump. As he shows skill at jumping with two hands held, I fade to one and then no hands held.

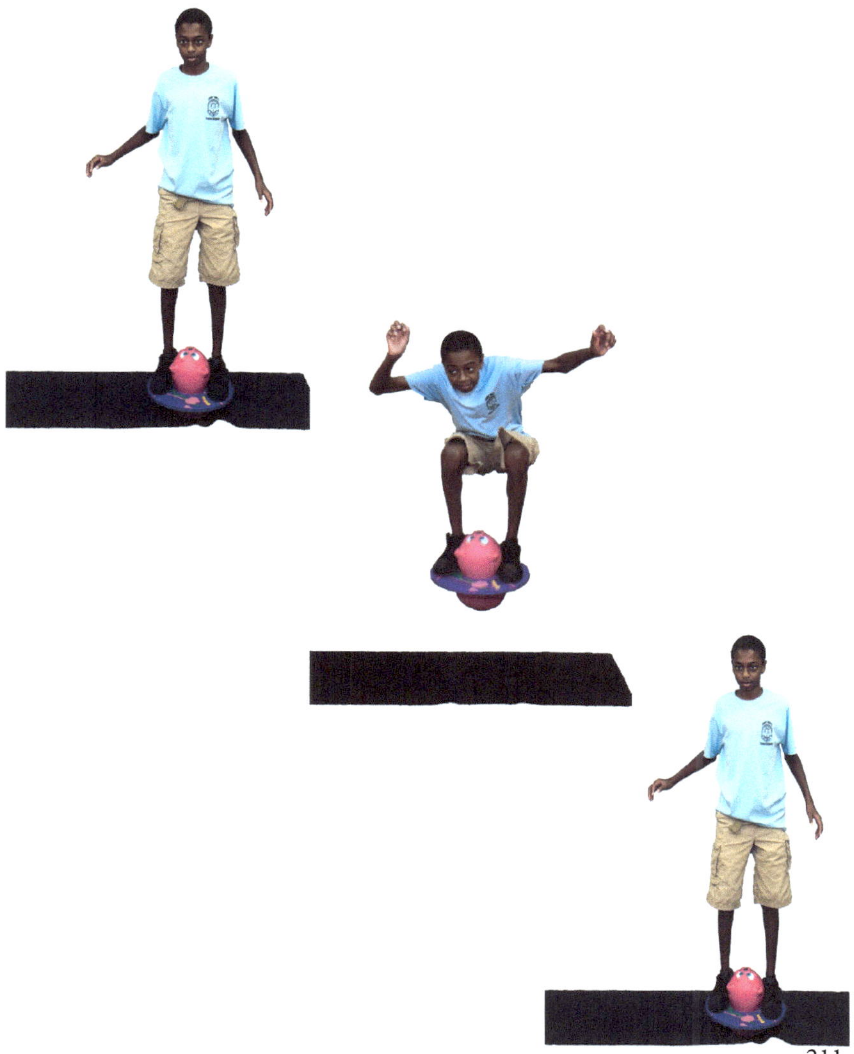

47. SCOOTERBOARD SITTING SIDE TO SIDE SLIDE

This is a challenging exercise. I stabilize the feet or make a spot for my client to keep her heels on. I have the child move the scooterboard sideways. I make a line for her to move the scooterboard along or mark two spots for her to move the scooterboard between.

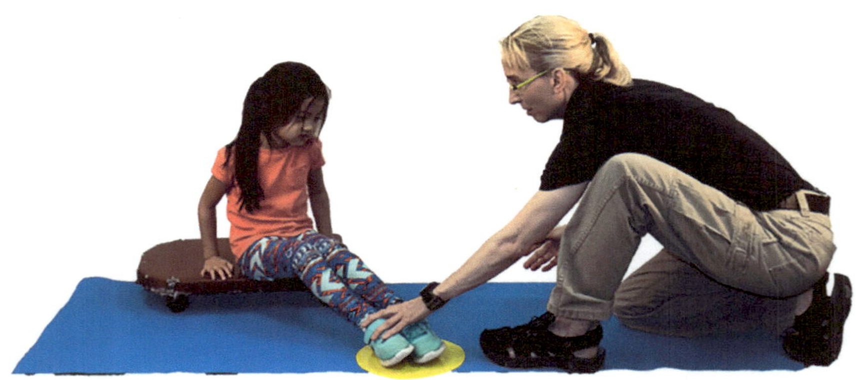

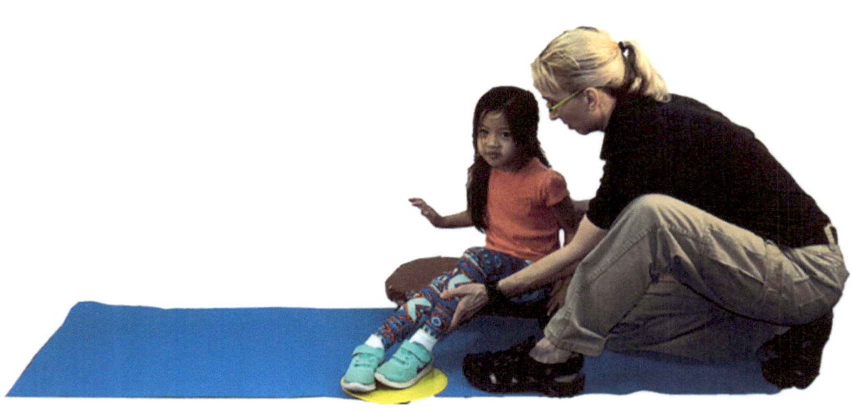

48. CRAB WALK SIDEWAYS

This is a nice way to get abduction with hip extension; however, I usually have to constantly cue the child to get him to keep his hips up/ extended if that is my aim. For the kids who can take the challenge, I like playing soccer in this position. I position the child in crab position in front of a goal that he has to protect by moving side to side. I am also in crab position. I kick the ball and try and get the ball in the goal. After five to ten trials and a break, we switch roles.

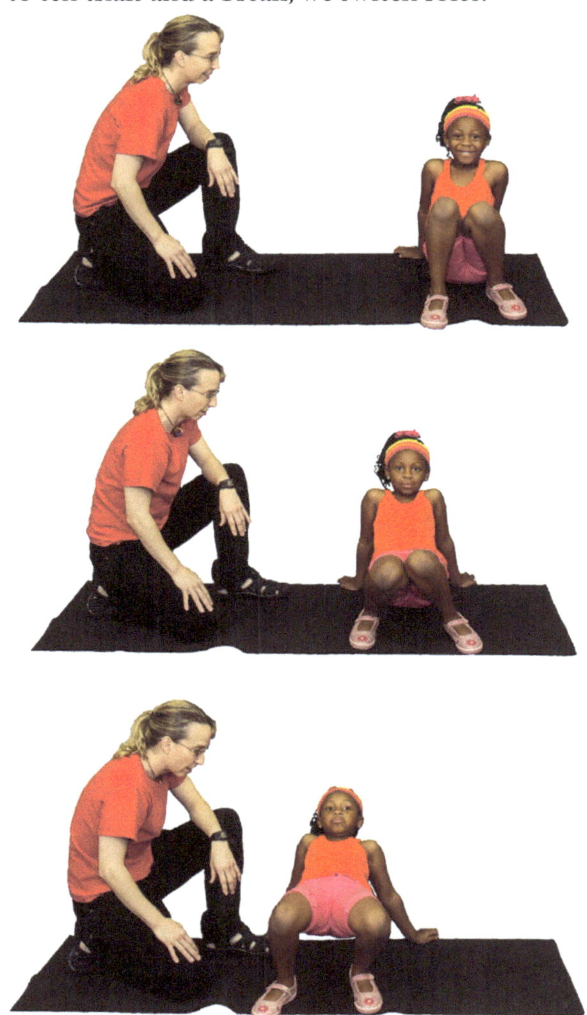

49. SUPINE HANG BY ARMS AND LEGS

I don't typically set this up this way. Usually I hold one end of the stick and the parent holds the other end. We lift together, so it is not quite as back breaking. I think you actually get more adduction when I use the bolster swing instead of a stick. I don't have to do any lifting when I use the bolster swing so that is actually how I set this up 99% of the time. I have the child lay down on her stomach on top of the bolster swing. She hugs it with her arms and squeezes tight with her legs, and then rolls over so that she is hanging upside down. Make sure the swing is reasonably close to the floor and a mat is protecting the ground. I usually swing the bolster swing as wild as I think the child can tolerate and let her try to stay on. Often I will sing a song like "Engine Engine Number 9" or "Cinderella Dressed in Yellow" and the goal is to try to make it through to the end. I let the child take turns either with me or a sibling. She swings the swing and tries to knock the rider off. This is always big fun. I usually get tired well before the child does.

If you use the bolster swing version of this game, make sure the swing hook up in the ceiling is professionally installed and inspected regularly. If not installed correctly, eye bolts in the ceiling can shear and the child fall without warning.

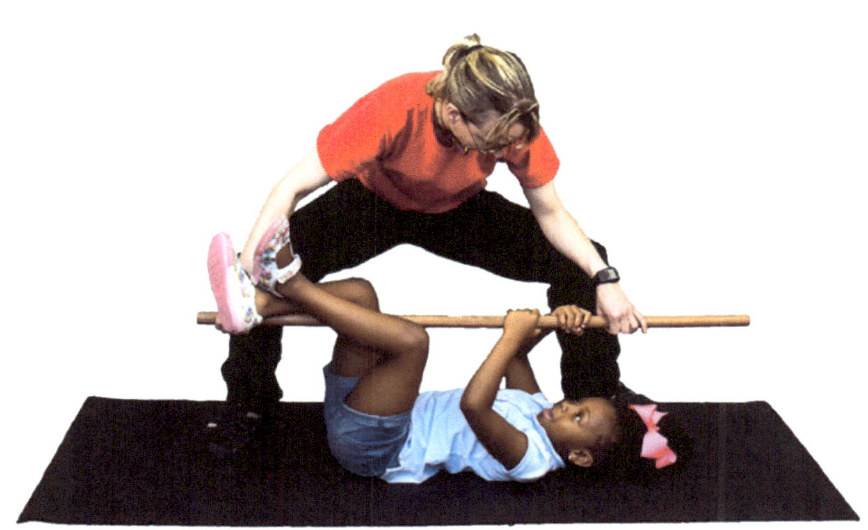

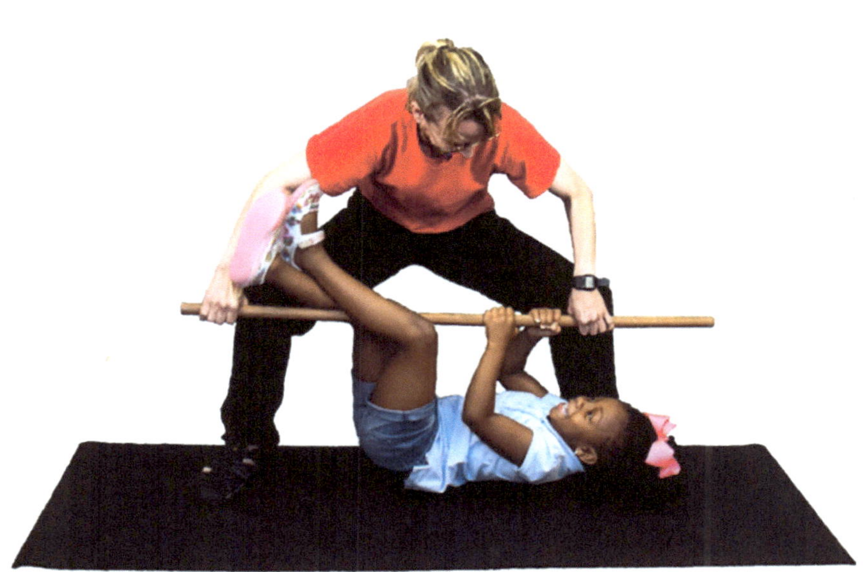

V. HIP EXTERNAL ROTATION

* * *

THE HIP EXTERNAL ROTATORS SPIN the femur laterally away from the other knee or from midline. These movements are in the transverse plane. The hip external rotators are important in lower leg alignment in walking, running, and sports related movements. Weakness or tightness in the hip external rotators will decrease the efficiency of gait and increase the likelihood of injury to the hip, knee or ankle. Weakness in hip external rotators has been linked to knee valgum related injuries.

1. SUPINE EXTERNAL ROTATION

This is one of the easier external rotation exercises. Some clients need a pillow or wedge under their head to be able to see their feet for this exercise. I tend to start with the hip internally rotated and then have my client externally rotate. I reference wind shield wipers so my client understands the movement. With clients who need work on this, I typically am able to resist moving from an internally rotated position to neutral and then have to assist progressively in the range from neutral to an externally rotated position.

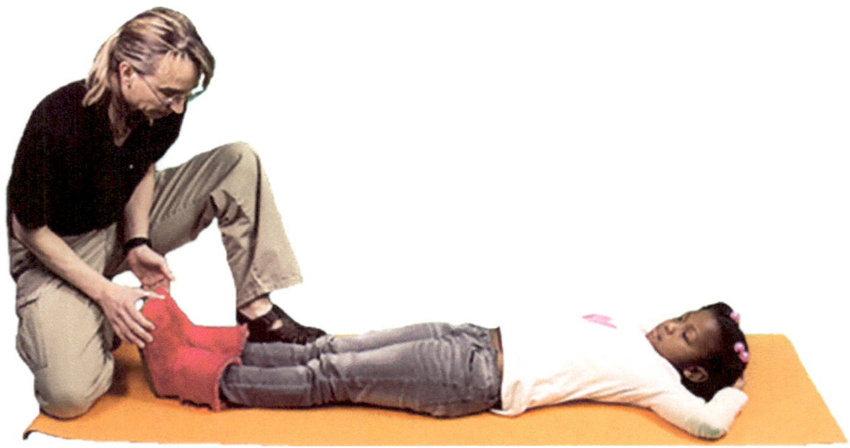

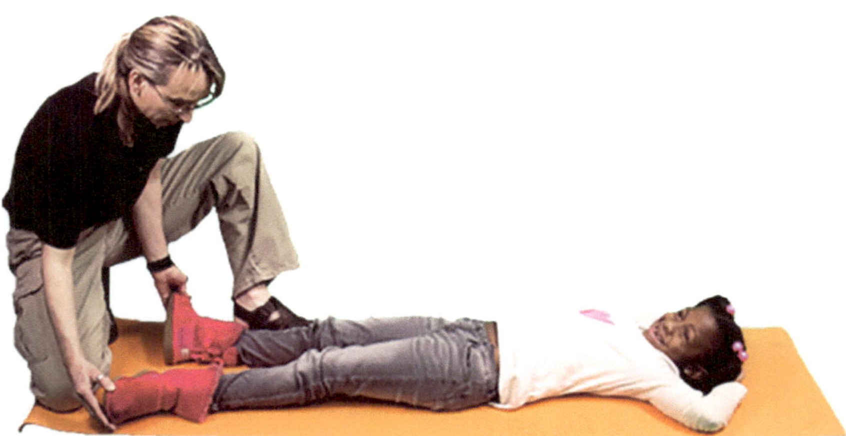

2. PRONE LEGS TOGETHER EXTERNAL ROTATION

When my client needs the visual feedback, I let her look in a mirror. Many kids need a little help, especially when I first work on external rotation. If the child has a better side, this exercise allows the less involved side to assist. Many clients tend to get movement of the entire pelvis helping with rotation as well. This exercise is easier to motor plan than both legs going into internal rotation and external rotation simultaneously, i.e., having them both out and then both in at the same time. See which works better for your client. Clients who have difficulty generating hip rotation, usually also have difficulty sustaining knee flexion. I often hold the client in knee flexion so she can focus on the rotation. I often facilitate/assist part of the movement and resist other parts of this movement.

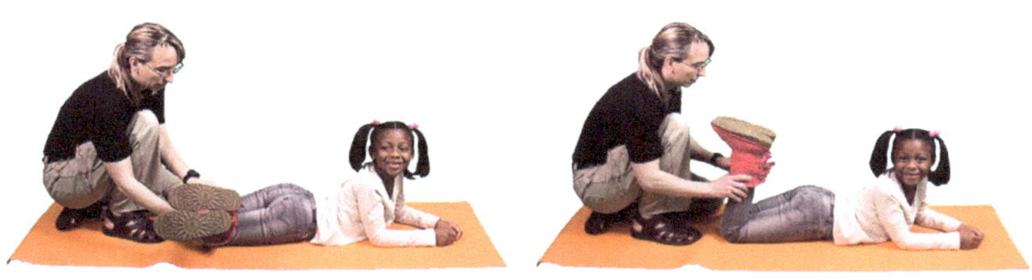

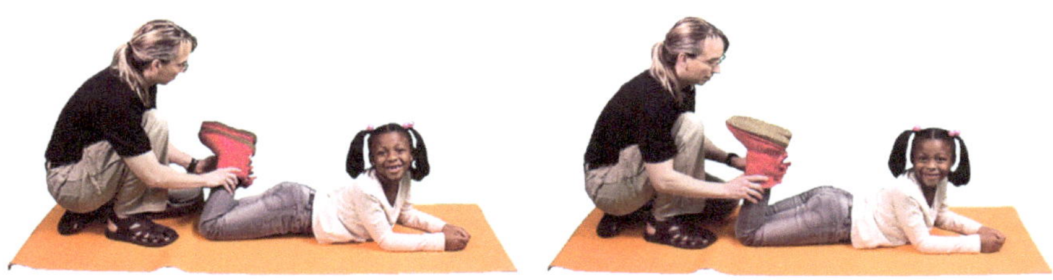

3. PRONE UNILATERAL EXTERNAL ROTATION

Here I am isolating only one leg. I use a mirror when possible to help the client see the movement.

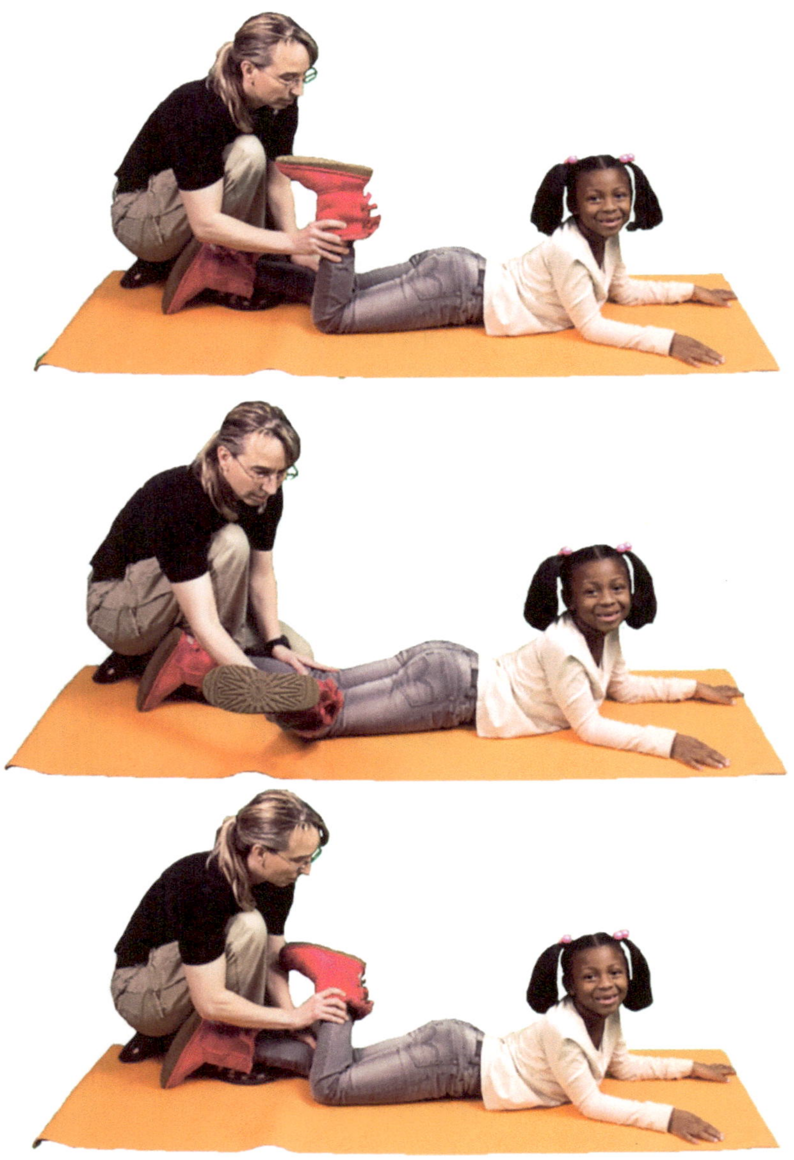

4. PRONE BILATERAL EXTERNAL ROTATION

I tend to start with the hip internally rotated and then have my client externally rotate. By moving two legs at a time, I tend to get less substitution/cheating.

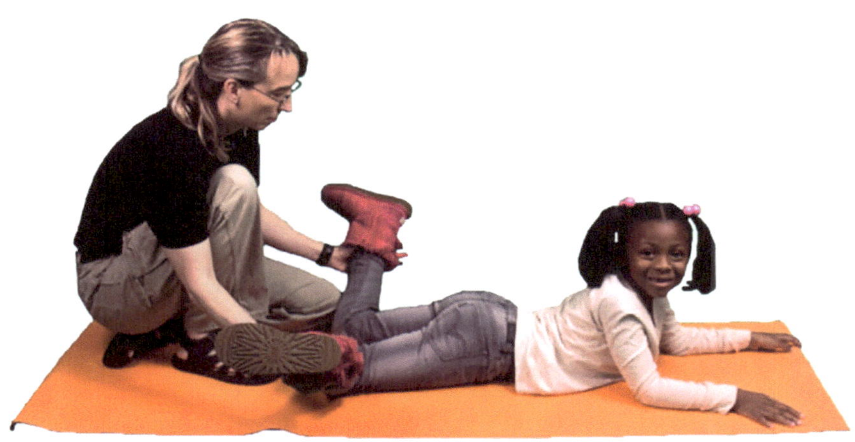

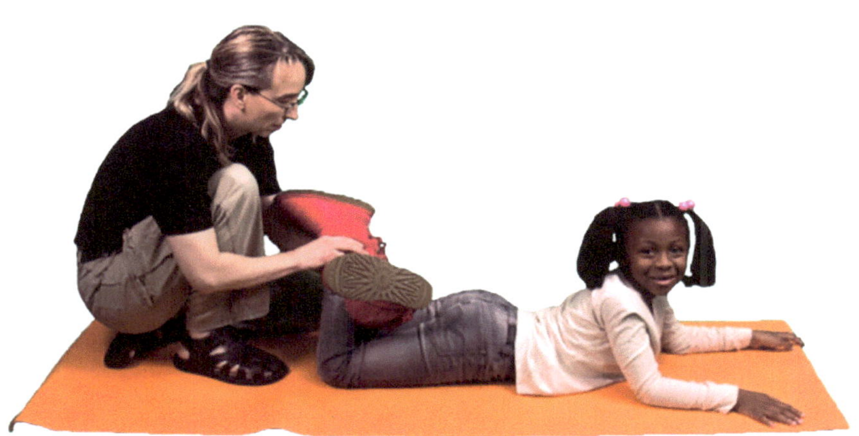

5. BALL HANDS AND KNEES TO SIDESIT HANDS ON BENCH

The ball has a great deal of degrees of freedom of movement, so spot your client closely if you have any concerns regarding his safety. Make sure you start with the ball under the knees in the quadruped position. This activity is harder the further I have my client go to the side. This model was capable of going far enough to touch his hips down on each side. This is really hard work. I have trouble doing it too!

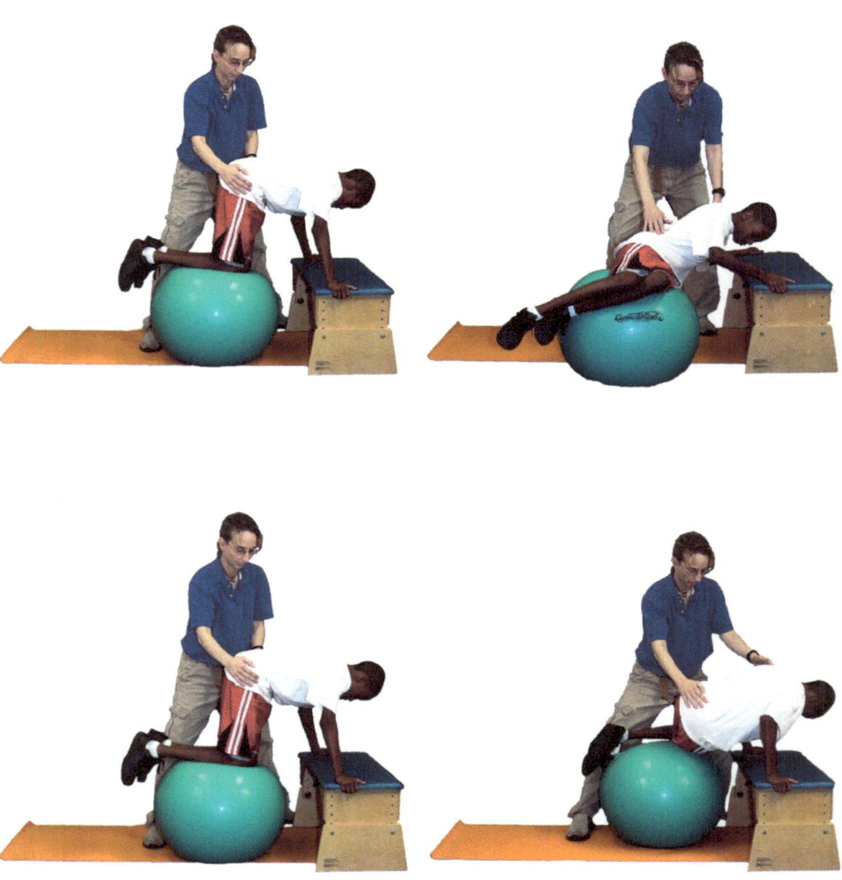

6. HIP EXTERNAL ROTATION LONG SITTING

I like that my client is in an excellent position to watch the movement of her feet. If my client needs back support, I allow her to lean on a wall or furniture. Sunbather's position (as seen here) or long sitting work as well.

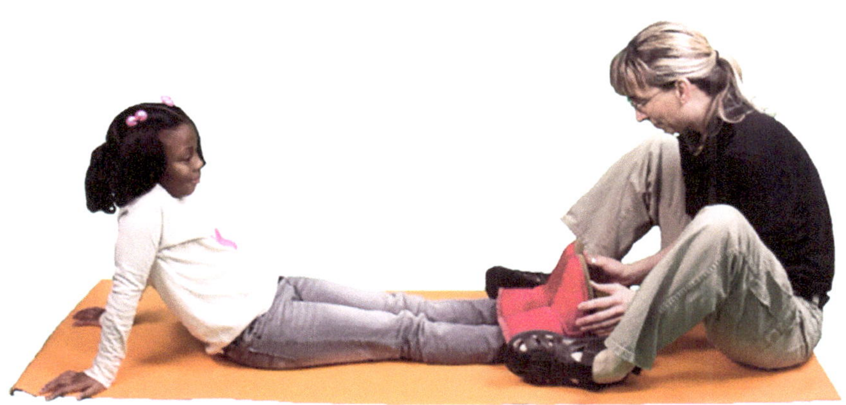

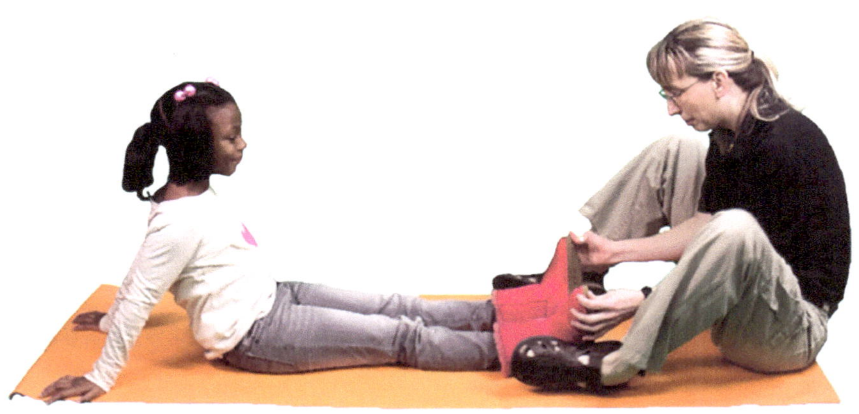

7. SIDESIT PROGRESSIVELY NARROW

I usually start with my client in a wide sidesit where the knees don't overlap at all. I have him clap his hands ten times (to discourage hands down). If he is successful, I inch his knees closer together. This in turn tilts the pelvis, and he has to work harder to maintain the position. I continue until my client can't hold the position any longer or until the knees are on top of each other.

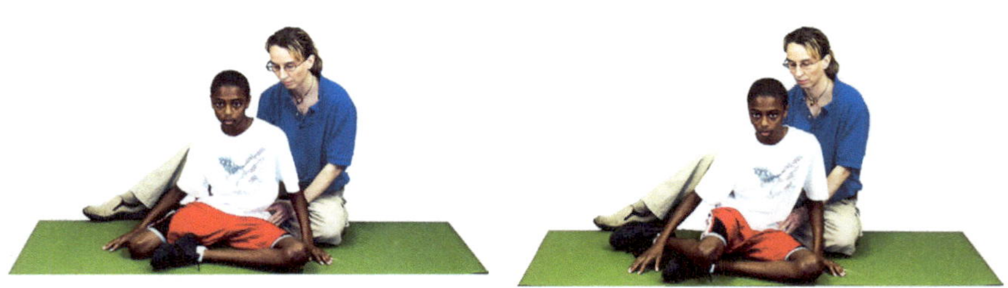

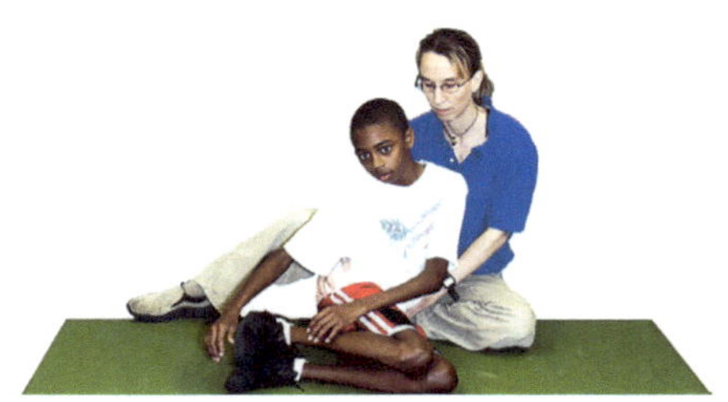

8. SIDESIT TO TALL KNEEL

Here one leg is internally rotating, the other is externally rotating. This can be a difficult transition for my clients. I allow him to sit down on pillows or a low bench if going to the floor is too difficult. If you need to challenge your client more, have him cross his arms on his chest.

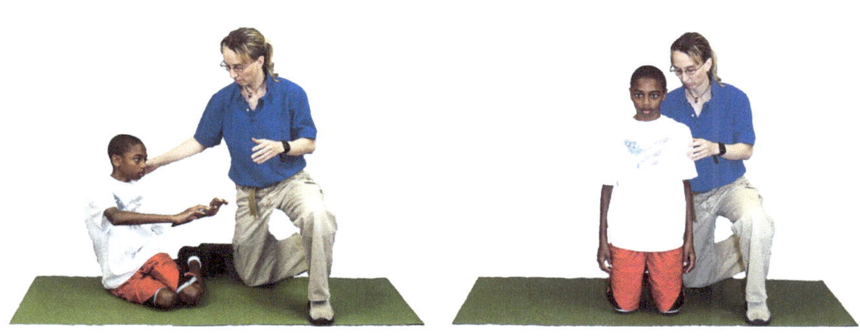

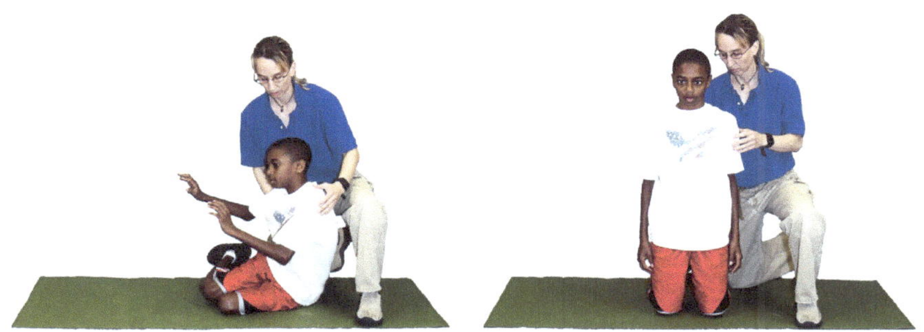

9. FEET ON SCOOTER SIDE TO SIDE SLIDE

I have a few clients who have no idea how to move in rotation at the hips. This exercise allows me to teach the motion with resistance minimized. Often my clients who need this work have trouble keeping the knee flexion. They extend their knees as they attempt to perform hip rotation. So I put down a chalk or Velcro line and explain that the scooterboard must stay behind the line. A skate board as opposed to a scooterboard may be better for the clients who have a hard time performing hip rotation. Having two legs on the scooter/skateboard allows cheating with the other leg, but some of my clients with diplegia need to cheat initially to figure out the movement.

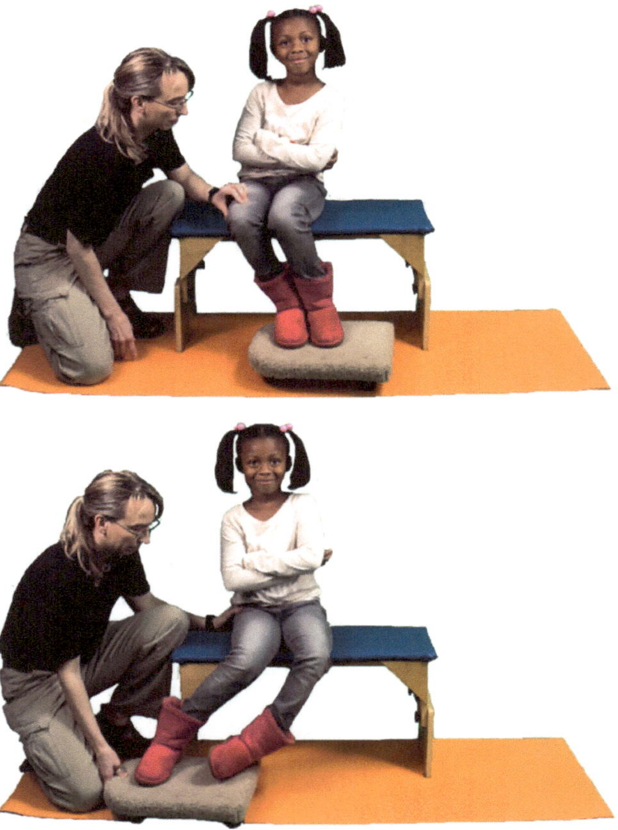

10. FOOT ON SCOOTER SIDE TO SIDE SLIDE

This exercise is the one leg version of the previous exercise. Having only one leg on the scooter/skateboard eliminates cheating with the other leg.

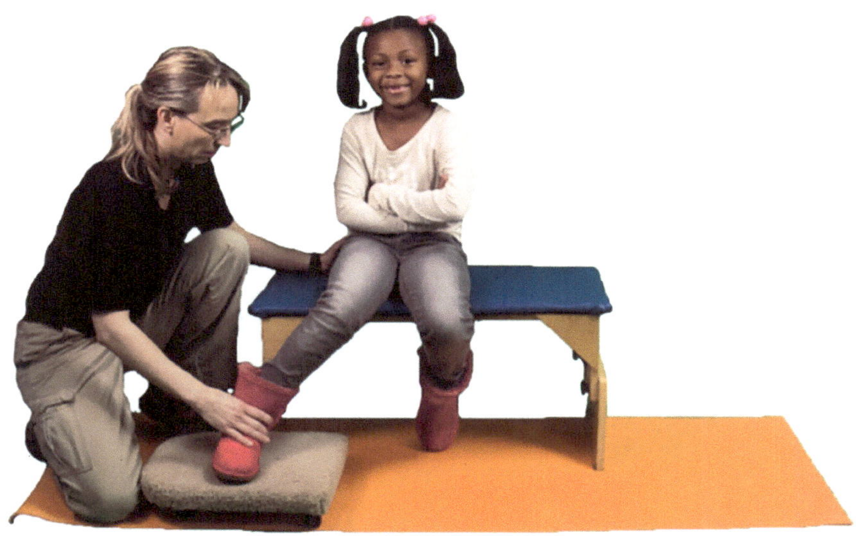

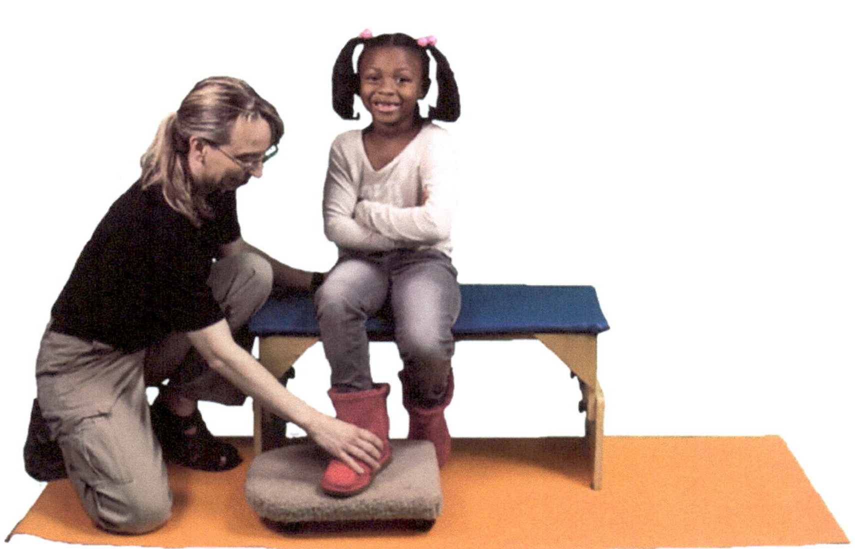

11. SITTING BALL PICK UP

This exercise gets hip flexion, hip abduction, inversion, abdominals and hip external rotation. Have your client lift the ball with knees apart to get more external rotation. Often I have him lift the ball and put it in a hoop I hold.

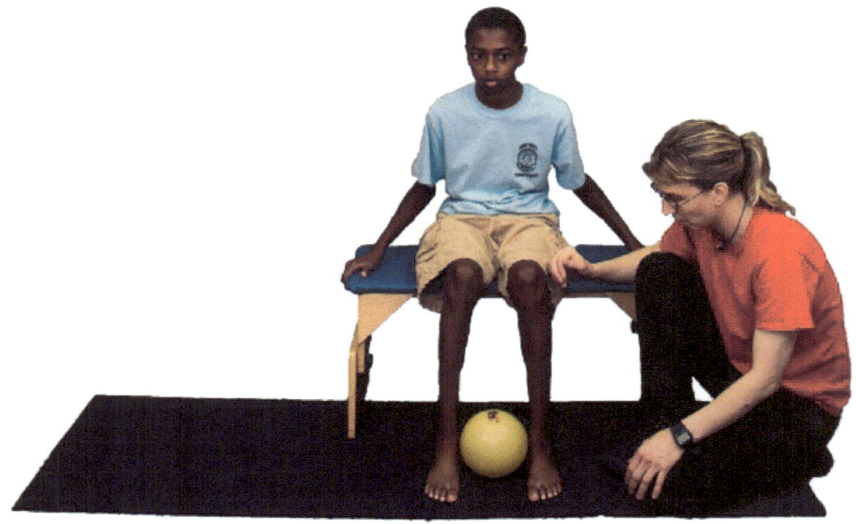

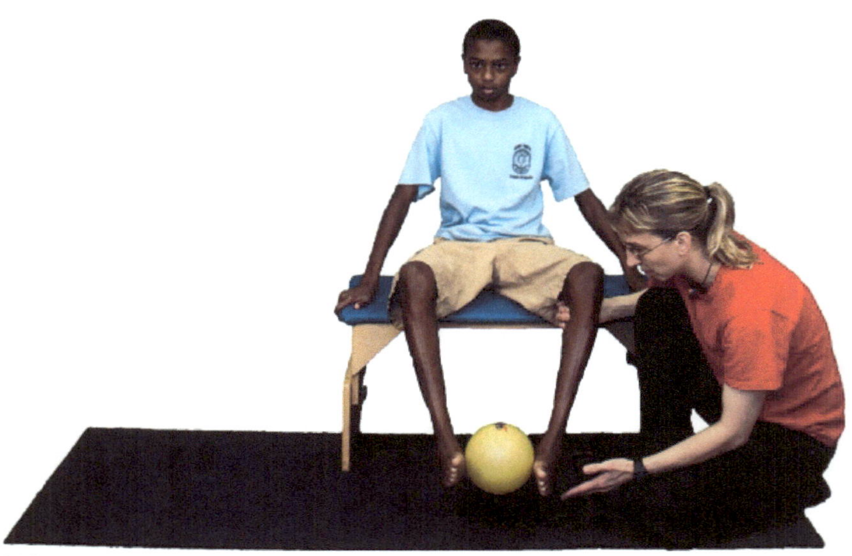

12. HALF KNEEL TOSS

Kids with diplegia have such a hard time holding half kneel, especially with dynamic challenges. They fail by having the raised knee fall into internal rotation and adduction. Finding ways to work on this is key to giving my clients the stability at the hips needed for standing balance and hip control for ambulation.

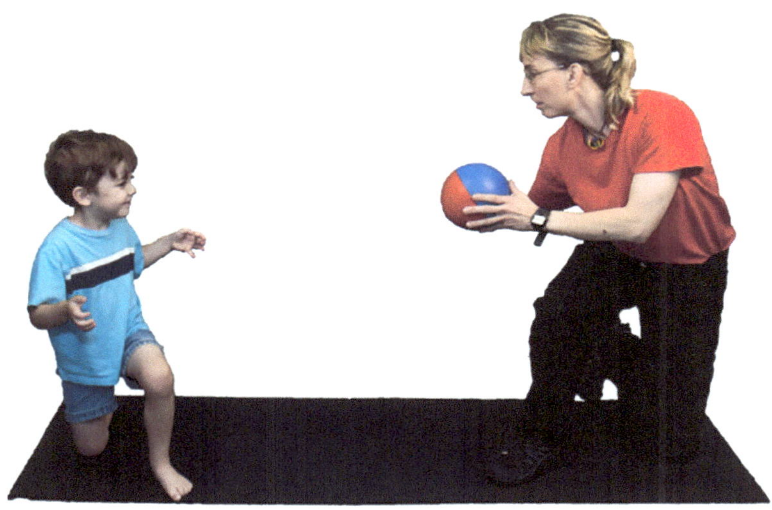

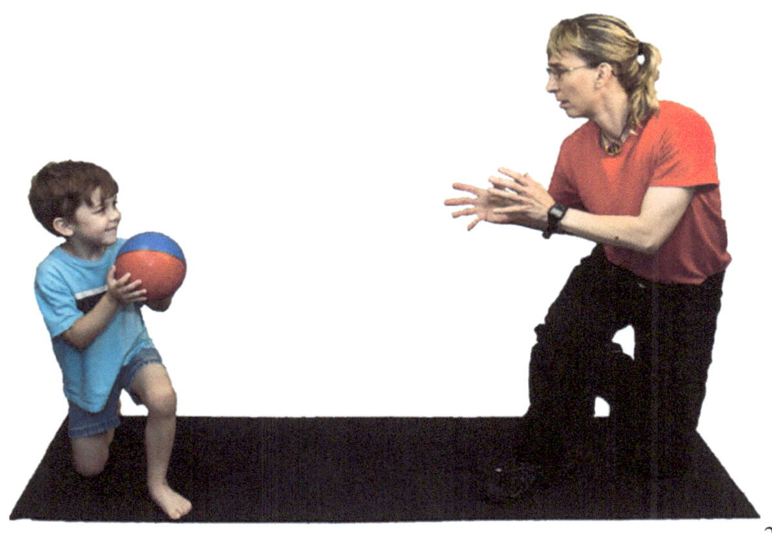

13. STAND WITH KNEES APART

Often when a person stands or walk with knees together, there is a weakness in both abductors and external rotators as well as poor biomechanical alignment. Here I simply work on standing with knees out. I put my hand between her knees and say keep your knees off my hands. When your client is ready for a challenge, add dynamic challenges like sit to stand transfers without knees touching. I may put a small electronic keyboard between my client's knees to give auditory cues for when the knees fall back together. I also love to put my clients on the trampoline and play the same game. I have some wall grips that my client can hold onto. I bounce her and challenge her to her knees apart for ten seconds or however long I feel like counting. Sometimes we go for records of minutes at a time with knees apart.

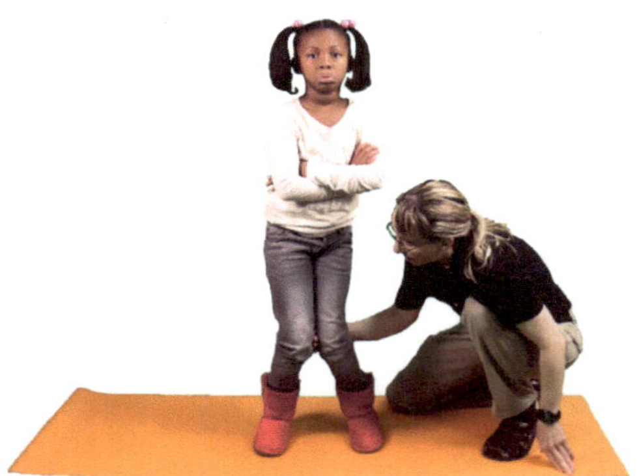

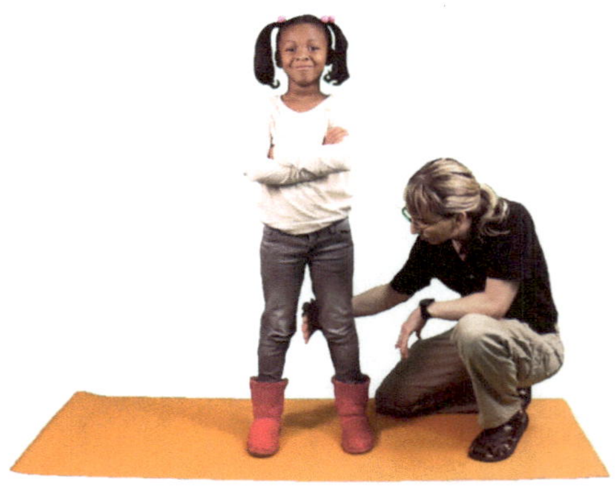

14. STAND SPINNING FEET IN AND OUT

I have some kids simply work on spinning their knees/feet in and out. I have a client with muscular dystrophy that stands so internally rotated that one foot is pointing backward. We do lots of this work. This is easiest in socks on slick floor like vinyl, tile or hardwood floors and harder on the carpet or in shoes. If your client can hold static standing with external rotation, try dynamic challenges. For example, I may have her hit a balloon back and forth while maintaining knees out. Sometimes, I draw a chalk line up the middle of a treadmill and have my client practice walking without turning in her feet. Faster speeds are harder.

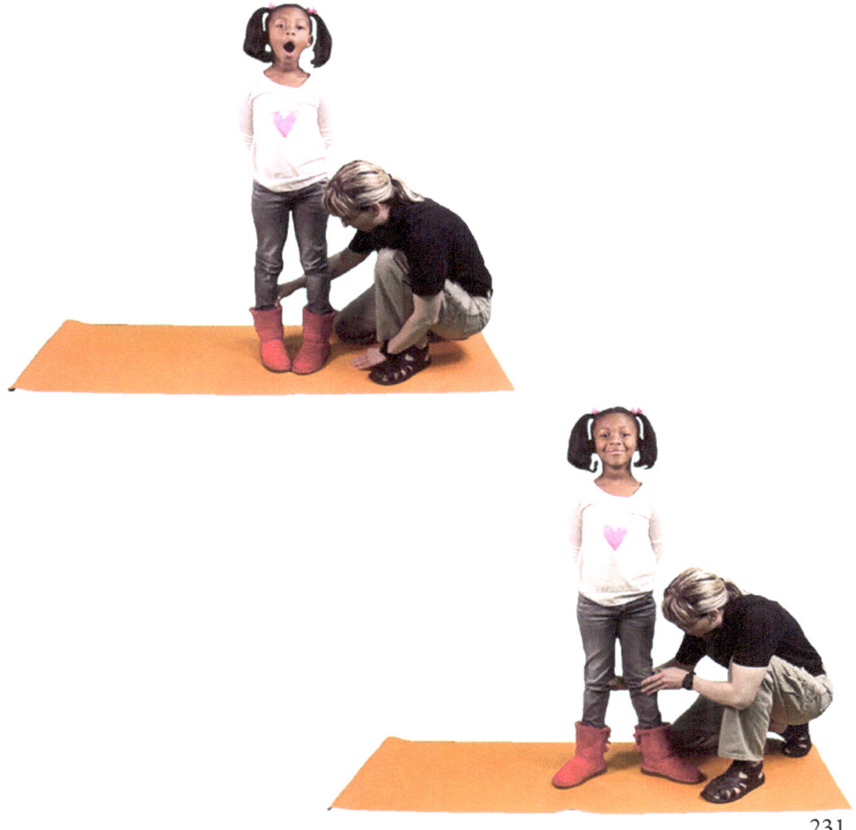

15. STANDING BOLSTER ROLL

This exercise requires some standing balance unless of course you hold a hand or two. Choose the bolster carefully. If the bolster is too small, it is harder to roll. It if it is too large, my clients have trouble getting their foot on top. The client simply rolls the bolster side to side.

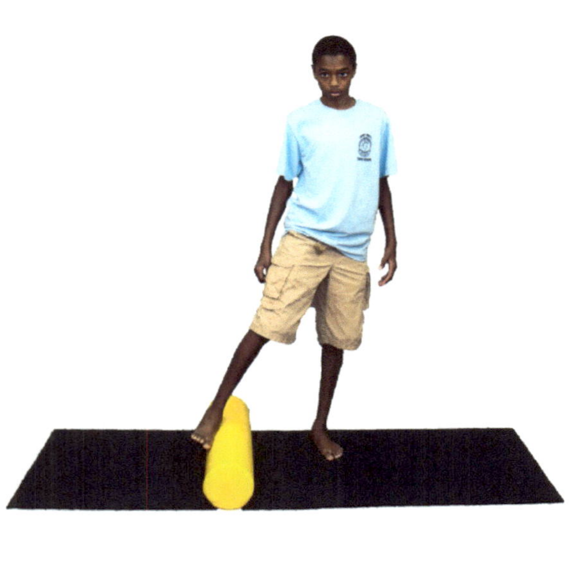

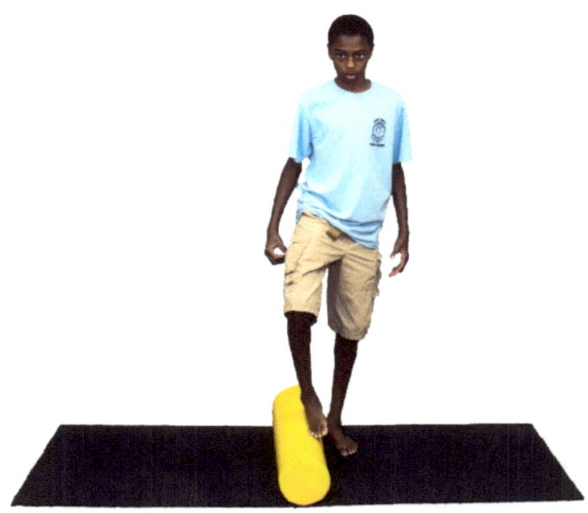

16. GET STICKER ON BOTTOM OF FOOT

This exercise also gets hip and knee flexion and inversion and if performed properly, also achieves hip external rotation. I have done this exercise in sitting and in standing. I use sitting when the client doesn't have the balance to perform it in standing. In sitting I encourage more hip external rotation by manually blocking the knee from coming up too high into hip flexion.

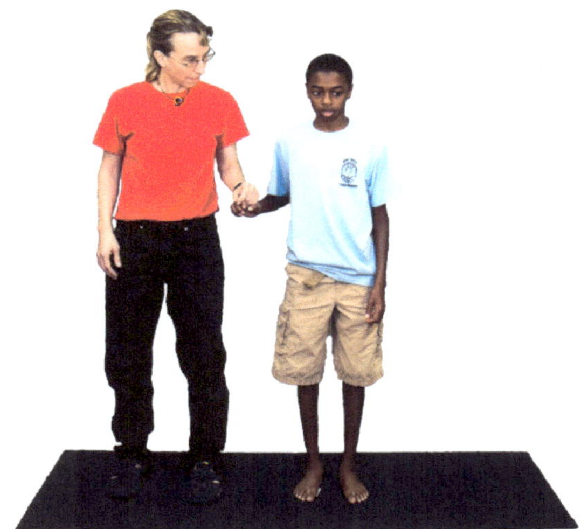

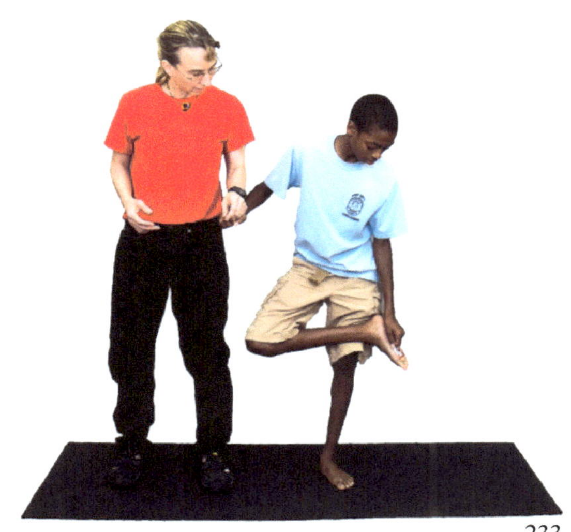

VI. HIP INTERNAL ROTATION

* * *

THE HIP INTERNAL ROTATORS SPIN the femur medially toward the other knee or toward midline. These movements are in the transverse plane. The hip internal rotators are important in lower leg alignment in walking, running and sports related movements. Weakness or tightness in the hip internal rotators will decrease the efficiency of gait and increase the likelihood of injury to the hip, knee or ankle. Limited hip internal rotation range has been linked to shortened stride and compensations for the weakness at the knee and foot.

1. KICK IN VAULT

Add a ball and most activities become more fun. I roll the ball and the client kicks it back. This is exquisitely hard for even my high functioning clients with cerebral palsy. If this is too hard, have the child in vault on a single, double or triple thick mat, with the kicking foot off the mat on the floor. This makes it dramatically easier. To emphasize hip internal rotation, I tell my client to kick the ball with the bottom of her foot.

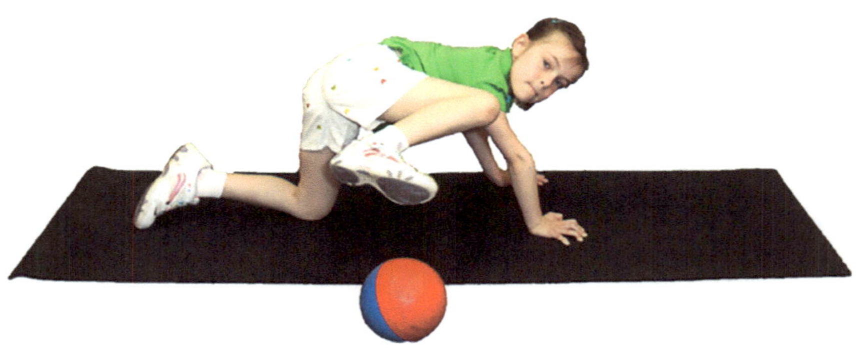

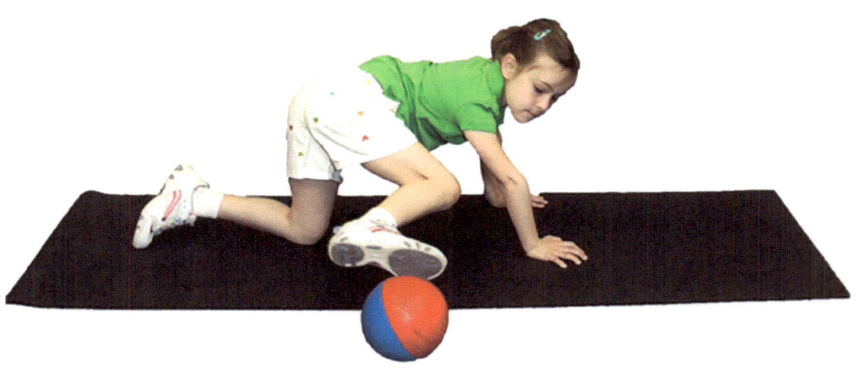

2. KICK TO THE SIDE WITH INTERNAL ROTATION SITTING

Make sure you stabilize the knee so the target is kicked with rotation and not abduction. Empty two liter soda bottles are good targets too. I usually take the child's leg through the available range to see how far the child's leg has the potential to move, and then I place the block. Or alternatively you can place the block an inch/centimeter away from her foot starting position, and then progressively move the target further away with success.

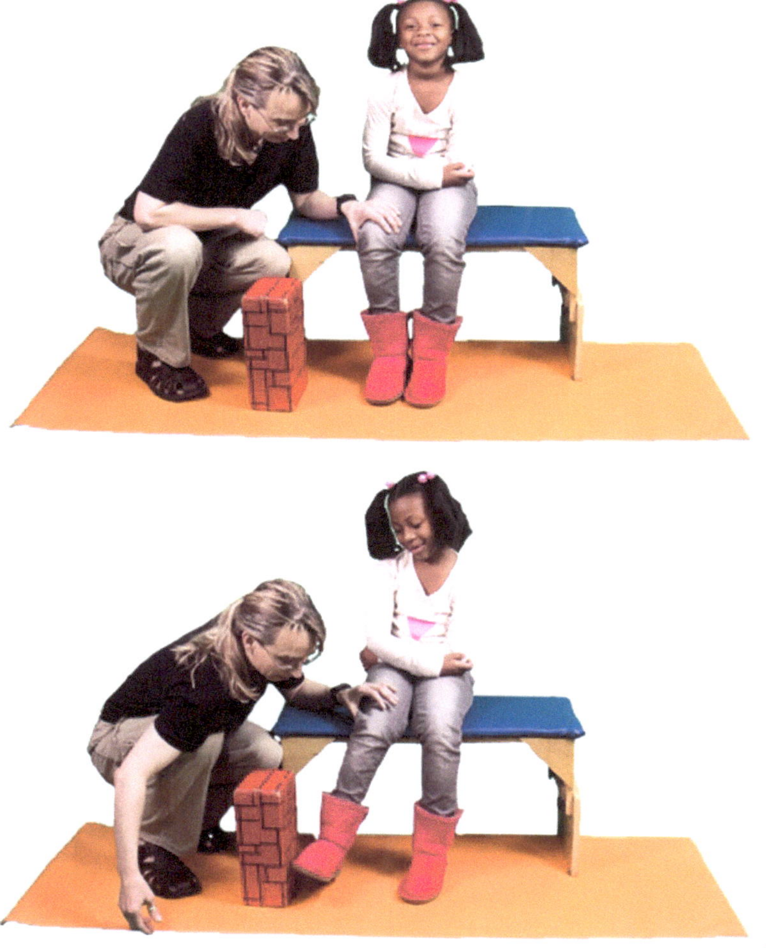

3. STANDING UNILATERAL INTERNAL ROTATION

Watch to make sure the movement is coming from the hip and not the knee or ankle. I love using a piece of paper under the shoe/foot to decrease the resistance for movement. This exercise is easier on a hard floor like vinyl, tile or hardwood than on a mat or carpeting. The paper makes this activity possible even if you have carpeting. Sometimes to make the activity easier, I put some baby powder down on the floor to decrease the resistance even more. For the clients who need this activity, it is not uncommon for me to have to passively move the leg first and fade toward more active movement. He may also need upper extremity support so he can concentrate on the lower extremity movement instead of the standing balance required.

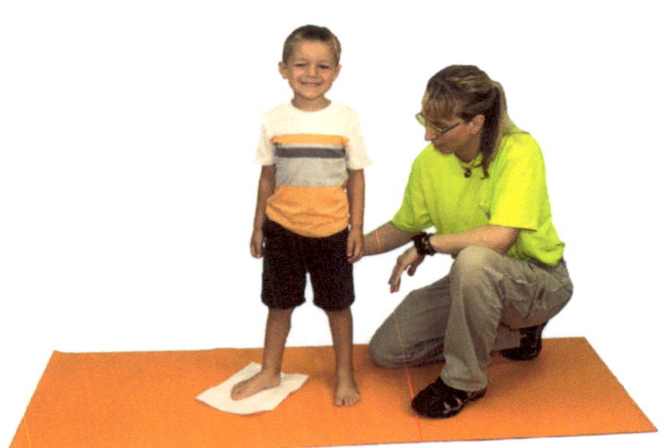

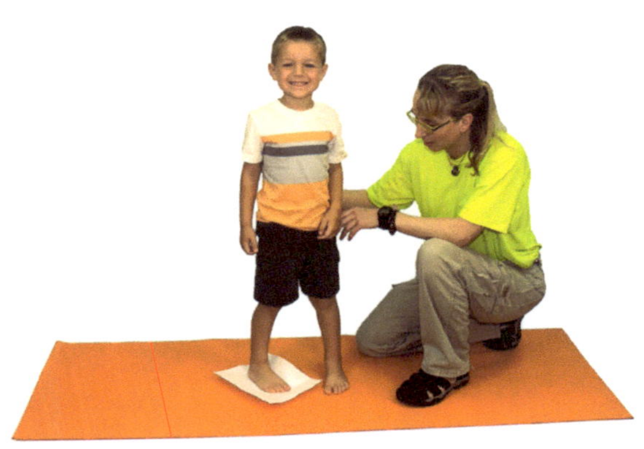

4. STANDING SPINNING LEGS IN AND OUT

This is easiest in socks on slick floor like vinyl, tile or hardwood floors and harder on the carpet or in shoes. The sole of the shoe makes a big difference with this activity. Athletic rubber shoes tend to grip more and are harder to turn. Darker, harder soles tend to slide more easily. If you put each shoe on a piece of paper or a small carpet square, then the shoe glides so much easier.

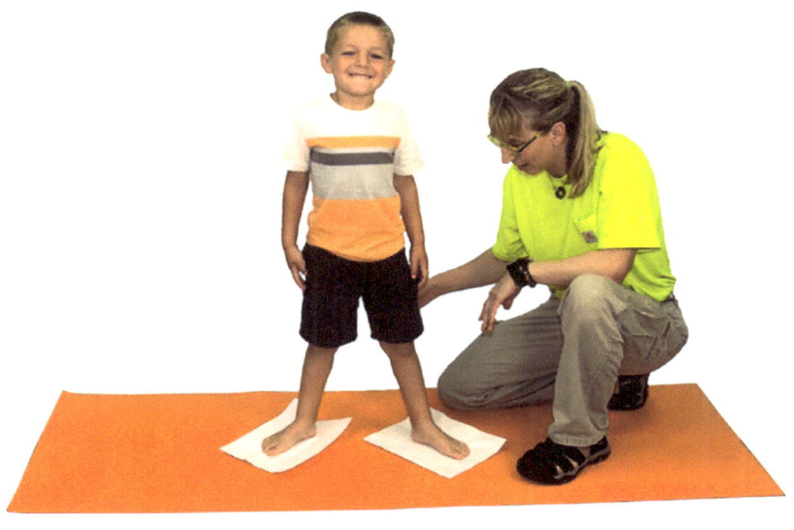

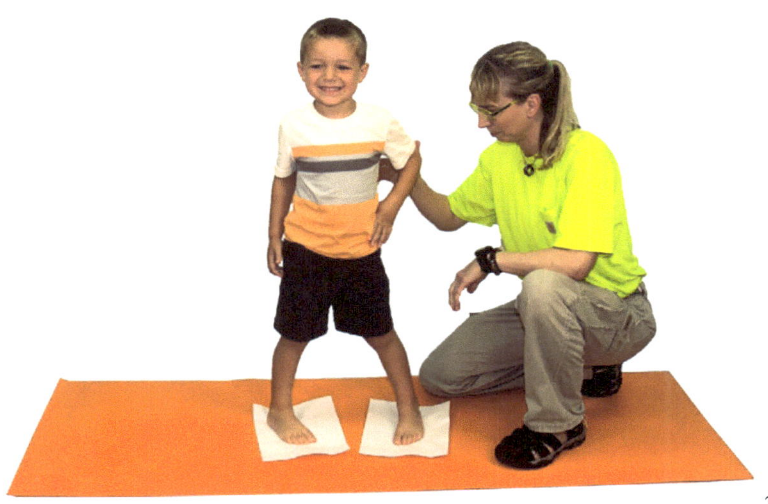

5. SUPINE HIP INTERNAL ROTATION

This is one of the easier internal rotation exercises. A pillow or wedge under her head allows her to see her feet with this exercise. I start with the hip externally rotated and have my client internally rotate. I reference wind shield wipers so my client knows the movement. It is not uncommon that I resist her moving from an externally rotated position to neutral and then have to assist progressively in the range from neutral to internal rotation.

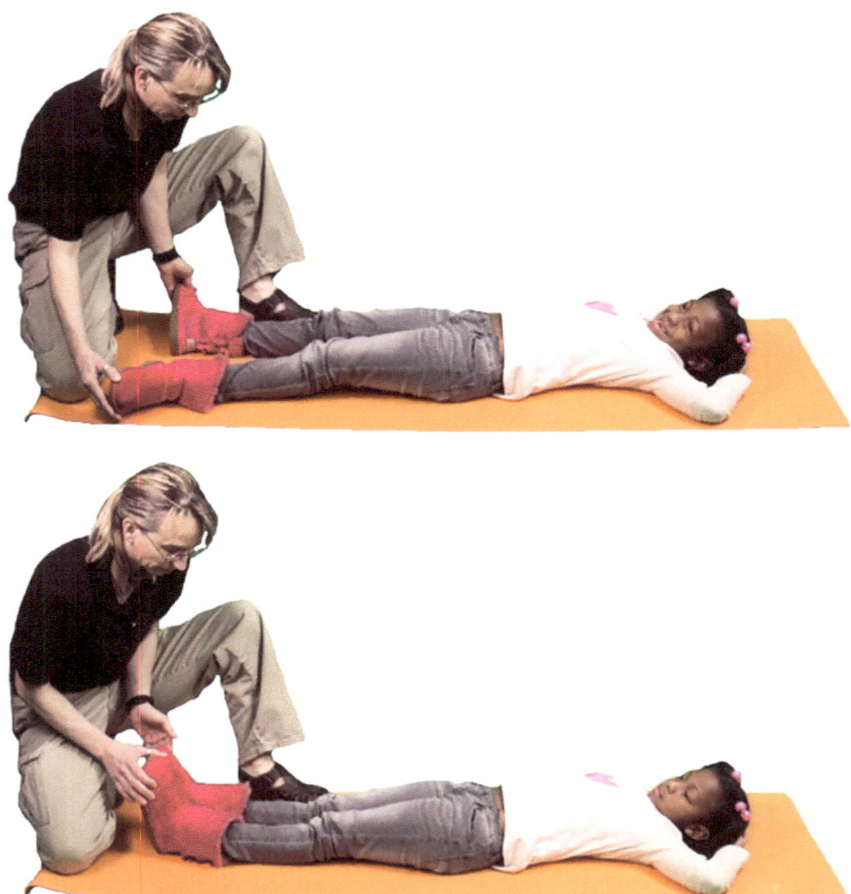

6. PRONE HIP INTERNAL ROTATION LEGS TOGETHER

I go to this exercise when I know my client needs to cheat a little to have success. The other leg can help in the movement. My clients tend to get movement of the pelvis helping with the effective movement of the legs into internal and external rotation. My clients rarely have the needed knee flexion strength to hold this position, so I often have to block the knees into flexion as well.

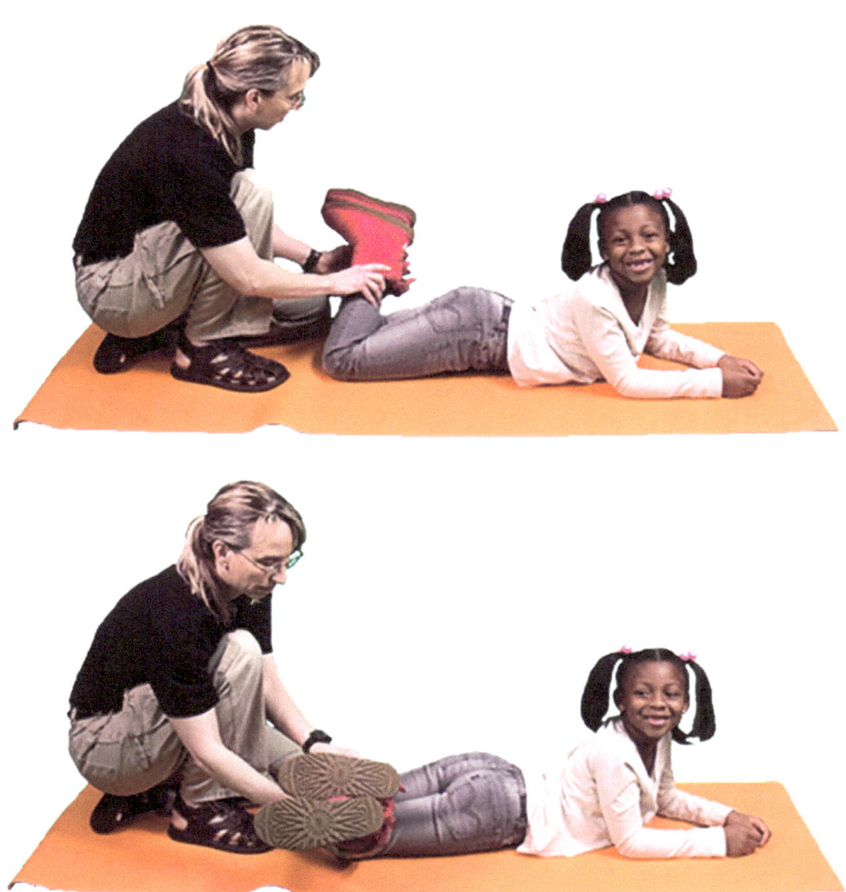

7. PRONE UNILATERAL INTERNAL ROTATION

I typically resist moving from an externally rotated position to neutral, and then assist progressively in the range from neutral to an internal rotation. This exercise minimizes a great deal of the substitutions seen in the previous exercise.

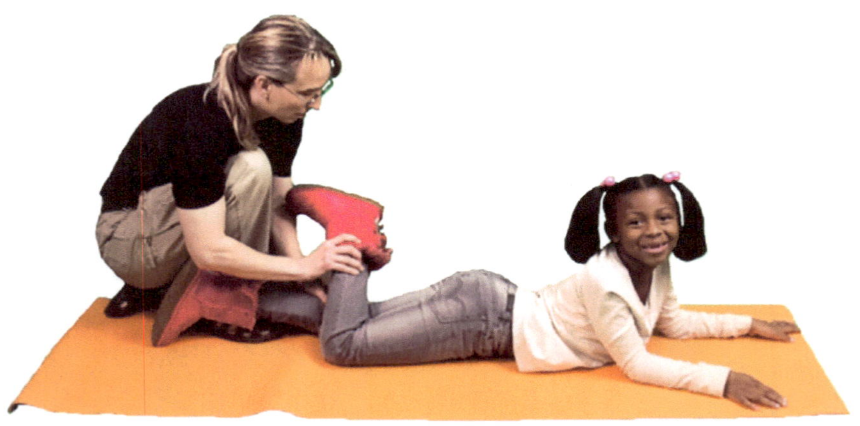

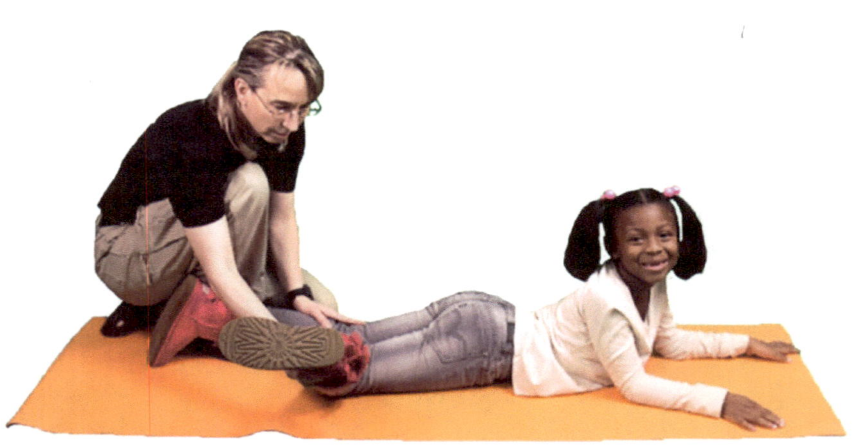

8. PRONE BILATERAL HIP INTERNAL ROTATION

By moving two legs at a time both simultaneously in internal and external rotation, I tend to get even less substitution/cheating. This one requires some coordination for my kids. I often need to help my clients passively with this movement before they can do it actively.

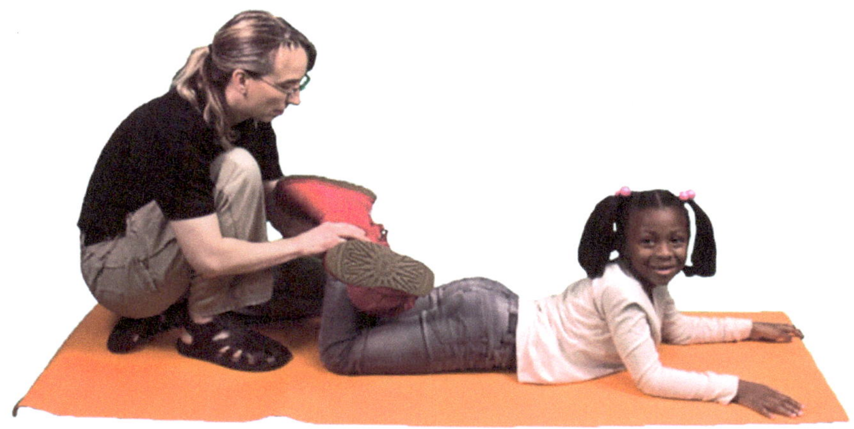

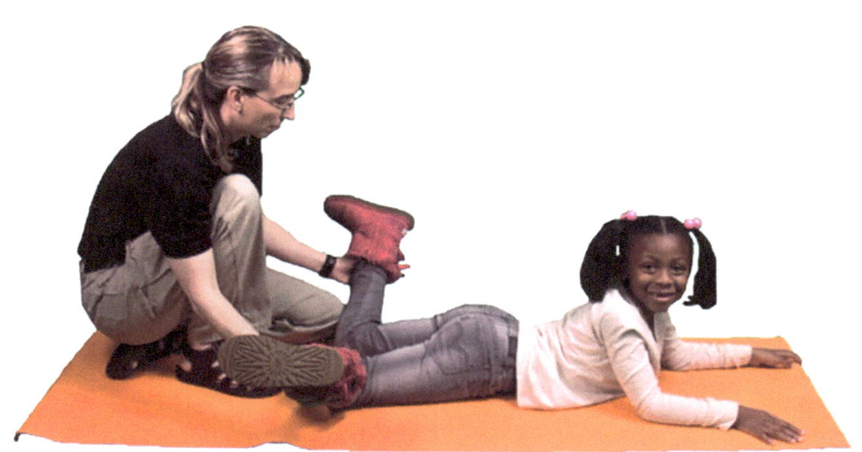

9. BALL SIDE SIT TO QUADRUPED

This activity is harder with a bigger range of movement. I tend to do all the reps on one side before working the other side. When children alternate from one side to the other, I see a loss of control. I like seeing my client control the stop at the top of the movement.

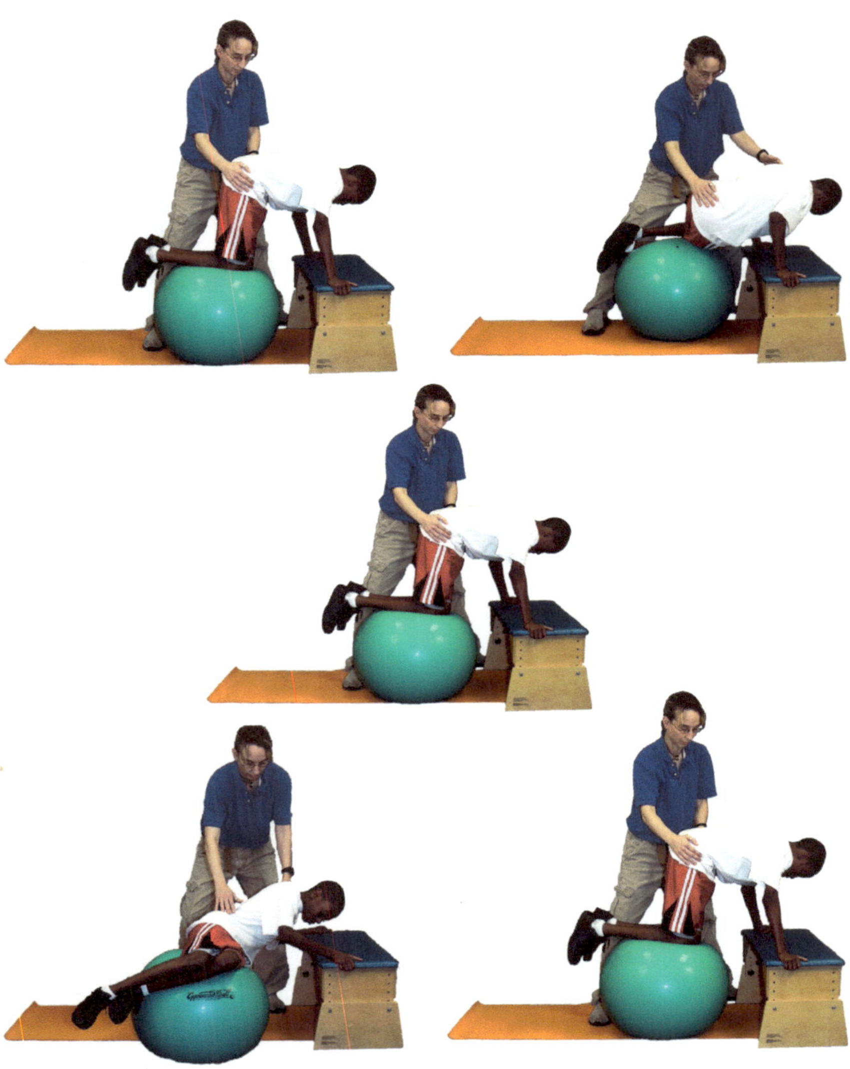

10. INTERNAL ROTATION LONG SITTING

For my clients who need internal rotation work, I'll work it in multiple positions back-to-back, i.e., long sitting, supine, and sitting with end range hip flexion. Long sitting is one of the easier ways to work internal rotation. I provide assistance/resistance according to the needs of the client.

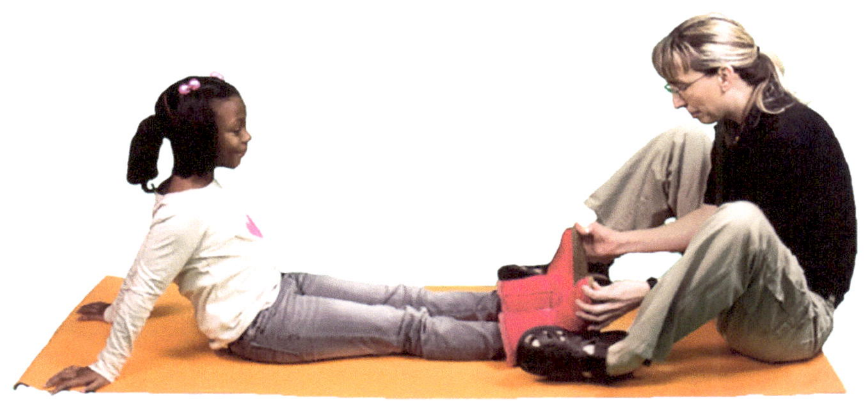

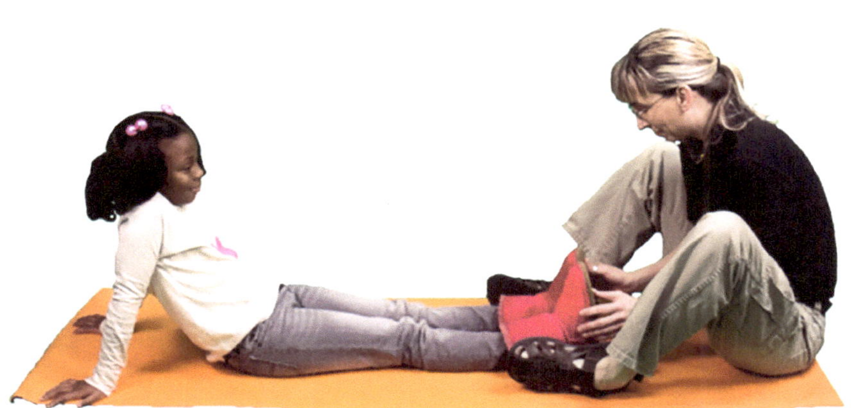

11. SIDE SIT PROGRESSIVELY NARROW

This exercise takes advantage of simple biomechanics. If a child sits side sit with his knee spread wide, the pelvis is fairly level. As the child puts his knees closer together, the pelvis becomes more tilted. When the knees are completely on top of each other, the pelvis is very angled. The more angled the pelvis is the more challenging a position the side sit is to hold. More lateral flexion, hip internal/external rotation and abduction/adduction strength are required depending on the leg referenced. I typically start the child with his knees very wide. I see what kind of support the child requires to hold this position and for how long.

I start with two hands held, then one hand held, then two hands propping on the floor, then one hand propping on the floor, then hands free. Once a child can hold a position for ten seconds, have the child move his knees a little closer. Sometimes instead of counting to ten, I ask the child to clap his hands ten times. I continue until the child can no longer hold the position or is successful with full knee overlap.

For more challenge, I sit the child on a trampoline, rockerboard, ball or even a platform swing, so I can bounce/rock/swing the child to make it more dynamic. If I am performing the activity on a dynamic surface, I usually find what level of leg overlap is challenging. Then I make sure the child can hold the position for ten seconds. Next I say, "I'm going to bounce (or rock/swing) you ten times small. See if you can hold it without falling over." If the child is successful with small bounces/rocks/swings, I progress to medium, large and then extreme. This usually ends in hysterics, with the child begging and pleading to do it again.

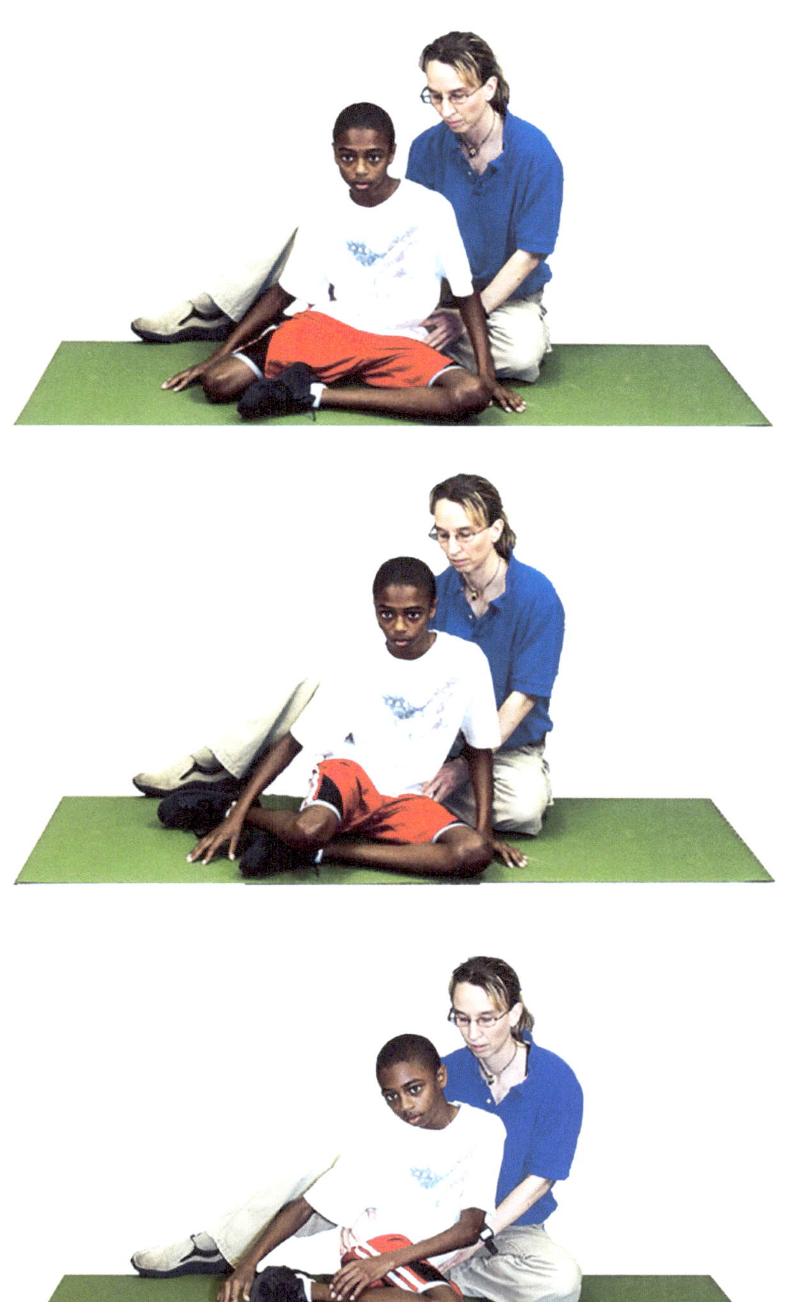

12. SIDESIT TO TALL KNEEL

This is an overlooked hip rotator work out. Obviously while one leg is internally rotating the other is externally rotating. Often this is a very difficult transition for my clients. I may put a four inch (10 cm) bench or pillow down for the client to sit down to from tall kneel to make it easier. I work progressively lower until he can go down to the floor. This exercise is quite hard in general, but if you need to challenge your client more, have him cross his arms on his chest.

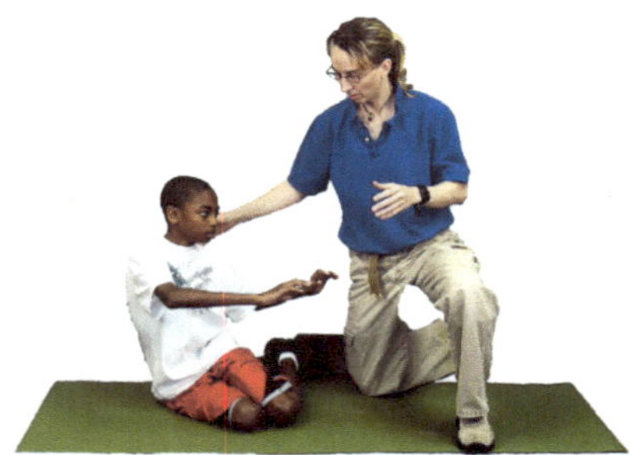

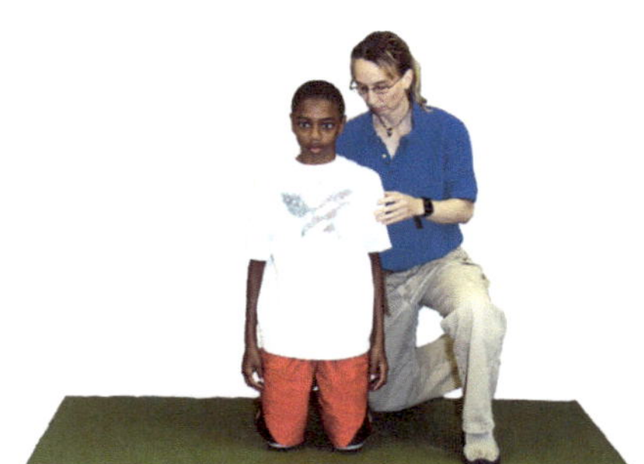

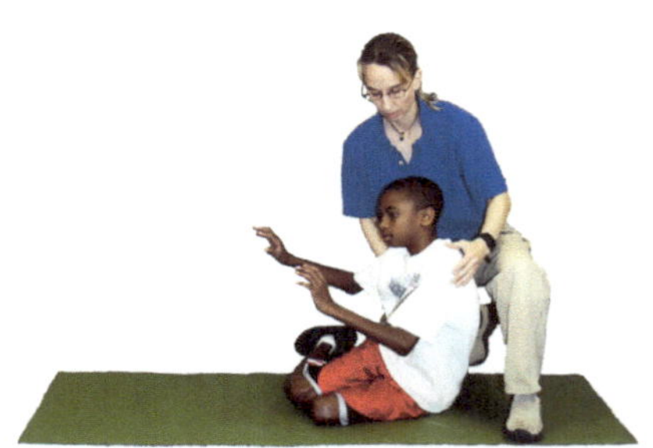

13. SIDE TO SIDE FEET ON SCOOTERBOARD

In the activity pictured, the model is working both internal and external rotators depending on the leg and direction. I could have placed a large block to knock down on the target side to add some entertainment value. Fortunately my model here was content to just do the movement. With both feet on the scooter, it is possible that the child can cheat wildly by using primarily one leg and minimally with the other. I have since discovered that a skateboard is best for the children who have a really hard time activating the internal rotators. With the scooterboard, I tend to get a great deal of knee extension in the child's attempts to internally rotate. Watch for cheating of whole body movement or abduction/adduction. You may need to stabilize the knees to discourage these two cheats.

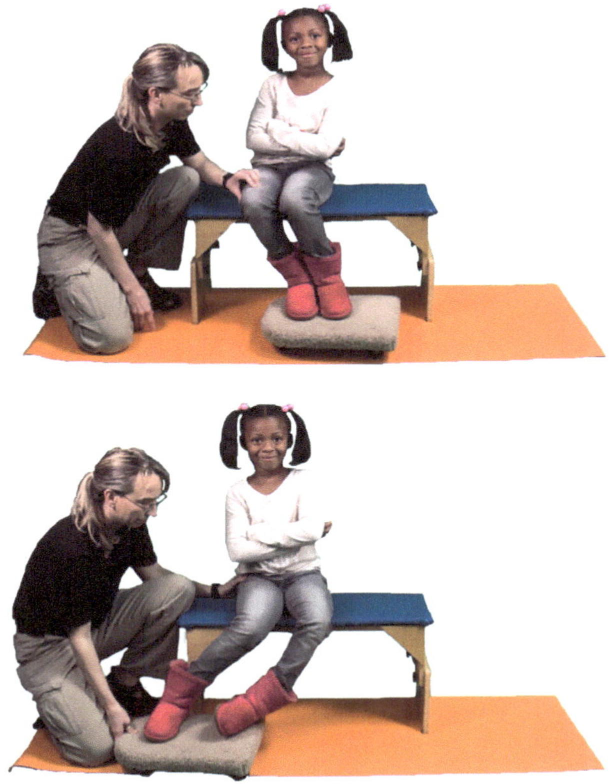

14. SIDE TO SIDE FOOT ON SCOOTERBOARD

Using one leg prevents the cheating or assistance from the other leg. Sometimes I let a client use two legs first and then switch to the "tricky" leg.

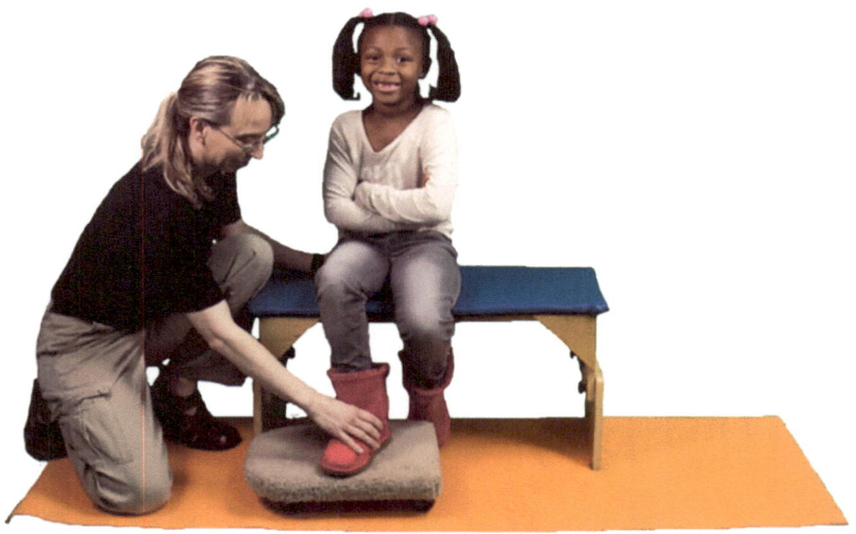

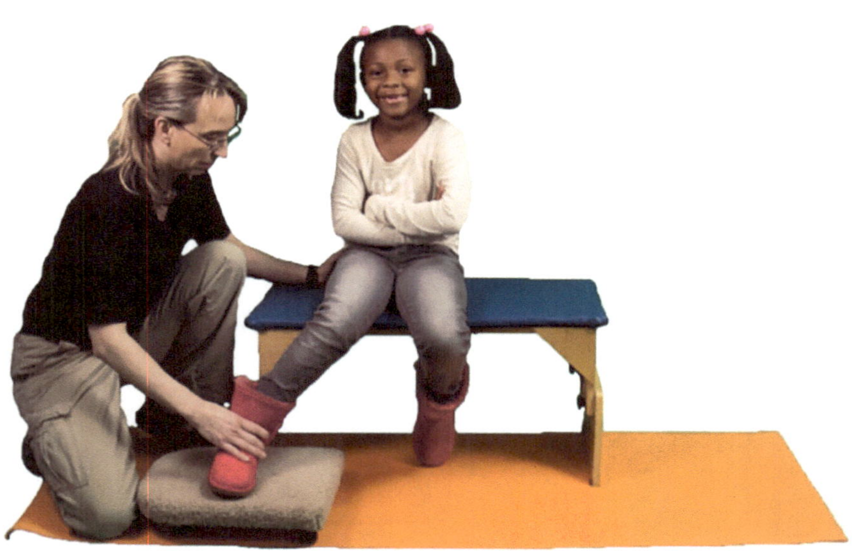

15. STANDING BOLSTER ROLL INTERNAL ROTATION

Have the client keeps his knee bent and his foot in contact with the bolster as he rolls it. If not, he gets more abduction/adduction than rotation.

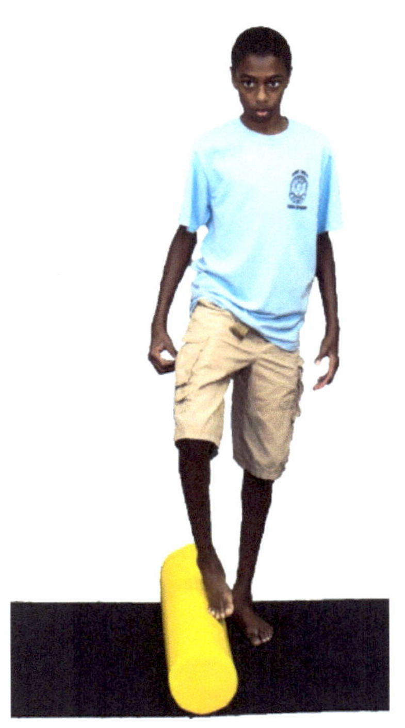

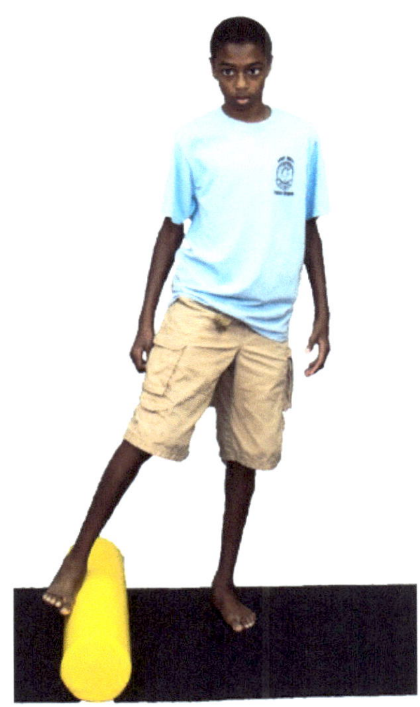

16. STANDING ROLL BALL UP INTERNAL ROTATION

Provide upper extremity support as needed for balance for this exercise. The right size bench is important. I like this 16 inch (40 cm) bench so I can sit on it too. I think my ten inch (25 cm) bench would work, but the four inch (10 cm) bench would be too small. A ball like a bumpy gerdy ball has a little traction or texture and is a little easier to control.

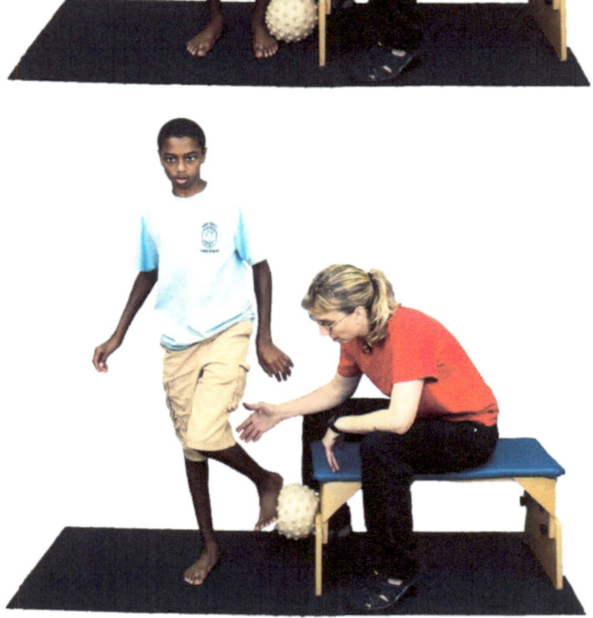

17. STANDING INTERNAL ROTATION KICK

Very nice exercise for clients with good balance to emphasize internal rotation. Of course you can hold a hand or two to minimize balance requirements. Make sure your client is close enough to the bench so that knee flexion and internal rotation is required. Kicking off a higher bench is harder.

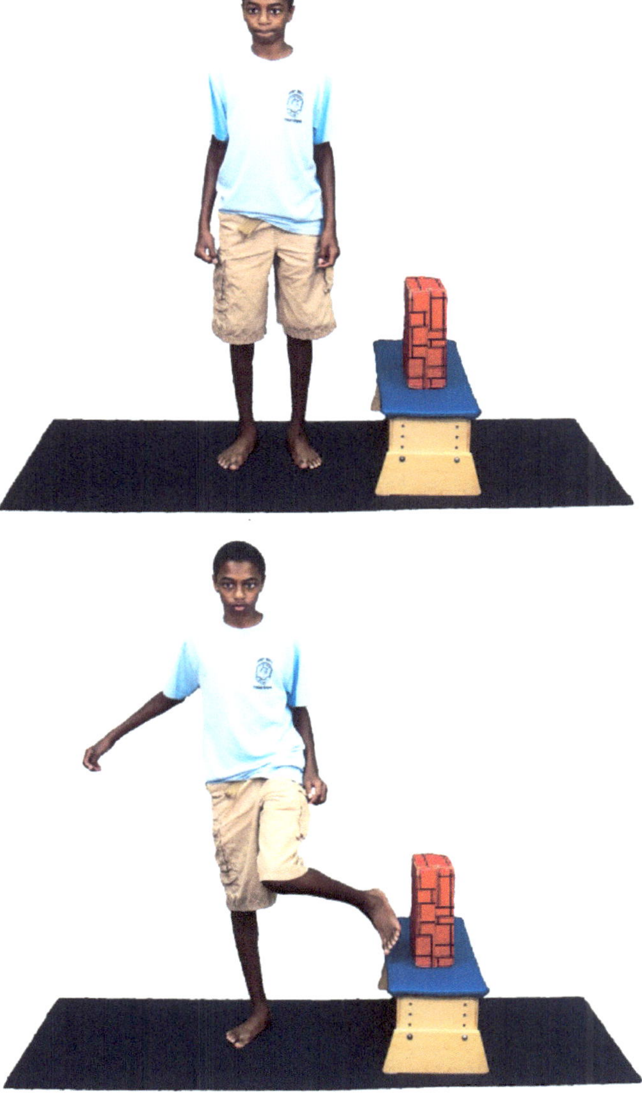

ABOUT THE AUTHOR

AMY STURKEY IS AN OUTPATIENT pediatric physical therapist at Child and Family Development in Charlotte, NC. Amy met an adorable boy with cerebral palsy and his family on a safari in Kenya. As she tried to help them, she realized that little information was available to help train pediatric therapists and to educate children and families about common childhood conditions and treatment options. After 30+ years of clinical experience, she decided she had information to share. Amy co-founded Gotcha Apps to produce educational products for pediatric therapists and their clients. She created an instructional Facebook page, a website, and a YouTube channel. Through these platforms, she releases weekly videos to instruct therapists and families of children with developmental challenges. This is her fourth book. Her previous books are "A is for Autism," "D is for Down Syndrome." and "C is for Cerebral Palsy." "A is for ADHD" is soon to be released. Her books are available on Amazon, Kindle, Audible and in the Apple Library. Amy won Outstanding Physical Therapist for North Carolina for 2016.

www.PediatricPTexercises.com

OTHER OFFERINGS BY THE AUTHOR

A is for Autism: A Child's View
D is for Down Syndrome: A Child's View
C is For Cerebral Palsy: A Child's View
Pediatric Physical Therapy Strengthening Exercises for the Knees

Coming Soon:
A is for ADHD: A Child's View

Blog:
www.PediatricPTexercises.com

YouTube Channel:
Pediatric Physical Therapy Exercises

Facebook page:
Pediatric Physical Therapy Exercises

Instagram page:
Pediatric PT Exercises

Pinterest page:
amysturkey/pediatric-physical-therapy

www.ingramcontent.com/pod-product-compliance
Lightning Source LLC
Chambersburg PA
CBHW040126270326
41926CB00005B/84
* 9 7 8 0 9 9 8 1 5 6 7 3 6 *